Medication Safety during Anesthesia and the Perioperative Period

Medication Safety during Anesthesia and the Perioperative Period

Alan Merry
University of Auckland and Auckland City Hospital

Joyce Wahr
University of Minnesota

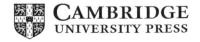

CAMBRIDGE
UNIVERSITY PRESS

University Printing House, Cambridge CB2 8BS, United Kingdom

One Liberty Plaza, 20th Floor, New York, NY 10006, USA

477 Williamstown Road, Port Melbourne, VIC 3207, Australia

314–321, 3rd Floor, Plot 3, Splendor Forum, Jasola District Centre, New Delhi – 110025, India

79 Anson Road, #06-04/06, Singapore 079906

Cambridge University Press is part of the University of Cambridge.

It furthers the University's mission by disseminating knowledge in the
pursuit of education, learning, and research at the highest international levels of excellence.

www.cambridge.org
Information on this title: www.cambridge.org/9781107194106
DOI: 10.1017/9781108151702

© Cambridge University Press 2021

First published 2021

Printed in the United Kingdom by TJ Books Limited, Padstow Cornwall

A catalogue record for this publication is available from the British Library.

Library of Congress Cataloging-in-Publication Data
Names: Merry, Alan, author. | Wahr, Joyce, 1952- author.
Title: Medication safety during anesthesia and the perioperative period/Alan Merry, Joyce Wahr.
Description: New York : Cambridge University Press, 2020|Includes bibliographical references and index.
Identifiers: LCCN 2020026694 (print) | LCCN 2020026695 (ebook)|ISBN 9781107194106 (hardback)|ISBN 9781108151702 (ebook)
Subjects: MESH: Anesthetics--adverse effects | Medication Errors--prevention & control | Anesthesia--methods | Anesthesia--adverse effects | Perioperative Period
Classification: LCC RD82.2 (print) | LCC RD82.2 (ebook) | NLM QV 81|DDC 615.7/81--dc23
LC record available at https://lccn.loc.gov/2020026694
LC ebook record available at https://lccn.loc.gov/2020026695
ISBN 978-1-107-19410-6 Hardback

Cover image caption

On first looking at the image on the cover of this book, one can readily imagine an anesthesiologist, wearing a mask, taking care in drawing up a medication from a vial for intravenous injection into a patient in the operating room. On close inspection, failures in safety can be identified. Thus, this image symbolizes the serious need for improvement in medication safety in anesthesia and the perioperative period, in the system and also in the practices of many of the clinicians who work within it.

This book is for the patients whom we as a profession have harmed through medication errors and for their loved ones, particularly those who are bereft forever because of these errors. It is also for those idealistic, dedicated, and compassionate people who (like us) work in healthcare and who (like us), in spite of their very best efforts and to their deep distress, have inadvertently harmed the very patients they have been trying so hard to help. We hope it will contribute to making the use of medications in anesthesia and the perioperative period a little safer for everyone.

The Snow Vaporizer, Mark II

John Snow was the first physician to specialize in the administration of anesthesia. He carefully investigated the first 100 deaths due to chloroform and performed an in-depth analysis of the vaporization characteristics of chloroform. He found a very narrow margin between the concentration that provided anesthesia (5%) and the concentration that produced cardiac paralysis and death (10%). In his comments to the Westminster Medical Society on March 31, 1849, Dr. Snow described his attempt to improve anesthesia safety through better design: "In the inhaler which I employ, the compartment containing the chloroform is surrounded with cold water to limit the quantity of vapour taken up by the air, and the expiratory valve of the face piece is so adapted as to admit additional air to further dilute the vapour."

The pictured inhaler is termed the "Mark II," showing the water bath, and a stopcock to control the amount of vapor being administered. Only two examples of this inhaler survive today; this one is in the archives of the American Society of Anesthesiologists.

Image courtesy of the Wood Library-Museum of Anesthesiology, Schaumberg IL.

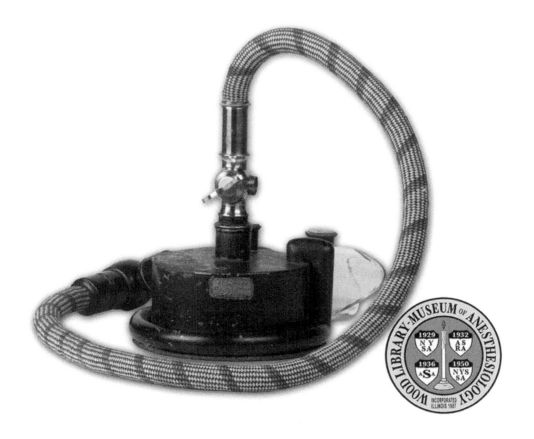

Contents

Foreword

In this day and age of hyperelectronic information feeds, 140-character tweets, viral YouTube videos, Instagram images and stories, and an endless conga line of podcasts, it is refreshing to find a full text that can capture and hold your attention. This is particularly true when the text provides remarkable insights into important issues. In this new text by Drs. Alan Merry and Joyce Wahr, we get the benefit of their years of astute observation and passionate leadership in perioperative patient safety. Their text, *Medication Safety during Anesthesia and the Perioperative Period*, is keenly written, sharply pointed, and laser-focused on the broad issues impacting and impacted by medication safety.

There are few important new texts written solo or by a small team of authors – and with this text, we get the benefit of a two-author tome that has a concise writing style, consistency in formatting, and a strong interlinking of principles from chapter to chapter. Common themes are interwoven through the diverse chapters, providing bundled insights that build on each other in a way that few multiauthored texts do. This stacking of ideas and observations augments their observations and strengthens their recommendations. It is an ideal approach for two authors who bring so much knowledge and expertise to their writing.

Drs. Merry and Wahr observe locally but think globally. They have a wealth of national as well as international experiences, with each having spent their professional lives engaged in the promotion of anesthesia and perioperative patient safety. Their observations have involved the local development of medication safety initiatives and the trials and tribulations associated with implementing them in their own institutions. In addition, each author has extensive experience in national and international leadership positions and has learned the difficulties – and appreciated the joys – associated with successful implementation of medication safety initiatives. Their authenticity rings true throughout the text.

The text is unique in that it includes crucial chapters that address the long-term sequelae and impact of medication safety issues, including errors, on patients and families as well as healthcare professionals who work in the perioperative period. Their use of case studies to illustrate the impact of patient harm on everyone involved is both clinically relevant and personally moving. Overall, it is a text that tells a compelling story of the impact of medication errors and systematic problems that arise within the complexities of medication administration.

Drs. Merry and Wahr have provided us with the insights and information we need to excel locally as well as within larger-scale health systems to improve medication safety. This text is a tribute to their expertise, their real-life experiences in patient safety, and their remarkable storytelling. Our patients deserve our best efforts, and this text provides us with the knowledge to make a difference in their safety. Hearty congratulations to Drs. Merry and Wahr!

Mark A. Warner, MD, President
Anesthesia Patient Safety Foundation

Acknowledgments

We are very grateful to Mia Jüllig, of Paper Dog Ltd (www.paperdog.co.nz), for creating clear, accurate, and usable illustrations from various sources including, in particular, our own somewhat arcane suggestions. We would also like to express our very sincere thanks to the following people who have each made invaluable contributions to this book, through support, advice, discussion, the provision of information, and the review of chapters: Professor Michael Wall, Dr. Karen Domino, Professor Robin Ferner, Mr. John Mead, Dr. John Villiger, Dr. Matthew Moore, Mrs. Debbie Beaumont, and Mr. Michael Merry. We are grateful to Dr. Mark Warner for providing us with such an excellent Foreword. We would particularly like to thank our publisher, Jessica Papworth, who has been amazingly understanding, helpful, and encouraging during the prolonged gestation of this book. Finally, we cannot adequately express our gratitude to Dennis Wahr, Sally Merry, and many other members of our two families for their unfailing support of this project.

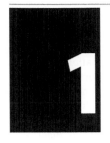

Introduction to Medication Safety in Anesthesia and the Perioperative Period

1.1 Introduction

Medication errors are believed to be a leading cause of avoidable harm to patients around the world, with an estimated cost of US$42 billion per year worldwide. In the end, human error is inevitable, but many of these errors actually reflect failures in the design and resourcing of the system within which medications are administered to patients, and some reflect violations of safe medication practices. Thus, much could be done to improve medication safety. To this end, the World Health Organization (WHO) recently launched its third global patient safety challenge, "Medication Without Harm." Its goal is to reduce the level of severe, avoidable harm related to medications by 50% over 5 years, globally (1,2).

It has been estimated that 5% of all patients who are admitted to a hospital experience a medication error, and that an average hospital will have one medication error every 22.7 hours or every 19.7 admissions. These data come from a very large study, where 1116 hospitals reported 430,000 medication errors, of which 17,338 adversely affected patient outcomes (3). In a recent study from the United States, 5.3% of medication administrations during anesthesia involved an error, an adverse medication event, or both, and 79% were considered preventable (4). Medication errors are the most common of all medical errors (5,6) and pose a tremendous emotional and physical cost to patients and economic burden to our health system (7,8). Clearly, medication error is a major source of risk and adverse events for our patients.

Occasionally, medication errors have devastating consequences and generate national attention (Box 1.1). However, these seriously harmful events come from a tiny fraction of the vast number of medications administered every day. Could one argue, then, that this harm is simply the cost of doing business, that errors will happen, and that attempting to eliminate these errors is not worth the tremendous effort required to understand and rectify the processes that make us vulnerable to both error and harm? Certainly, the majority of errors that are either reported or observed are minor, many do not reach the patient, and of those that do, most are essentially harmless. Indeed, in a study of intensive care unit medication errors reported to the *United States Pharmacopeia*'s MED-MARX and to the United Kingdom's National Reporting and Learning System, only 3.4%–5% of all medication errors reported involved harm to a patient, and only 0.03%–0.1% resulted in death (9). A central theme of this book is that, to the contrary, the fact that most medication errors are of little consequence has unjustifiably given rise to a culture of dangerous complacency. An argument of this type provides no answer for the young mother who died when bupivacaine for an epidural injection was given intravenously (this case is discussed in detail in Chapters 10 and 13) (19), the 153 young patients who died of vincristine administration errors (Box 1.1) (18), the babies lost to heparin overdoses (20), and 18-month-old Josie King and her lethal opioid administration (21) – in each of these examples, a medication error cost a patient's life and left behind a devastated family who will never forget that their loss was preventable.

1.2 A Road Map to the Book

In this book we explore the landscape of medication errors as we understand it today, with a focus on advancing the cause of safe medication management for patients as they traverse a pathway from living in the community, preparing for a surgical operation, being admitted to a ward and then an operating room, going back to a ward, and then returning to their community. Of course, medication errors in

Box 1.1 The tragic story of vincristine

Discovered in the 1950s by Canadian scientists Robert Noble and Charles Beer, vincristine, vinblastine, and other vinca alkaloids have saved countless lives. These were among the earliest, and are among the most effective, chemotherapeutic agents available; they have been used in the battle against breast cancer, osteosarcoma, Hodgkin lymphoma, small-cell lung cancer, and brain tumors, to name but a few. But these agents are incredibly aggressive vesicants: they become merciless killers when delivered via the wrong route. Although vincristine is not typically used during anesthesia and the perioperative period, many of the points illustrated by the vincristine story are of general relevance to medication safety, and the story serves as an excellent introduction to the themes of this book.

A typical regimen for brain cancer includes methotrexate given intrathecally, with vincristine given intravenously. A typical chemotherapy visit would have a young patient come to an outpatient setting, where the pharmacy delivers both the methotrexate and the vincristine, all too often in very similar syringes. The perceptive reader should now have a sense of dread.

The first case of fatal ascending myeloencephalopathy and death caused by inadvertent administration of vincristine into the intrathecal space was reported in 1968 (10). It was learned that intrathecal vincristine initiates a uniquely horrifying scenario: The young patient, told of the error, knows that he or she faces a rapidly progressing neuropathy, and an ascending encephalopathy that will lead inevitably and painfully progress to paralysis, coma, and then death. Over the subsequent 50 years, it is estimated that 135 patients have died (11), with the most recent case reported in 2018 (12). The true incidence is not known. Despite multiple safety alerts and highly publicized criminal prosecutions of some of the doctors involved in these tragedies, patient after patient has continued to die as a consequence of this known, predictable, and *preventable* medication error. And each skilled and compassionate physician who made this error while trying to do the right thing will have been beset by incredible guilt, and potentially even suicidal thoughts, as they are forced to watch a young patient, whom they hoped to save, die from this error (13).

The provision of vincristine and methotrexate, *both in syringes and both with white labels*, fits perfectly what James Reason has described as an error trap.

The MD Anderson Cancer Center in the U.S. designed and implemented a solution to this devastating error in 1980, dispensing vincristine only in 50-mL minibags, and never in syringes. Unfortunately, the involved pharmacists did not publish this method widely. In 2001, Trissel and colleagues published a paper (14), accompanied by an editorial (15), encouraging all to adopt this practice. Shortly thereafter, the Institute for Safe Medication Practices Canada (ISMP Canada) published a safety bulletin endorsing this approach. This safety bulletin was followed by a sentinel event alert from The Joint Commission in 2005 (which has now been retired and updated), and one from the WHO in 2015 (16). Despite a clear mechanism to decrease the risk of this tragic event, an international survey in 2012 reported that a third of institutions overall, and 45% of United States hospitals, continued to deliver vincristine in a syringe (17).

In 2010, Noble and Donaldson wrote of the "classic systems error which has proved intractable for nearly 40 years" (18). The failures to learn from history, to communicate safety solutions, and to develop robust physical design changes that they cite are central themes to this book.

We acknowledge the incredible loss and pain that these errors have inflicted. This is a prime case of *there but for the grace of God go I*. Most of us who practice in anesthesia and perioperative medicine live in fear of one day committing an error that causes serious harm to a patient entrusted to our care. This book is for the patients that we as a profession have harmed through medication errors and their loved ones, particularly those who are bereft forever because of these errors. It is also for those idealistic, dedicated, and compassionate people who (like us) work in healthcare and who, in spite of their very best efforts, to their deep distress, have inadvertently harmed the very patients they have been trying so hard to help. Medication safety is not easy. We hope that this book can contribute, at least in a small way, to making healthcare safer for patients and also for their caregivers.

particular and errors in general are not confined to this perioperative period. However, this tends to be a period of increased complexity in any patient's care. It is characterized by changes in routine medications before, during, and after surgery, and the additional administration of potent medications for the provision of anesthesia, for the postoperative relief of pain, for the prevention of nausea and vomiting, and for various other aspects of postsurgical patient care. In general, then, our focus is on data from the perioperative period, but from time to time we extend the boundaries of our exploration to include data from other clinical contexts because some studies mingle medical and surgical populations, and some studies that do not include surgical patients are of general relevance.

In this introductory chapter, we outline the extent of the problem of medication error in general and explain why we have chosen to focus on medication error in anesthesia and the perioperative period. We provide an outline of the book's contents. Substantial variation in terminology about different types of events related to the use of medications is to be found in the literature, so in the interests of clarity, we next present definitions that we use in this book. We move to a discussion of measurement in the context of medication safety. Measurement is generally held to be important for improving any aspect of healthcare, but once again, there has been substantial variation in the way this has been done in the studies reviewed for this book. Our hope is that this discussion may be useful not only for readers who need to interpret this literature but also for those who are planning future research in this field.

In Chapters 2 and 3, we consider failures in medication safety before the patient reaches the operating room, in the operating room, in the intensive care unit (ICU) and in the postoperative ward. In Chapter 4, we explore the effects these errors have on patients and their families. In this book, we use the term "family" to mean all those people who are close to and important to the patient. Some of these might be relations of the patient by blood or marriage and others might not. The boundaries to which harm from an adverse medication event extends are wide. In fact, these boundaries often extend to include the practitioners responsible for the care of the patient at the time an adverse medication event occurs. We discuss this important and rather complex issue in Chapter 5. We largely reject terminology that extends the concept of being "a victim" from the injured patient to those who were actually responsible for providing that patient with safe care. At the same time, we acknowledge that the consequences to such a practitioner may at times be out of proportion with any degree of blameworthiness pertaining to the event, and that managing

these consequences is important for the effective and safe provision of ongoing patient care.

In Chapter 6, we discuss the complexity that underpins the seemingly simple processes of medication management in anesthesia and the perioperative period and consider how these processes can at times go wrong. In Chapter 7, we look at the human element within the system, the nature of human error, and the reasons why admonitions to simply try harder or be more careful are generally useless. In Chapter 8, we introduce the subject of violations, distinguish violations from errors, and argue that minor violations are endemic in healthcare and are a substantial contributor to avoidable adverse medication events. The importance of violations in the generation of adverse medication events is a second key theme of the book, closely aligned with the theme of a dangerous complacency about medication errors. Improving medication safety depends on redesigning the system to reduce the likelihood of error, but system redesign will only occur if administrators and clinical leaders decide that investing in medication safety is a priority and will only be effective if practitioners take advantage of such investment by following safe practices conscientiously.

In Chapter 9, we move to solutions. We present some examples of front-line interventions and process changes that have been shown to reduce the likelihood of errors as well as interventions that seem obvious as critical steps toward improved safety. In Chapter 10, we extend this discussion to aspects of medication safety in special contexts, given the large gap between medication practices (and safety) and the economic resources to address them in high-income countries and also in low- and middle-income countries.

Chapters 11 and 12 are devoted to the question of accountability for medication safety. On the face of it, medication safety should be a given in our hospitals as much as sterilization of surgical instruments. However, it often seems that the law is less than effective in proactively ensuring safe practices in healthcare, and the litigation or prosecution that may occasionally follow a catastrophic medication event sometimes seems only to make terrible situations worse without substantially reducing the risk of similar events in the future. We consider some of the legal and regulatory approaches that operate in various countries today and discuss changes that would support a "just culture" and thereby contribute effectively to improving medication safety.

The challenge lies not so much in knowing what to do to improve medication safety as in actually doing it. In Chapter 13, we acknowledge that change is hard to achieve, and ask why, for example, so many hospitals have resisted adopting a safer way to prepare vincristine and methotrexate for administration to patients (18). Nearly 20 years ago, Merry and colleagues described a multifaceted approach to safe medication delivery during anesthesia (that included barcoding) (22), and several studies have subsequently demonstrated the potential of such an approach to reduce medication errors in anesthesia (23–27). The Australian and New Zealand College of Anaesthetists published the first edition of its professional document "PS51 Guidelines for the Safe Management and Use of Medications in Anaesthesia" over 10 years ago (28). Ten years ago, the Anesthesia Patient Safety Foundation published its "New Paradigm" for medication safety during anesthesia (29). Certain core concepts of medication safety underpin all three of these approaches, and these have been captured in two systematic reviews (30,31). Given all of this, we ask why it is that only a handful of hospitals around the world have implemented these principles, even in wealthy countries.

In Chapter 14, we return to our patients' stories, and to why medication safety in anesthesia and the perioperative period matters so much. We discuss a multilevel framework within which greater efforts could be made to manage the numerous domains of the medication process within safe limits. We finish with a call to arms, concluding that concerted action is long overdue to ensure that patients undergoing surgery receive safe management of their medications during anesthesia and the perioperative period.

1.3 Some Definitions and Concepts

Throughout this book, we use the term "medication" rather than "drug," as the term "drug" includes nonprescribed substances that alter physiology, while "medication" defines the smaller subset of drugs that are given for the express purpose of diagnosing or treating a disease state. Thus, when medications are involved, although the term "adverse drug event" (ADE) is in common use, we use the more specific term "adverse medication event" (AME).

1.3.1 Definitions of Medication Error

One of the challenges in understanding the nature and rate of medication error lies in the multiplicity of relevant definitions. This variation in definition contributes to a substantial variability in the reported rate of medication errors, which is compounded by variation in the methods used in different studies. Several authors have attempted to analyze these differences and synthesize a uniformly accepted set of definitions (32–35). Unfortunately, that has not yet occurred. Although some of the definitions set out by societies and agencies are quite similar, a uniform terminology has not been widely adopted by researchers. Lisby and colleagues (36) reviewed 45 studies that provided definitions of medication errors and found 26 different forms of wording in relation to errors. Among these studies, the cited rate of "medication error" ranged from 2% to 75%, in large part because of varying definitions.

For the purposes of this book, we use the following definitions, adopted or modified from various sources (27–34,37–39).

Drug: Any substance other than food that, when inhaled, injected, smoked, consumed, absorbed via the skin, or dissolved under the tongue, causes a physiological change in the body. Drugs include medications and other agents taken to effect a physiological change in an individual. Vodka is an example of a drug that is not a medication; ketamine, owing to its recreational potential, can be both a medication and a drug.

Medication: A legal drug that is intended for use in the diagnosis, cure, mitigation, treatment, or prevention of disease. Medications may be prescribed by clinicians, directly administered by clinicians without prescription, or obtained over the counter without prescription. Many AMEs in anesthesia and the perioperative period involve medications of the first two categories, but even over-the-counter medications can cause harm, including through interactions with prescribed medications. The term "drug-drug interaction," unlike the term "medication-medication interaction," includes interactions involving substances often taken by patients such as marijuana, alcohol, and herbal remedies that are not medications.

Error: An error is unintentional; it involves either the use of a flawed decision or plan to achieve an aim, or the failure to carry out a planned action as intended.[1]

Violation: A violation is an intentional – but not malevolent and not necessarily reprehensible – deviation from those practices deemed necessary (by designers, managers, or regulatory agencies) or appreciated by the individual as advisable to maintain the safe operation of a potentially hazardous system.[2]

Harm: Impairment of the physical, emotional, or psychological function or structure of the body, including pain.

Medication incident: Any irregularity in the process of medication management.[3]

Adverse medication event (AME): A response to a medication that is undesired and causes harm. AMEs can be avoidable (e.g., an allergic reaction after giving penicillin to a patient with a known allergy) or unavoidable (e.g., an allergic reaction after giving penicillin to a patient with no prior history of adverse reaction to penicillin). Undesired or harmful effects of the failure to administer an indicated medication should be included in AMEs.

Medication error: An error[4] in any part of the medication process, irrespective of whether it reaches the patient or of its outcome.[5]

Figure 1.1 presents a schematic of the various types of incidents associated with the medication process. Figure 1.2 presents a similar schematic, this time with real data from the observational study of intraoperative medication events by Nanji et al. (4).

We already noted that the majority of medication incidents involve errors or minor violations that cause little or no harm. In fact, many have no

---

[1] See Chapter 7 for discussion of this definition.
[2] See Chapter 8 for discussion of this definition.
[3] This definition has been modified from a definition of an incident by Morimoto et al. in 2004 (40) by adding the word "medication" to indicate that its scope is confined to the context of this book; as discussed later in this chapter, the general concept of an incident is much broader.
[4] As defined earlier.
[5] The term "near miss" is often used to describe a medication error that does not reach the patient, but some people view such events as "near hits" and prefer the term "close calls": see www.youtube.com/watch?v=zDKdvTecYAM, accessed January 25, 2020 (personal communication, Professor Jan Davies).

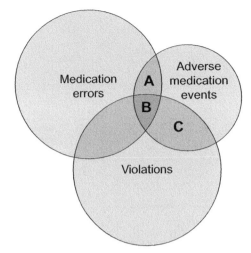

Figure 1.1 Relationship between adverse medication events (AMEs), medication errors, and violations of safe practices. All errors and violations associated with the management of medications create the potential for an AME, but many are in fact without consequence (i.e., those not within intersects A, B, and C). Not all AMEs arise from errors or violations. Those that do (i.e., those within intersects A, B, and C) are potentially preventable, particularly those arising from violations. Note that violations predispose to errors, so some errors arise, at least in part, from violations. The term "medication incident" includes any irregularity in the process of medication management (i.e., any error, violation, or AME). The sizes of the circles are not intended to accurately represent the relative frequencies of these various categories of incidents (see Figure 1.2). Inspired by a figure from Morimoto et al. 2004 (40).

serious potential to cause harm, such as administering acetaminophen instead of ibuprofen to a patient in the absence of a contraindication to acetaminophen (including the recent previous administration of acetaminophen, perhaps under a different brand name). Medication errors are at least theoretically preventable, and violations are certainly avoidable. Some adverse medication events arise from the innate properties of a medication, perhaps in conjunction with particular characteristics of a patient, and are not preventable other than through advances in pharmacology (e.g., a Stevens–Johnson reaction in a patient without any history of sensitivity). Importantly, many AMEs may be ameliorable. We discuss the relevance of this to medication safety in later chapters.

1.4 Levels of Harm from Medication Errors

There are various taxonomies in the literature to describe the level of harm associated with a

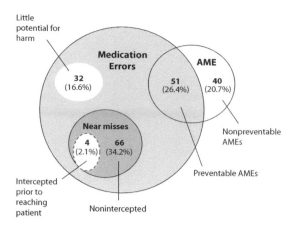

Figure 1.2 The 193 events detected in a study by Nanji et al. (4) included 153 (79.3%) medication errors (MEs) and 91 (47.2%) adverse medication events (AMEs). Nanji et al. used the term "adverse drug events"; we updated the figure per our definition. A single event could involve both an error and an AME. Of these events, 40 (20.7%) were AMEs that did not involve a ME, 51 (26.4%) were MEs that led to an observed AME, 70 (36.3%) were MEs with the potential for an AME (4 intercepted and 66 not intercepted), and 32 (16.6%) were MEs with little potential for harm. No attempt was made in this study to explicitly identify violations. Reprinted with permission from Nanji et al. 2016 (4).

medication error. In the early 2000s, on the heels of the publication of *To Err Is Human*, MEDMARX, which was established to facilitate electronic and anonymous reporting of medication incidents, was adopted by the United States Department of Defense as the incident reporting system for all military hospitals. MEDMARX initially had just three levels of harm: near miss; error, no harm; error, harm. This quickly expanded to more complex standardized taxonomy with definitions (see Table 1.1), established by the National Coordinating Council for Medication Error Reporting and Prevention (NCC MERP). This severity index scale provides granularity for hospitals to understand their own error landscape and to compare their events with those in other institutions around the United States. Although many studies use the NCC MERP definitions, there are still many reports that use their own unique definitions of levels of harm. Indeed, we, like others, have chosen not to adopt all the definitions recommended by the NCC MERP, notably in relation to defining a medication error (Box 1.2). Given that the NCC MERP definition is strongly recommended and widely used, it is worth

Table 1.1 National Coordinating Council for Medication Error Reporting and Prevention Index for Categorizing Medication Errors. Harm is "impairment of the physical, emotional, or psychological function or structure of the body and/or pain resulting therefrom." Monitoring is "to observe or record relevant physiological or psychological signs." Intervention "may include change in therapy or active medical/surgical treatment." Intervention necessary to sustain life "includes cardiovascular and respiratory support (e.g. CPR, defibrillation, intubation, etc.)."

Error?	Harm?	Category
No error occurred	No harm occurred	**A:** Circumstances present or events occurred that have the capacity to cause error
An error occurred		**B:** An error occurred but did not reach the patient[a]
		C: An error occurred that reached the patient but did not cause patient harm
		D: An error reached the patient and required monitoring to confirm that it resulted in no harm to the patient and/or required intervention to preclude harm
	Harm less than death occurred	**E:** The error may have contributed to or resulted in temporary harm to the patient and required intervention
		F: The error may have contributed to or resulted in temporary harm to the patient and required initial or prolonged hospitalization
		G: The error may have contributed to or resulted in permanent patient harm
		H: The error required an intervention to sustain life
	Death occurred	**I:** The error may have contributed to or resulted in the patient's death

Source: This table is derived from the diagram at www.nccmerp.org/sites/default/files/indexColor2001-06-12.pdf with some modification.
Note: An Algorithm for Categorizing Medication Errors according to this index is available at www.nccmerp.org/sites/default/files/algorColor2001-06-12.pdf.
[a] In the diagram from which this table is derived, a comment in parentheses states, "An error of omission does not reach the patient." We disagree in that the consequences of such an error may well reach the patient and cause harm (e.g., awareness if an anesthetic agent is omitted). Similarly, in category D, it is arguable whether the requirement for an intervention is or is not a form of harm.

> **Box 1.2 The National Coordinating Council for Medication Error Reporting and Prevention definition of a medication error (38).** The definition used in this book differs from this definition in that this definition would include violations and the malevolent use of a medication with intent to harm, both of which are excluded by ours; our definition also replaces the listed possibilities with the phrase "any part of the medication process" (which is arguably more inclusive) and emphasizes that the definition of an error does not depend on outcome.

> A medication error is any preventable event that may cause or lead to inappropriate medication use or patient harm while the medication is in the control of the healthcare professional, patient, or consumer. Such events may be related to professional practice, healthcare products, procedures, and systems, including prescribing, order communication, product labeling, packaging, nomenclature, compounding, dispensing, distribution, administration, education, monitoring, and use.

explaining our reasons for this. In practice, there is considerable overlap between our definition and that of the NCC MERP, and it is likely that for many purposes the same events would be captured using either definition. However, there are some important differences, which are explained in the caption of Box 1.2.

The harm typically reported or observed with medication errors is usually overt, tightly coupled with the medication error (coupling is discussed in Chapter 6), and closely related to it temporally (e.g., cerebral hemorrhage in an infant who received a 10-fold overdose of heparin) (20). However, overt harm may represent only the tip of the iceberg, because much of the harm from medication errors is actually covert. Covert harm may occur some considerable time after the relevant error and may not be tightly coupled to that error. A classic example of this is a surgical site infection occurring days after a missed redosing of prophylactic antibiotics intraoperatively, an error that may or may not have contributed to this complication. An even more covert example is that of a fall precipitated by unsteadiness induced by a mild overdose of pain medication or sedation. These

covert errors are not usually captured in studies on AMEs, in part because the people making them are often not aware of having done so, and therefore do not report them.

1.5 Measurement and Medication Safety in Anesthesia and the Perioperative Period

From the earliest days of anesthesia, there has been interest in measuring the harm that may arise specifically from the use of potent and potentially dangerous medications that is intrinsic to this specialty. Interest in measuring medication errors on the ward and in intensive care units during the perioperative period has tended to be aligned with investigations into medication errors in general. The third safety challenge of the WHO (mentioned earlier) extends even further, beyond the boundaries of the hospital into primary care settings. A patient undergoing surgery may experience a failure in the safe management of medications in any of these contexts, but very little research has attempted to capture the totality of this experience in a single study.

1.5.1 Early Days of Measuring Harm Associated with Anesthesia

The first documented death from anesthesia was that of Hannah Greener at the age of 15 years, during the administration of chloroform for the removal of an infected toenail on January 28, 1848. Discussion over the exact cause of this death has continued until recent times, but a fatal arrhythmia associated with the use of chloroform is certainly a likely possibility. A likely alternative possibility was aspiration (41). Within 15 months of Hannah Greener's death, Dr. Snow published the first study of anesthetic deaths (42). He attributed most of the deaths associated with chloroform in this study to what he called "cardiac paralysis" and later described how vaporization of chloroform, being distinctly different than that of ether, had an extremely narrow margin of error between the concentration of chloroform required for anesthesia (5%) and that resulting in death (10%) (43).

Despite Dr. Snow's recognition that deaths were often due to too high a concentration of chloroform and preventable with proper instruments, the prevailing view between the 1850s and the end of World War II was that the occasional "anesthetic death" was an inevitable concomitant of the medications used for anesthesia (44). In 1948, Robert Macintosh, Nuffield Professor of Anesthesia at Oxford, published a scathing challenge to this concept. He stated that "there should be no deaths due to anaesthetics" and advocated that attention should be diverted from developing new anesthetic drugs to training young "anaesthetists" (i.e., anesthesiologists) in "the care of the unconscious patient and in the correct administration of the time-proved anaesthetics readily to hand in any hospital" (45). A few years later, in the Crawford Long Memorial Lecture during the Fourteenth Annual Postgraduate Course in Anesthesiology at Atlanta, Georgia, Arthur Keats challenged what he called an excessive emphasis on mistakes in anesthetic practice (46). He reminded his audience (and subsequently his readers) that many of the medications (and techniques) used in anesthesia are potent and potentially lethal. He argued that AMEs (which he called ADEs) were not always preventable, that pharmacologic advances were important, and most importantly that great care should be taken in attributing the cause of any death associated with anesthesia. He suggested that only 10% of anesthetic deaths were attributable to error and provided an early warning against too ready a tendency to assign blame when things go wrong.

The first substantial investigation into anesthetic mortality in the era after World War II was undertaken in the United States by Beecher and Todd, who conducted a detailed examination of the results of 599,548 anesthetics given at 10 institutions between 1948 and 1952. Their objective was to establish the rate of death primarily attributable to anesthesia (which they found to be 1 in 2680 cases) and in which anesthesia was an important factor (1 in 1560 cases) (47). They were also interested in why these deaths occurred and in their relationship to various medications used during anesthesia (including, among others, curare, the vapors and gases of that day, and local anesthetic agents administered spinally). Further studies followed from Dripps et al. (48), Clifton and Hotten (49), and others. Unfortunately, differences in definition and methodology made it difficult to compare results between studies and therefore difficult to be sure about improvement over time in anesthetic

safety (50,51). A systematic review by Bainbridge et al. (52), conducted 10 years later, provided clear evidence of dramatic improvements in anesthetic mortality over time, particularly in high-income countries (the risk in low-income countries is often two to four times higher.) Nevertheless, these authors still comment on disparate definitions between studies, even in relation to the time frame for data collection. The one source of data collected on anesthetic mortality longitudinally in a consistent manner is to be found in Australia.

In Australia, in 1959, Ross Holland persuaded the Government of New South Wales to establish the Special Committee Investigating Deaths Under Anaesthesia (SCIDUA). The work of this committee was extended around Australia and then to New Zealand and now continues under the overall coordination of the Australian and New Zealand College of Anaesthetists, which publishes a triennial report containing epidemiologic data and recommendations for improved safety. There is no doubt from these reports that the safety of anesthesia has improved dramatically over the years since SCIDUA was first established. The most recent of these reports gives an estimated rate of anesthesia-related mortality of 1 per 57,023 cases or 2.96 deaths per million population per annum. Furthermore, the vast majority of the deaths in today's era involve elderly patients (87% were over 60 years of age) and patients with comorbidities (93% were ASA III-V). Interestingly, in light of the likely causes of Hannah Greener's death, of the 23 deaths where it was "reasonably certain" that the cause was anesthesia, 6 were due to cardiac arrest and 6 to aspiration. A further 7 were due to anaphylaxis, 2 to hypoxia following the loss of the patient's airway, and 2 to strokes following accidental arterial placement of central venous catheters. Many comments in the report address aspects of management of medications used by anesthesiologists. The average number of contributory factors per death is now very low indeed, at 1.03, suggesting high standards of care overall (53).

This picture is one in which improvements have occurred in all aspects of the provision of anesthesia. Snow and Keats were correct: Many of the medications and techniques used in anesthesia did carry inherent risk in their day, and even after much development, they still do. Macintosh was also correct in calling for better training of anesthesiologists. The standard of this training in high-income countries is now excellent. However, even well-trained anesthesiologists using modern medications and equipment can and do make mistakes, and systemic factors can and do contribute to adverse events in healthcare. The understanding of the importance of these factors in safe medication management in anesthesia and perioperative medicine owes its origins to leaders such as Jeff Cooper and Dave Gaba, among others (54–61). In an important initiative in 1987, Jeep Pierce led the formation of the Anesthesia Patient Safety Foundation, with the mission that "no patient shall be harmed by anesthesia" (61–63). All the reports referred to in this section, including the most recent, emphasize the need for ongoing improvement if this mission is to be fulfilled.

1.5.2 Metrics for Measuring the Rate of Medication Errors

It is a widely held tenet that measurement is fundamental to improvement. Medication errors turn out to be quite difficult to quantify. Some investigators have used the terms "incidence" and "prevalence" in attempting to do this. "Incidence" is generally understood to be the number of new cases per population that develop a certain condition in a given time period; "prevalence" is the proportion of a population who have a specific characteristic in a given time period. Given that a medication error is an event rather than a condition, that a single patient may experience more than one of these events during a particular clinical episode, and that the likelihood of this may be influenced by the number of medications administered to him or her within a particular clinical episode as well as the number of clinical episodes, "rate" is probably a better term for describing how often medication error occurs. Even then, the denominator needs to be defined. Possibilities include the rate of errors per medication administration, rate per anesthetic, rate per hospital day, rate per hospital admission, and many others.

One of the most rigorous metrics used to report rates of medication error uses the total opportunities for error (TOE) as its denominator (see Table 1.2). TOE is defined as the total number of doses given, whether correct or incorrect, plus any omitted doses, or as the total number of doses scheduled plus any extra doses given (64). TOE rates are

Table 1.2 Some metrics used to measure rates of medication error

Metric	Comments
Medication errors per total opportunities for error	Total opportunities for error may be defined in various ways: • Total doses due + total as-needed doses • With or without timing error • Can include each medication as a single opportunity for error, or as presenting an opportunity for error at each phase • Can count only a single error per opportunity (each medication is thus binary) or count multiple errors (e.g., in prescribing phase, used dangerous abbreviation *and* omitted dose)
Medication errors per patient	• Can be binary (e.g., a patient does or does not have at least one error during his or her stay) • Can be cumulative (how many errors any given patient experienced, from 0 on up)
Medication errors per 1000 patient days	• All reported errors normalized for total number of patient days in the study period

often presented as "with timing errors" or "without timing errors" (64). The rationale for this reporting scheme is that nurses often give medications early in order to complete all administrations prior to going off shift or because they have so many to give that some are necessarily late. As we discuss in Chapter 3, these minor variations in timing seldom cause harm to a patient, so there may be an argument for omitting these particular events, or for setting limits of tolerance within which timing variations are deemed to be acceptable.

A common metric used in calculating rates of error is that of overall medication errors, where each dose or prescription can be judged only correct or incorrect. This metric can be applied across the entire medication process from prescription through monitoring, or to any single phase of the process. Another metric is the total number of errors (TNE), where a single medication administration could have multiple errors, including improper preparation or dilution, wrong dose, wrong time, or even wrong documentation. Even when precise definitions of this type are used, variability continues to be seen in reported rates. For example, systematic reviews over the years have reported error rates based on TOE ranging from 1.7% to 72.5% (64), because of wide variations in the definitions of error, in who performed the observations, and in local processes and procedures.

A difficulty in reporting medication errors during anesthesia arises from the fact that the number of medication administrations, or alternatively the TOE per case, varies considerably. There is thus a good argument for reporting the rate by administration or by TOE rather than by anesthetic. However, the data points are not independent with any of these metrics, and particularly not with the first two. Thus, treating administrations or TOE as independent will inflate the statistical power of any tests comparing rates between groups (25). To understand this point, it is useful to consider the 30 (or more) intravenous medication administrations made on a particular night by a particular anesthesiologist working with a particular surgeon during a single difficult emergency cardiac case, and compare these with 30 administrations divided among several anesthesiologists managing various different minor elective procedures during the day. The first 30 administrations share many features that may influence the likelihood of error, whereas the second 30 are more independent of each other. Ideally, potentially confounding factors should be included in statistical analyses used to compare medication error rates between groups or over time, and as a minimum these should include case and anesthesiologist.

Having decided on metrics, the next choice to be made is in the research method used to estimate the rate of medication error. This has been done using various distinct methods, each with its own strengths and weaknesses.

1.5.3 Incident Reporting in the Study of Medication Errors

Perhaps the easiest method for studying medication errors is voluntary incident reporting. Incident reporting had its genesis in the work of Flanagan (65), who in 1954 published an insightful analysis of the "critical incident technique" that had been used throughout World War II to understand and reduce critical events among pilots during training. One of the first studies of medication error, published in 1960 (66), used research methods based on Flanagan's technique. In 1978, Cooper and colleagues published their seminal study in which they used a modified critical incident reporting technique to examine the nature of human error and equipment failure in anesthesia practice: "syringe swap" errors were one of the three most frequent categories of incident identified (54). Incident reporting methods vary from single surveys of practitioners (e.g., asking "have you ever made a medication error in your career?"), to annual or more frequent inquiries (e.g., asking "did you have a medication error in the past year?"), through the provision of ongoing opportunities for an individual who commits, who participates in, or who observes an error or incident to voluntarily report it to a central databank or research group, either anonymously or confidentially. Flanagan noted in his original description that contemporaneous inquiry, where events or incidents are reported immediately after they occur, significantly increases the number and quality of incidents collected (65). Although surveys can provide high-level information, such as how many anesthetists make medication errors over a lifetime, detailed information about the nature of individual incidents and about potential contributing or mitigating factors will be more comprehensive and more reliable when collected in real time. A particularly successful example of a national anesthesia reporting system with real-time reporting of medication-related incidents in anesthesia was the Australian Incident Monitoring Study, established in the 1990s by Runciman and others, in anesthesia services across Australia and New Zealand (67–73).

Voluntary incident reporting and surveys are inexpensive and allow for thousands or even millions of participants. This increases the likelihood that even very rare events will be captured. Incident reporting is best used to describe the nature of medication errors and events. It can also show changes in the patterns of reported incidents over time. For example, on the basis of an analysis of the 1000 most recent reports to the Australian Incident Monitoring Study in 2007, Williamson et al. were able to note that "unrecognised oesophageal intubation is now extremely rare" (74). This presumably reflected the benefit of technological developments in anesthesia, notably in relation to the establishment of monitoring with pulse oximetry and capnography as the standard of care in anesthesia (75).

Incident reporting systems have been credited with significantly improving anesthesia safety (as well as safety in aviation and other industries) (58). However, voluntary incident reporting does have certain limitations. The anonymous nature of these reports, considered necessary to encourage reporting, means that further details usually cannot be obtained after the report has been submitted, which often leaves an incomplete picture of the incident. Furthermore, this methodology does not permit an accurate rate of medication error to be determined, in part because memories are faulty, and many incidents are not reported. In fact, as observed previously, many medication errors are simply unrecognized by the practitioner, particularly if no harm occurs (e.g., the omission of a scheduled antibiotic). There may also be difficulties in obtaining denominator data accurately. It is possible to obtain some general information on denominators, such as the number of anesthesiologists surveyed or the number of cases or patient days studied, for example, but it is more difficult to precisely obtain the TOE or the total number of medication administrations in the study. Electronic record keeping may assist with this, but during anesthesia at least, it may still be uncertain whether every bolus of medication administered has actually been recorded.

One way of substantially improving the collection of both numerator and denominator data with incident reporting has been called "facilitated incident reporting." This approach is the least memory-dependent method of incident reporting. In facilitated incident reporting, practitioners are asked to complete a form at the end of every relevant encounter with a patient (e.g., every anesthetic) regarding whether or not an incident occurred. The question can be made even more direct and ask whether a particular type of incident, such as a medication error, occurred. Typically, the requested answer is simply a choice between "yes" and "no," with more detailed information collected only when the answer is "yes" (76). Facilitated incident reporting tends to identify much higher rates of error than voluntary reporting. We suspect that many practitioners may feel insufficient motivation to go to the trouble of making an incident report if the alternative is to do nothing, but once a report has to be submitted anyway, and they have

actually begun the process of doing so, this hurdle has been overcome, so their full participation seems to become much more likely.

Facilitated reporting is particularly useful in capturing anesthesia-related medication errors, as each case is discrete and typically is of a limited duration. Facilitated reporting has also been used in studies of prescribing errors, whereby a pharmacist reviews each prescription as part of daily work duties, and codes each as with an error or without an error. It is feasible that facilitated reporting could also be used in the ICU or on the ward, where nurses could be queried at the end of every shift, but we have not found publications describing facilitated reporting in any setting other than anesthesia and pharmacy.

The increasing use of electronic medical records allows for prompts to report incidents and can also enforce reporting after every case, in line with facilitated incident reporting. Notable examples of this are online reporting registries such as webAIRS (www.anzca.edu.au/fellows/safety-and-quality/incident-reporting-webairs, accessed January 2, 2020), developed and supported by the Australian and New Zealand Tripartite Anaesthetic Data Committee, and the Anesthesia Incident Reporting System (AIRS) managed by the Anesthesia Quality Institute (AQI) of the American Society of Anesthesiologists (see https://qualityportal.aqihq.org/AIRS-Main/AIRSSelectType/0, accessed January 2, 2020). Importantly, as well as allowing for ease of reporting, these electronic systems make it much easier to collate and analyze the reports. Because they are supported by major anesthesia organizations, they have also been set up with the express purpose and capability of generating authoritative recommendations for improvement in anesthesia safety. To this end, regular articles of educational value are published as "AIRS cases" in the ASA Monitor from the AQI system, and regular reports are published in the newsletters of the parent organizations of webAIRS. Both systems also support workshops at major anesthesia conferences and have informed various peer-reviewed publications (77–80).

Many of the events reported to these anesthesia-oriented systems concern medication safety. More generally, many large-scale, multidisciplinary, national-level medication incident reporting systems exist that offer practitioners opportunities to voluntarily report medication errors or incidents from any area of healthcare. One such system, MEDMARX, was initiated in 1993 by the *United States Pharmacopeia* (USP) and is currently maintained by Quantros. It is a privately maintained, subscription-based voluntary reporting system, focusing solely on medication errors to allow hospitals to report, track, and share medication error data in a standardized format (9). Currently, this database has over 1.2 million records of medication incidents from more than 860 facilities across the United States. Another national reporting system is the National Reporting and Learning System (NRLS), managed by the United Kingdom's National Health Service (NHS), which collects incident reports from NHS trusts in England and Wales (81). Since its inception, over 5.5 million incident reports have been submitted to the NRLS, of which approximately 9% have been medication related (9). It is interesting that in a recent review of 227 medication administration errors resulting in death reported to the NRLS arising from acute care between 2007 and 2016, only one report seems to have involved anesthesia (81).

As with any voluntary system of incident reporting, these large, national, voluntary incident reporting systems depend on individuals taking the initiative to report an incident. It is well recognized that the number of incidents reported varies by profession, with nurses and pharmacists having a high rate of reporting, while physicians report rarely (82,83). In one study, 89% of errors were reported by nurses, while only 1.9% were reported by physicians (84). It may be that physicians tend to fear shame and possible damage to job status and respect that may follow reporting an error (85). Furthermore, in the operating room, medication errors by an anesthesia provider are usually easily hidden and thus often ignored. Although the NRLS reporting was made mandatory in 2010, one can question the effectiveness of such a mandate, which may simply result in better hiding of events. On the other hand, reports from the NRLS are used to inform policy for patient safety in the NHS (86), whereas the anesthesia-specific systems do not seem to have formed comparable links with government agencies responsible for the safety of healthcare. Various comparable medical incident reporting systems exist in Australia and New Zealand, Switzerland, Denmark, Japan, Thailand, and many other countries.

1.5.4 Observational Studies of Medication Safety

A more rigorous method of studying medication safety involves "prospective observation." In these studies, trained researchers undertake prospective, direct observation of any or all parts of the medication process. This method has been used in the operating room (4,25), in the ICU (87), and on the wards (88). These studies provide more rigorous and detailed capture of medication errors and typically identify a much higher frequency of errors than voluntary reporting (4,25). Observational studies permit collation of the number of errors associated with medication administration to a patient over the course of a hospitalization, over an episode of care (such as an anesthetic), or with a single prescription of medication. The accuracy of determining the medications actually given can be improved by collecting used ampules and vials and by reconciling medications before and after each case (25). However, observational studies are highly resource intensive (25). Because of the expense and time required, observations are typically confined to short periods of time, meaning that rare but potentially devastating events, which would have been captured with an ongoing incident reporting system, can be missed. For example, it is unlikely that an observational study would have captured any of the 153 vincristine errors that have been reported worldwide, or the well-known medication error in which bupivacaine intended for an epidural infusion was given intravenously, causing the death of a young parturient (this tragic event is discussed in more detail in Chapters 10 and 13) (19).

1.5.5 Chart Review and Medication Errors

A third method of studying medication errors involves retrospective reviews of patients' charts or electronic records, including records of prescriptions or other aspects of the medication process.

Chart review has been used to study the incidence of adverse events in general, and these studies have typically uncovered large numbers of adverse medication events (5,6,90–92). Chart review has been used for all parts of the medication process but is particularly useful when studying prescription errors. A limited number of trained reviewers is required, strict definitions of what constitutes an error are needed, and the method is expensive. Interrater reliability may be quite low, and a degree of subjectivity is inevitable when evaluating records made for clinical purposes rather than for the purposes of research (e.g., in deciding whether a given dose of an opioid is appropriate for the subject's age and physical status). More recently, on wards and in intensive care units, electronic algorithms have been used to automatically capture and report erroneous doses, medication-medication interactions, and so on. One way of doing this is by using "trigger tools" (93). These electronic approaches are further explored in Chapter 3.

1.5.6 Simulation-Based Studies of Medication Safety

Finally, various forms of simulation have been used to study different aspects of medication safety, varying from screen-based interactive applications (94) to highly realistic simulations in which practitioners use real medications to manage complex scenarios (95).

Simulation allows challenging clinical situations to be created in which error becomes more likely, and it not only lends itself to observation but also permits video recording and debriefing to gain greater insights into the factors that influence medication safety (95). Other advantages of simulation include the minimization of medicolegal and ethical challenges associated with research into errors and violations. Evidence to support the validity of simulation for research applicable to clinical practice is growing (26,96), but simulation, like observational clinical studies, is highly resource intensive.

1.6 Conclusions

In the next chapters, we attempt the enormous task of making any sort of sense of the myriad reports on failures in medication safety in the literature. Almost every study that has been published on the topic of medication safety has used its own, slightly different definitions of what constitutes a medication error (to determine the numerator), and different definitions of what constitutes an *opportunity* for error (to determine the denominator). Studies have often focused on only a single phase

of the medication process, on a particular location (e.g., only ICUs or only wards, or combinations of the two), on one specialty (e.g., pediatrics, cardiovascular), or on a certain type of medication (e.g., high-risk medications, which also can be variously defined). However, one thing that is clear from virtually all of these studies is that the problem of failures in medication safety is substantial, notably during anesthesia and the perioperative period.

After reading Chapters 2 and 3, readers may conclude, as have the authors, that our understanding of either the rate or the nature of medication errors is imprecise. In the end, different research questions lend themselves to different research methodologies. In evaluating evidence to inform recommendations on medication safety, it is necessary to triangulate information from different studies, but to this end, it is important to understand the precise definitions used in each study and each study's strengths and limitations. It is our hope that the present chapter will provide a deeper understanding of the complexities of this problem to the appraisal of this literature and allow readers to be better equipped to interpret the results of the relevant research and apply them to their own institutions.

References

1. Donaldson LJ, Kelley ET, Dhingra-Kumar N, Kieny MP, Sheikh A. Medication without harm: WHO's third global patient safety challenge. *Lancet*. 2017;389(10080):1680–1.

2. World Health Organization (WHO). Medication without harm. WHO's third global patient safety challenge. 2017. Accessed January 3, 2020. https://www.who.int/patientsafety/medication-safety/medication-without-harm-brochure/en/

3. Bond CA, Raehl CL, Franke T. Medication errors in United States hospitals. *Pharmacotherapy*. 2001;21(9):1023–36.

4. Nanji KC, Patel A, Shaikh S, Seger DL, Bates DW. Evaluation of perioperative medication errors and adverse drug events. *Anesthesiology*. 2016;124(1):25–34.

5. Brennan TA, Leape LL, Laird NM, et al. Incidence of adverse events and negligence in hospitalized patients – results of the Harvard Medical Practice Study I. *N Engl J Med*. 1991;324(6):370–6.

6. Leape LL, Brennan TA, Laird N, et al. The nature of adverse events in hospitalized patients – results of the Harvard Medical Practice Study II. *N Engl J Med*. 1991;324(6):377–84.

7. Choi I, Lee SM, Flynn L, et al. Incidence and treatment costs attributable to medication errors in hospitalized patients. *Res Social Adm Pharm.* 2016;12(3):428–37.

8. Cranshaw J, Gupta KJ, Cook TM. Litigation related to drug errors in anaesthesia: an analysis of claims against the NHS in England 1995–2007. *Anaesthesia.* 2009;64(12):1317–23.

9. Wahr JA, Shore AD, Harris LH, et al. Comparison of intensive care unit medication errors reported to the United States' MedMarx and the United Kingdom's National Reporting and Learning System: a cross-sectional study. *Am J Med Qual.* 2014;29(1):61–9.

10. Schochet SS Jr, Lampert PW, Earle KM. Neuronal changes induced by intrathecal vincristine sulfate. *J Neuropathol Exp Neurol.* 1968;27(4):645–58.

11. Gilbar PJ. Inadvertent intrathecal administration of vincristine: time to finally abolish the syringe. *J Oncol Pharm Pract.* 2020;26(2):263–6.

12. Dabrowska-Wojciak I. The death of an infant after the unfortunate intrathecal injection of vincristine. *Clin Pract.* 2018;15:438–41.

13. Bain PG, Lantos PL, Djurovic V, West I. Intrathecal vincristine: a fatal chemotherapeutic error with devastating central nervous system effects. *J Neurol.* 1991;238(4):230–4.

14. Trissel LA, Zhang Y, Cohen MR. The stability of diluted vincristine sulfate used as a deterrent to inadvertent intrathecal injection. *Hosp Pharm.* 2001;36:740–5.

15. ISMP Canada. Healthcare Insurance Reciprocal of Canada (HIROC). Published data supports dispensing vincristine in minibags as a system safeguard. ISMP Canada; 2001. Accessed January 19, 2020. https://www.ismp-canada.org/download/safetyBulletins/ISMPCSB2001-10Vincristine.pdf

16. World Health Organization. *Information Exchange System Alert, No. 115.* Geneva: World Health Organization; 2007. Accessed January 19, 2020. https://www.who.int/patientsafety/highlights/PS_alert_115_vincristine.pdf

17. Greenall J, Shastay A, Vaida AJ, et al. Establishing an international baseline for medication safety in oncology: findings from the 2012 ISMP International Medication Safety Self Assessment for Oncology. *J Oncol Pharm Pract.* 2015;21(1):26–35.

18. Noble DJ, Donaldson LJ. The quest to eliminate intrathecal vincristine errors: a 40-year journey. *Qual Saf Health Care.* 2010;19(4):323–6.

19. Smetzer J, Baker C, Byrne FD, Cohen MR. Shaping systems for better behavioral choices: lessons learned from a fatal medication error. *Jt Comm J Qual Patient Saf.* 2010;36(4):152–63.

20. Arimura J, Poole RL, Jeng M, Rhine W, Sharek P. Neonatal heparin overdose – a multidisciplinary team approach to medication error prevention. *J Pediatr Pharmacol Ther.* 2008;13(2):96–8.

21. Kennedy P, Pronovost P. Shepherding change: how the market, healthcare providers, and public policy can deliver quality care for the 21st century. *Crit Care Med.* 2006;34(3 suppl):S1–6.

22. Merry AF, Webster CS, Mathew DJ. A new, safety-oriented, integrated drug administration and automated anesthesia record system. *Anesth Analg.* 2001;93(2):385–90.

23. Webster CS, Merry AF, Gander PH, Mann NK. A prospective, randomised clinical evaluation of a new safety-orientated injectable drug administration system in comparison with conventional methods. *Anaesthesia.* 2004;59(1):80–7.

24. Webster CS, Larsson L, Frampton CM, et al. Clinical assessment of a new anaesthetic drug administration system: a prospective, controlled, longitudinal incident monitoring study. *Anaesthesia.* 2010;65(5):490–9.

25. Merry AF, Webster CS, Hannam J, et al. Multimodal system designed to reduce errors in recording and administration of drugs in anaesthesia: prospective randomised clinical evaluation. *BMJ.* 2011;343:d5543.

26. Merry AF, Hannam JA, Webster CS, et al. Retesting the hypothesis of a clinical randomized controlled trial in a simulation environment to validate anesthesia simulation in error research (the VASER study). *Anesthesiology.* 2017;126(3):472–81.

27. Bowdle TA, Jelacic S, Nair B, et al. Facilitated self-reported anaesthetic medication errors before and after implementation of a safety bundle and barcode-based safety system. *Br J Anaesth.* 2018;121(6):1338–45.

28. Australian and New Zealand College of Anaesthetists. *PS 51 2018 Guidelines for the Safe Management and Use of Medications in Anaesthesia.* Melbourne: Australian and New Zealand College of Anaesthetists; 2018. Accessed April 26, 2019. http://www.anzca.edu.au/resources/professional-documents

29. Eichhorn J. APSF hosts medication safety conference: consensus group defines challenges and opportunities for improved practice. *APSF Newsletter.* 2010;25(1):1–7. Accessed January 3, 2020. https://www.apsf.org/article/apsf-hosts-medication-safety-conference/

30. Jensen LS, Merry AF, Webster CS, Weller J, Larsson L. Evidence-based strategies for preventing drug administration errors during anaesthesia. *Anaesthesia.* 2004;59(5):493–504.

31. Wahr JA, Abernathy JH 3rd, Lazarra EH, et al. Medication safety in the operating room: literature and expert-based recommendations. *Br J Anaesth.* 2017;118(1):32–43.

32. Aronson JK. Medication errors: definitions and classification. *Br J Clin Pharmacol.* 2009;67(6):599–604.

33. Ferner RE, Aronson JK. Clarification of terminology in medication errors: definitions and classification. *Drug Saf.* 2006;29(11):1011–22.

34. Pintor-Marmol A, Baena MI, Fajardo PC, et al. Terms used in patient safety related to medication: a literature review. *Pharmacoepidemiol Drug Saf.* 2012;21(8):799–809.

35. Lisby M, Nielsen LP, Brock B, Mainz J. How should medication errors be defined? Development and test of a definition. *Scand J Public Health.* 2012;40(2):203–10.

36. Lisby M, Nielsen LP, Brock B, Mainz J. How are medication errors defined? A systematic literature review of definitions and characteristics. *Int J Qual Health Care.* 2010;22(6):507–18.

37. Anesthesia Patient Safety Foundation. Medication safety in the operating room: Time for a new paradigm. Anesthesia Patient Safety Foundation; 2010. Accessed July 11, 2020. https://www.apsf.org/videos/medication-safety-video/

38. National Coordinating Council for Medication Error Reporting and Prevention. About Medication Errors: What Is a Medication Error? National Coordinating Council for Medication Error Reporting and Prevention. Accessed January 12, 2020. https://www.nccmerp.org/about-medication-errors

39. Wikipedia contributors. Drug. Wikipedia, The Free Encyclopedia; 2020. Accessed January 12, 2020. https://en.wikipedia.org/w/index.php?title=Drug&oldid=934040601

40. Morimoto T, Gandhi TK, Seger AC, Hsieh TC, Bates DW. Adverse drug events and medication errors: detection and classification methods. *Qual Saf Health Care.* 2004;13(4):306–14.

41. Knight PR 3rd, Bacon DR. An unexplained death: Hannah Greener and chloroform. *Anesthesiology.* 2002;96(5):1250–3.

42. Snow J. On the fatal cases of inhalation of chloroform. *Edinb Med Surg J.* 1849;72(180):75–87.

43. Snow J. On chloroform and other anesthetics: their action and administration. *Br J Anaesth.* 1957;29(3):142–4.

44. Runciman WB, Merry AF. A brief history of the patient safety movement in anaesthesia. In: Eger E II, Saidman L, Westhorpe R, eds. *The Wondrous Story of Anesthesia.* New York, NY: Springer; 2014:541–56.

45. Macintosh R. Deaths under anaesthetics. *Br J Anaesth.* 1948;21:107–36.

46. Keats AS. What do we know about anesthetic mortality? *Anesthesiology.* 1979;50(5):387–92.

47. Beecher HK, Todd DP. A study of the deaths associated with anesthesia and surgery: based on a study of 599, 548 anesthesias in ten institutions 1948–1952, inclusive. *Ann Surg.* 1954;140(1):2–35.

48. Dripps RD, Lamont A, Eckenhoff JE. The role of anesthesia in surgical mortality. *JAMA.* 1961;178:261–6.

49. Clifton BS, Hotten WI. Deaths associated with anaesthesia. *Br J Anaesth.* 1963;35:250–9.

50. Lagasse RS. Anesthesia safety: model or myth? A review of the published literature and analysis of current original data. *Anesthesiology.* 2002;97(6):1609–17.

51. Cooper JB, Gaba D. No myth: anesthesia is a model for addressing patient safety. *Anesthesiology.* 2002;97(6):1335–7.

52. Bainbridge D, Martin J, Arango M, Cheng D; Evidence-based Peri-operative Clinical Outcomes Research (EPiCOR) Group. Perioperative and anaesthetic-related mortality in developed and developing countries: a systematic review and meta-analysis. *Lancet.* 2012;380(9847):1075–81.

53. McNicol L, ed. *Safety of Anaesthesia in Australia. A Review of Anaesthesia Related Mortality 2006 to 2008.* Melbourne: Australian and New Zealand College of Anaesthetists; 2017.

54. Cooper JB, Newbower RS, Long CD, McPeek B. Preventable anesthesia mishaps: a study of human factors. *Anesthesiology.* 1978;49(6):399–406.

55. Newbower RS, Cooper JB, Long CD. Learning from anesthesia mishaps: analysis of critical incidents in anesthesia helps reduce patient risk. *QRB Qual.* 1981;7(3):10–16.

56. Cooper JB, Long CD, Newbower RS, Philip JH. Critical incidents associated with intraoperative exchanges of anesthesia personnel. *Anesthesiology.* 1982;56(6):456–61.

57. Cooper JB, Newbower RS, Kitz RJ. An analysis of major errors and equipment failures in anesthesia management: considerations for prevention and detection. *Anesthesiology.* 1984;60(1):34–42.

58. Cooper JB. Toward prevention of anesthetic mishaps. *Int Anesthesiol Clin.* 1984;22(2):167–83.

59. Cooper JB. Anesthesia can be safer: the role of engineering and technology. *Med Instrum.* 1985;19(3):105–8.

60. Gaba DM, Maxwell M, DeAnda A. Anesthetic mishaps: breaking the chain of accident evolution. *Anesthesiology.* 1987;66(5):670–6.

61. Pierce EC, Jr. The 34th Rovenstine Lecture. 40 years behind the mask: safety revisited. *Anesthesiology.* 1996;84(4):965–75.

62. Eichhorn J. The APSF at 25: pioneering success in safety but challenges remain. *APSF Newsletter.* 2010;25(2):1, 23–4, 35–9.

63. Cooper J. Patient safety and biomedical engineering. In: Kitz R, ed. *This Is No Humbug: Reminiscences of the Department of Anesthesia at the Massachusetts General Hospital.* Boston: Department of Anesthesia and Critical Care, Massachusetts General Hospital; 2002:377–420.

64. Keers RN, Williams SD, Cooke J, Ashcroft DM. Prevalence and nature of medication administration errors in health care settings: a systematic review of direct observational evidence. *Ann Pharmacother.* 2013;47(2):237–56.

65. Flanagan JC. The critical incident technique. *Psychol Bull.* 1954;51:327.

66. Safren MA, Chapanis A. A critical incident study of hospital medication errors. *Hospitals.* 1960;34:32–4; passim.

67. Barker L, Webb RK, Runciman WB, Van der Walt JH. The oxygen analyser: applications and limitations – an analysis of 2000 incident reports. *Anaesth Intensive Care.* 1993;21:570–4.

68. Cockings JGL, Webb RK, Klepper ID, Currie M, Morgan C. Blood pressure monitoring – applications and limitations: an analysis of 2000 incident reports. *Anaesth Intensive Care.* 1993;21:565–9.

69. Fox MAL, Webb RK, Singleton R, Ludbrook G, Runciman WB. Problems with regional anaesthesia: an analysis of 2000 incident reports. *Anaesth Intensive Care.* 1993;21:646–9.

70. Holland R, Webb RK, Runciman WB. Oesophageal intubation: an analysis of 2000 incident reports. *Anaesth Intensive Care.* 1993;21(5):608–10.

71. Kluger MT, Tham EJ, Coleman NA, Runciman WB, Bullock MF. Inadequate pre-operative evaluation and preparation: a review of 197 reports from the Australian incident monitoring study. *Anaesthesia.* 2000;55(12):1173–8.

72. Currie M, Mackay P, Morgan C, et al. The Australian Incident Monitoring Study. The "wrong drug" problem in anaesthesia: an analysis of 2000 incident reports. *Anaesth Intensive Care.* 1993;21(5):596–601.

73. Currie M, Webb RK, Williamson JA, Russell WJ, Mackay P. Clinical anaphylaxis: an analysis of 2000 incident reports. *Anaesth Intensive Care.* 1993;21:621–5.

74. Williamson J, Runciman B, Hibbert P, Benveniste K. AIMS anaesthesia: a comparative analysis of the first 2000 and the most recent 1000 incident reports. *ANZCA Bulletin.* 2008:13–15. Accessed January 4, 2020. http://www.anzca.edu.au/documents/anzca-bulletin-2008-mar.pdf

75. Eichhorn JH, Cooper JB, Cullen DJ, et al. Standards for patient monitoring during anesthesia at Harvard Medical School. *JAMA.* 1986;256(8):1017–20.

76. Webster CS, Merry AF, Larsson L, McGrath KA, Weller J. The frequency and nature of drug administration error during anaesthesia. *Anaesth Intensive Care.* 2001;29(5):494–500.

77. Gibbs NM, Culwick M, Merry AF. A cross-sectional overview of the first 4,000 incidents reported to webAIRS, a de-identified web-based anaesthesia incident reporting system in Australia and New Zealand. *Anaesth Intensive Care.* 2017;45(1):28–35.

78. Gibbs NM, Culwick MD, Merry AF. Patient and procedural factors associated with an increased risk of harm or death in the first 4,000 incidents reported to webAIRS. *Anaesth Intensive Care.* 2017;45(2):159–65.

79. Leslie K, Culwick MD, Reynolds H, Hannam JA, Merry AF. Awareness during general anaesthesia in the first 4,000 incidents reported to webAIRS. *Anaesth Intensive Care.* 2017;45(4):441–7.

80. Guffey PJ, Culwick M, Merry AF. Incident reporting at the local and national level. *Int Anesthesiol Clin.* 2014;52(1):69–83.

81. Harkanen M, Vehvilainen-Julkunen K, Murrells T, Rafferty AM, Franklin BD. Medication administration errors and mortality: incidents reported in England and Wales between 2007–2016. *Res Social Adm Pharm.* 2019;15:858–63.

82. Gallagher TH, Waterman AD, Ebers AG, Fraser VJ, Levinson W. Patients' and physicians' attitudes regarding the disclosure of medical errors. *JAMA.* 2003;289(8):1001–7.

83. Sarvadikar A, Prescott G, Williams D. Attitudes to reporting medication error among differing healthcare professionals. *Eur J Clin Pharmacol.* 2010;66(8):843–53.

84. Nuckols TK, Bell DS, Liu H, Paddock SM, Hilborne LH. Rates and types of events reported to established incident reporting systems in two US hospitals. *Qual Saf Health Care.* 2007;16(3):164–8.

85. Perez B, Knych SA, Weaver SJ, et al. Understanding the barriers to physician error reporting and disclosure: a systemic approach to a systemic problem. *J Patient Saf.* 2014;10(1):45–51.

86. Tingle J. Improving the National Reporting and Learning System and responses to it. *Br J Nurs.* 2018;27(5):274–5.

87. Valentin A, Capuzzo M, Guidet B, et al. Errors in administration of parenteral drugs in intensive care units: multinational prospective study. *BMJ.* 2009;338:b814.

88. al Tehewy M, Fahim H, Gad NI, El Gafary M, Rahman SA. Medication administration errors in a university hospital. *J Patient Saf.* 2016;12(1):34–9.

89. Orser BA, Byrick R. Anesthesia-related medication error: time to take action. *Can J Anaesth.* 2004;51(8):756–60.

90. Davis P, Lay-Yee R, Briant R, et al. Adverse events in New Zealand public hospitals I: occurrence and impact. *N Z Med J.* 2002;115(1167):U271.

91. Wilson RM, Runciman WB, Gibberd RW, et al. The quality in Australian health care study. *Med J Aust.* 1995;163:458–71.

92. Gawande AA, Thomas EJ, Zinner MJ, Brennan TA. The incidence and nature of surgical adverse events in Colorado and Utah in 1992. *Surgery.* 1999;126(1):66–75.

93. Rozich JD, Haraden CR, Resar RK. Adverse drug event trigger tool: a practical methodology for measuring medication related harm. *Qual Saf Health Care.* 2003;12(3):194–200.

94. Cheeseman JF, Webster CS, Pawley MD, et al. Use of a new task-relevant test to assess the effects of shift work and drug labelling formats on anesthesia trainees' drug recognition and confirmation. *Can J Anaesth.* 2011;58(1):38–47.

95. Merry AF, Weller JM, Robinson BJ, et al. A simulation design for research evaluating safety innovations in anaesthesia. *Anaesthesia.* 2008;63(12):1349–57.

96. Weller J, Henderson R, Webster CS, et al. Building the evidence on simulation validity: comparison of anesthesiologists' communication patterns in real and simulated cases. *Anesthesiology.* 2014;120(1):142–8.

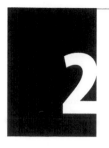

Failures in Medication Safety during Anesthesia and the Perioperative Period

2.1 Introduction

It is estimated that some 300 million surgical operations are performed worldwide every year (1). The clinical pathway of a typical surgical patient can be construed as beginning with the transition of care from primary care clinicians to hospital clinicians and ending with the transition of care back to the same primary care clinicians (see Figure 2.1). Within the hospital, surgical patients undergo further transitions of care from the ward into the operating room, perhaps via a holding area, then to a postanesthesia care unit (PACU) or possibly to an intensive care unit (ICU) or high-dependency unit (HDU), back to the ward (or possibly a different ward), and then back to their home. Many of the physical transitions also involve transfer of care between care teams. Each patient undergoing surgery will receive many medications during this continuum of care, and every medication administration exposes him or her to risk, including the risk of error. The frequency and nature of failures in medication safety vary by the phase of surgical care, as preoperative preparation, intraoperative management, postoperative recovery, and transition to home involve their different tasks and workflows. Not all of these failures are attributable to error on the part of the clinicians at the sharp end of caring for patients. Some reflect violations, and some reflect deficiencies in the system, including failures of equipment.

In the preoperative phase, medication reconciliation is important. Common missteps include failure to accurately identify all the medications being taken by the patient, failure to note allergies, and neglect or mismanagement of anticoagulation, cardiac medications, and diabetic control. Intraoperatively, the anesthesiologist typically serves as a sole agent prescribing, dispensing, preparing, administering, documenting, and monitoring the effect of medications. This is done without the

usual safeguards, whereby a pharmacist verifies a prescribed medication as appropriate in action, dose, and route, and then a nurse repeats these checks before administering the medication. After surgery, at transfer to the PACU, and then to the ward, and finally to home from the hospital, the issues of medication reconciliation return into play, notably with a risk of failures in communication (including through documentation) of medications that have or have not been given, and then of failing to restart medications discontinued preoperatively (e.g., anticoagulation and antiplatelet medications).

Recently in the United States, the concept of a "patient-centered medical home" has been promoted, where a single primary care provider or personal physician is the overall coordinator of medical care (2). This concept is well established in the British tradition of medicine (which extends to many countries of the British Commonwealth), in which the "general practitioner" is expected not only to manage routine care but also to coordinate interactions with specialty consultants. However, the extent to which this concept translates into actual practice is variable. In particular, when patients enter the hospital for surgery, their primary care physicians almost always hand over their care to hospital-based physicians. Patients are thus disconnected not only from their familiar *family* home, but also from their familiar *medical* home. This carries the risk of losing the safeguard of a single provider responsible for coordinating all aspects of their care, including all their medications. In one view, the responsibility for the overall coordination of the care of surgical patients within the hospital passes to the surgeon, and some surgeons exercise that responsibility very conscientiously. However, surgical training is not necessarily the best preparation for managing complicated comorbidities and the associated medications at the same time

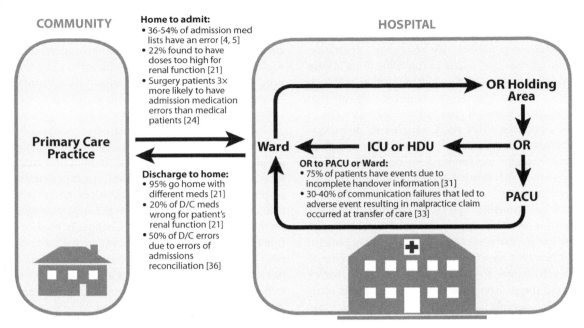

COMMUNITY

Home to admit:
- 36-54% of admission med lists have an error [4, 5]
- 22% found to have doses too high for renal function [21]
- Surgery patients 3× more likely to have admission medication errors than medical patients [24]

HOSPITAL

Primary Care Practice

OR Holding Area

Ward ← ICU or HDU ← OR

OR to PACU or Ward:
- 75% of patients have events due to incomplete handover information [31]
- 30-40% of communication failures that led to adverse event resulting in malpractice claim occurred at transfer of care [33]

PACU

Discharge to home:
- 95% go home with different meds [21]
- 20% of D/C meds wrong for patient's renal function [21]
- 50% of D/C errors due to errors of admissions reconciliation [36]

Figure 2.1 The clinical pathway followed by many surgical patients. OR = operating room, PACU = postanesthesia care unit, ICU = intensive care unit, HDU = high-dependency unit, D/C = discharge, meds = medications. Transfers of care (indicated by arrows) are strongly associated with medication errors, particularly those between the community and the hospital, during which changes in routine medication regimens may often be needed. Individual patients may follow slightly different pathways, and many variations are possible. The numbers in the figure may represent a single or multiple papers, with variable results, so they cannot be taken at face value. They do, however, indicate the risk for error at these transitions.

as coordinating the additional, often rather potent, medications needed to manage surgical recovery. Often, aspects of patients' care are given to various other physicians to manage, including hospitalists, internists, intensivists, and anesthesiologists. Anesthesiologists are well qualified to manage and coordinate the overall medical care of surgical patients, and over the past decade there has been a growing emphasis on their role as "perioperative physicians." From this perspective, anesthesiologists should at least be cognizant of, and ideally involved in, all phases of the extended perioperative period, from the decision for surgery until discharge from the hospital and even until the patient's full return to normal function. However, properly resourced formal arrangements to facilitate the exercise of these responsibilities may still be the exception rather than the norm. Thus, the challenge lies in ensuring that between the surgeons, the anesthesiologists, the intensivists, and the various other physicians who may become involved in a patient's perioperative care, this overall coordination is not lost. The key to all of this is, of course, communication, and the greatest challenge to communication lies at the transitions of care.

In some institutions, reconciliation of medications on admission to the hospital (and on discharge) has become routine and is often done by a pharmacist. Increasingly, institutions are adopting electronic prescribing and recording systems to facilitate the entire process of medication management, and these systems may include functions to assist with medication reconciliation. At least conceptually, these systems can link with electronic systems used by primary care practices and by pharmacies both in the hospital and in the community. However, comprehensive solutions of this type are difficult and expensive to establish and are still uncommon. For example, efforts to achieve this functionality at a national level have been ongoing for many years in New Zealand, the Netherlands, and Denmark, as well as other countries (3), but the current situation still falls well short of this ideal.[1]

---

[1] The New Zealand Health Quality and Safety Commission provides a useful overview of some of these issues: see www.hqsc.govt.nz/our-programmes/medication-safety/projects/medicine-reconciliation/, accessed July 14, 2019.

In this chapter and the next, we explore failures in medication safety in various phases of the perioperative period. We start our exploration with failures that occur in the transitions of care from home to hospital, while in hospital, and then back to home. We then move to the very different context of errors in medication management in the operating room itself, whether by anesthesia providers or by other clinicians in the operating room. Finally, in Chapter 3, we deal with medication errors in intensive or critical care units and on general wards.

The various examples in this section of the book are not intended to provide specific guidance for any particular aspect of medication management. Rather, they have been given to highlight some of the challenges to medication safety that characterize the preoperative period. Judgment is often needed, not just in managing patients through this period, but also in deciding whether a particular medication management decision represents an error, a violation, or good practice. In fact, nuanced decisions are less likely to result in harm than a failure to identify an obvious risk, such as that associated with the use of epidural or spinal anesthesia in the presence of anticoagulants.

2.2 Managing Medications during Surgical Patients' Transitions of Care

2.2.1 Transitions of Care between the Community and the Hospital

Transitions of care between the community and the hospital pose a significant risk to patients. It has been estimated that 54%–67% of admitted patients have at least one discrepancy between home medications and those noted at admission, and that 27%–59% of these discrepancies have the potential to cause harm (4,5). Inadequate medication reconciliation at admission may account for up to 20% of adverse medication events in hospitalized patients (6). This is not difficult to believe, as medication history taking and reconciliation are difficult processes and prone to error. Increasing age and the number of medications taken are both predictors of a medication error on admission (5). Many elderly patients and those with low health literacy frequently cannot list the names of their medications,

let alone their doses, strengths, or frequency of use. Linguistic and cultural barriers add substantially to risk, as does the sheer number of medications prescribed to many patients. Look-alike or sound-alike products further complicate medication history taking, as does unfamiliarity with particular medications on the part of the history taker.

Pharmacology is a field that never stands still, and the proliferation of new medications, notably agents based on monoclonal antibodies and antiviral medications, can baffle the most experienced of physicians, let alone a surgical or anesthesia trainee – or a patient. Discharge home provides further opportunity for error. Changes in medication regimens that have been made during the hospital stay (perhaps because the surgical treatment has altered the need for certain medications) have to be conveyed to the patient and the primary care physician, and prescriptions need to reflect the new regimen. The assumption that a patient will take the intended medications may itself be flawed, but accurate prescribing and clear instructions are obviously a prerequisite for this to occur.

2.2.2 Some Challenges to Medication Safety in the Presurgical Period

Patients presenting for surgery are often chronically ill with numerous medical comorbidities, which typically translate into complicated medication regimens. Presurgical medication management should begin at least 5–7 days before surgery, or even earlier, depending on the medication involved (e.g., adjusting the use of an immunosuppressant with a six-weekly dosing schedule would need a longer period). Decisions must be made on whether to continue or suspend certain medications (or other drugs such as herbal supplements) and, if so, whether to bridge with alternative medications. Coordination is required, and there is a considerable burden of communication with patients and between the various doctors involved in their care. If a medication is to be withheld or changed, clear instructions to the patient are needed, specifying exactly when to stop taking the medication (including both date and time for medications taken several times a day). Verbal instructions should be supplemented with written ones. Sadly, failures in communication with patients about their medications are common, both in this context and in general, and confusion on their part over which medication to suspend and when is common. This can result in cancellation on the day of surgery, or in harm if a misunderstanding is not detected (7).

These decisions should ideally be driven by evidence-based guidelines. However, guidelines change with regularity, and some medications (e.g., immunologic agents, which can alter immune status) have little evidence available to guide appropriate preoperative management. Furthermore, consensus on best practice changes as new evidence is published, and it is difficult even for experts to stay current. For example, beta-blockers were "probably recommended" for initiation in patients undergoing vascular surgery and in those with strong cardiac risk factors in 2007 guidelines from the American Heart Association (8), but this advice was reversed in the 2009 focused update (9), following the publication of data from the POISE I trial (10).

For many years, it was advised that angiotensin-converting enzyme (ACE) inhibitors and angiotensin-receptor blocking (ARB) agents be withheld prior to surgery because of the increased likelihood of hypotension with anesthesia. In 2014, however, the American College of Cardiology/American Heart Association recommendations stated that continuation of ACE inhibitors or ARB agents preoperatively is reasonable, especially in patients with chronic heart failure (class IIa, level of evidence B) (11). Frequent changes like these can increase the difficulty of ensuring that patients receive the latest evidence-based management, and the predominance of expert consensus over definitive evidence in developing guidelines adds to the difficulty of knowing what to do for individual patients in specific circumstances (12). Thus, it may sometimes be difficult to determine whether a particular decision was or was not an error.[2]

The perioperative management of coagulation is particularly challenging, with potentially grave consequences if mistakes are made. Patients may be on anticoagulation agents (vitamin K antagonists or novel oral anticoagulants such as direct thrombin inhibitors or anti–factor Xa agents) or antiplatelet agents (e.g., acetylsalicylic acid, clopidogrel, ticagrelor) or some combination of these classes of medication. Decisions about whether to stop, when to stop, and whether to bridge with other agents (e.g., heparin, enoxaparin) are driven by the underlying reason for anticoagulation (e.g., a mechanical heart valve, the presence of atrial fibrillation, a history of deep venous thrombosis), the presence of medical comorbidities, and the risk and potential consequences of surgical bleeding during the proposed procedure. These nuances are difficult to manage. The matter is made more difficult if there is an expectation for the idiosyncratic (rather than evidence-based) preferences of a particular surgeon to be accommodated. Many surgeons have widely differing preferences for coagulation management prior to surgery, even in relation to the same category of surgical procedure within the same institution.[3] In practice, it often falls to the patient's primary care physician to make decisions about whether to withhold anticoagulants and, if so, whether to bridge anticoagulation or not, typically without knowing either the surgeon or the specific implications of anticoagulation for the planned surgery. Inappropriate decisions can again lead to cancellation of surgery or to harm, notably excessive bleeding or preventable thromboembolism. Unsurprisingly, one of the more common errors in relation to the management of coagulation is that of simply overlooking the issue completely: In a survey of patients scheduled for spinal surgery, 19% of those on anticoagulants or antiplatelet agents were not instructed to withhold them before surgery, and so their operations were cancelled on the morning of surgery (7).

Opioid management presents its own profile of challenges and risks. Outpatients can be on transdermal, oral, or even nasal preparations. Calculation of a total oral morphine equivalent daily dose is critical for translation of doses into those suitable for parenteral opioids for intraoperative and immediate postoperative pain management. Errors in calculation and translation can result in underdosing (potentially resulting in withdrawal symptoms or excessive pain) or overdosing (potentially resulting in respiratory depression or death).

If it is difficult to manage medications for which best practice guidelines exist, it is even more difficult to manage medications for which there are few data and no guidelines related to the periop-

---

[2] We expand on the theme of errors of judgment in Chapter 7.

[3] Appropriate and inappropriate variation in clinical practice is discussed in detail in Chapter 8.

Box 2.1 An oversight followed by a difficult decision

A physician known to the authors of this book was scheduled for a dental implant in the community-based practice of a consultant oral surgeon. The dental implant was to be undertaken under local anesthesia, so no anesthesiologist was involved. At about the time this procedure was being planned, this patient was diagnosed through a separate process as having idiopathic osteoporosis and was started on a regimen of intravenous bisphosphonates. The one question that was not asked during the extensive internal medicine assessment of this patient was, "Are you considering having a dental implant?" Similarly, the oral surgeon did not ask about bisphosphonates (after all, it is common to think of osteoporosis as predominantly a disease of women rather than men). In fact, bisphosphonates are a relative contraindication to dental implants (13), but this turns out to be an excellent example of a topic on which advice has shifted somewhat over time and for which the evidence is still very limited.

On the day of surgery, the patient thought to mention the fact that he had recently received this treatment. This nearly resulted in postponement of the surgery for some months, but in the end, after considerable discussion and with informed consent, the procedure went ahead, and the postoperative course was uneventful. This case illustrates several points:

- One cannot judge an error by its outcome. In this case, there clearly was an error in history taking by each of the two specialist practitioners, which manifested as a failure to identify a relative contraindication to the planned surgery, but the ultimate outcome of the procedure was satisfactory.
- Furthermore, the outcome would presumably have been even more satisfactory if this error had been compounded by a complete failure to detect the issue (which very nearly occurred), because this would have eliminated the anxiety experienced by both the patient and the practitioner in having to make a decision on whether to proceed regardless of the potential risks of bone necrosis and failure of the implant.
- Even when an issue about the perioperative management of a medication is identified and carefully considered, the evidence to guide a decision may be limited.
- Patients can often play an important role in contributing to their own medication safety by asking whatever questions come to mind, even when these do not appear to have obvious relevance to their care.
- In situations of uncertainty, the properly informed view of the patient becomes particularly important in the making of clinical decisions.

---

erative period. A good example is to be found in the rapid proliferation of immune system suppressants, which may increase the risk of surgical site infection. These medications have dosing schedules that range from daily to once every 6 weeks, which makes scheduling of surgery difficult – even supposing that the surgeon or scheduler actually considers the implications of these medications. Another example is provided in Box 2.1.

2.2.3 Reconciliation of Medications at the Preoperative Clinic

Preoperative preparation for anesthesia ideally includes a clinic visit some time before admission to hospital, at which time a history is taken, a physical examination carried out, and appropriate investigations are initiated. This is the perfect opportunity both for a complete medication reconciliation to be conducted and for a plan to be formulated for any changes that might be needed in the patient's medications. Unfortunately, both these matters are often overlooked or inadequately addressed.

Adequate medication reconciliation includes verifying not only every medication *prescribed* (including its name, dose, frequency of administration, formulation, and route) but also how the patient is actually *taking* these medications (e.g., with or without food) and even whether the patient actually *is* taking them at all. This is particularly important for "as needed" medications, such as analgesics. In one study, congruence between patients' recall, the information in the primary care record, and the information recorded on hospital admission was found to be present in fewer than 10% of admitted patients (14). If a primary care physician has not embraced the concept of a medical home and taken responsibility for all prescribed medications, this general practitioner may not even know all the medications a patient is taking, and reconciliation will be made more difficult by the fragmentation of prescriptions among multiple consultant physicians. Truly accurate reconciliation may require telephone calls to various pharmacies, the primary care physician, and multiple consultants. The number of medications to be reconciled substantially influences the time required for the preoperative visit, with 12 medications predicting an evaluation time of nearly 45 minutes in one study (15). In addition to prescribed medications, which can be accurately verified by the relevant pharmacy, patients may be taking a plethora of over-the-counter drugs, such as vitamins and herbal supplements, which may or may not have been disclosed to the primary care physician (16). It may be very difficult to know the relevant potential drug-drug or drug-excipient interactions with any accuracy, as the U.S. Food and Drug Administration and other regulatory bodies have little say about these nonprescription agents.

Even if all normally prescribed and taken medications are accurately documented during reconciliation, changes may be made between the preoperative clinic visit and admission to the hospital either to accommodate surgery (e.g., anticoagulation holds, an altered amount of insulin taken the night before, etc.) or for other reasons (e.g., alterations in the patient's medical condition). These changes also need to be tracked. Therefore, when a patient is admitted to the hospital, another complete medication reconciliation should be done.

2.2.4 Medication Management for Outpatient or Same-Day Surgery

Patients who are managed as outpatients, or whose surgery is a same-day procedure, may or may not have been seen at a preoperative clinic. Arguably, they should have a formal medication reconciliation and review on admission and on discharge, but these steps may often be missed. In particular, it seems often to be simply assumed that these patients will resume their normal medication regiments postoperatively. This may not be justified. For example, some patients will have suspended or withheld anticoagulation agents or antiglycemic medications and should receive specific instructions at discharge about when and how to restart these. Patients who have been bridged with

enoxaparin may need explicit instruction about the need to continue bridging postoperatively until their international normalized ratio returns to a desirable level as warfarin is resumed. Often the surgeon will be the individual discharging these patients and may need to manage this issue. Some will be highly competent to do this, others less so. Sometimes it will be an anesthesiologist who discharges a patient from the recovery unit, but the reconciliation of discharge medications may or may not be explicitly recognized as part of an anesthesiologist's responsibilities in a day surgical unit. Often it is assumed that someone else (e.g., the primary care physician, or the practitioners at the "Coumadin Clinic") will manage these aspects of care. This may be appropriate, but clearly such an assumption should be verified and supported by appropriate communication. Interestingly, we found no studies of the incidence of medication errors related to the transitions of care in same-day procedure patients. Many of these patients may be on no medications at all, but the potential for errors in light of these various possibilities would seem to be considerable for those who are.

2.2.5 Medication Management for Surgical Patients Admitted to Hospital for One or More Nights

It seems to be widely accepted today that patients admitted to hospital with a planned stay of one or more nights after surgery require medication reconciliation and review on admission and at discharge. However, this is not always done well, or even at all. It is increasingly common for such patients to be admitted on the morning of the day of surgery, and this can create some pressure of time to get these important tasks completed. The matter is made more complicated by the need for different clinicians to be involved in the review of these patients' medications. The anesthesia team needs to identify issues such as the potential for drug-drug interactions during anesthesia, the likely approximate opioid requirement intra- and postoperatively given preoperative opioid dosing, and the routine medications (if any) that may need to be redosed during anesthesia. The surgical team needs to consider how to manage home medications while the patient is in the hospital. The preliminary medication reconciliation may be carried out by one or another of these teams, or by a separate practitioner, ideally a pharmacist. Clearly there should be a single source of truth about a patient's medications, but these duplications in process and involvement of multiple practitioners can all too easily undermine this objective. For example, one study found that 73% of all patient records have at least one discrepancy between anesthesia and surgery medication lists. Of the discrepancies, 23% had different allergy records, 56% had different medications, and 43% had different doses or dosing frequencies (17).

Looking across all types of admissions to the hospital, a detailed, pharmacist-performed review of admission orders found that 36% of patients had at least one wrong medication order entry. The vast majority (85%) of these errors originated in a wrong medication history being taken by the admitting physician, and most of these were omissions (i.e., the patient was taking a medication that the admitting physician missed) (5). In another study, a nurse-performed admission medication list was accurate only 16% of the time, and 13% of medication errors were classified as having the potential to cause moderate or serious harm (18). Other authors report that 53% of patients had at least one unintended discrepancy, of which 36% were felt to have the potential for moderate or serious harm (4). Among patients undergoing gastrointestinal and orthopedic surgery where reconciliation was done by the surgery team, a mean of 0.65 unintended medication discrepancies was found per patient (actual home medications versus the admission medication history) (19). Among patients admitted for spinal surgery, 36% failed to receive at least one appropriate medication: One-third of these failures were due to an omission at admission, and 60% were due to incorrect substitution of previously taken medications while in the hospital (7). Geriatric patients are more likely than others to have medication reconciliation errors at admission (with an estimated rate of 50%), with the most common error being omission (20). In another study, nearly 22.5% of patients had dosing that was inappropriate for their renal function, and nearly 19% had potential drug-drug interactions (21). The Screening Tool of Older People's Prescriptions (STOPP) criteria (22) are designed to identify potentially inappropriate prescribing in geriatric populations. STOPP has mostly been

used during medical rather than surgical admissions but clearly has potential value in the surgical context. Thus, the risk of medication error at admission increases with both polypharmacy and older age (23), and omission of a home medication seems to be, by far, the most common of these errors.

It is clear from these data that reconciliation of medicines on admission to the hospital is a very important element of medication safety for all patients, but particularly for those undergoing surgery. In one study that included both medical and surgical services, the rate of reconciliation error was significantly increased in the general surgical service (odds ratio 3.31) (24). This is understandable, because as we have discussed, surgery often creates a requirement for suspension or alteration of home medications, which increases the risk of error. In addition, some surgeons may understandably have less familiarity than internists with the vast array of medications used to treat even common maladies.

Pharmacists bring specific expertise to the task of medication reconciliation. In fact, their involvement can add greatly to the safety of every aspect of perioperative medication management (25–30), but often the resources to provide this support are limited.

2.2.6 Transfers of Care Within the Hospital

Few data exist about medication reconciliation during transfers of care within the hospital following admission. Certainly, a medication omitted at admission is unlikely to be noted at any successive transfer of care, as the receiving team will likely only reconcile to the admission medication list, and not repeat complete medication reconciliation with home medications. We know that transfers of care in hospitalized patients are fraught with errors due to incomplete communication and transfer of patient information, and that correct knowledge about a patient tends to degrade across the continuum of care, with each successive transfer of care providing less complete critical information (31). In a study by Nagpal et al., 75% of patients suffered clinical events due to incomplete transfer of patient information (31). Communication failures between caregivers, whether within a discipline (physician to physician) or across disciplines (physician to nurse), are well recognized as a leading cause of preventable adverse events (32) and are a common precipitating factor in medical malpractice lawsuits (33). In a study of surgical malpractice closed claims, 43% of communication failures occurred during a handoff, and 39% occurred with a transfer between locations (33). This study primarily concerned failures to notify a senior physician of a critical change in a patient's condition rather than medication errors, but it serves to highlight the dangers of transitions of care.

2.2.7 Discharge from Hospital to Home

Medication errors at discharge from hospital have been less well studied than medication errors on admission, but they are frequent (~40%), and many are clinically relevant (24,34). The number of medication errors per patient identified at discharge is likely to be even higher than at admission because many unrecognized errors in medication management at admission will carry through to discharge (35). Again, omission is common: In one study that compared patients' preadmission home medication lists with those at discharge, nearly 50% of discrepancies were attributable to omissions at admission (36).

Few patients go home from the hospital on the same medications they were on at admission, and surgical patients in particular are often discharged on new, additional medications. This opens the door for unrecognized drug interactions with ongoing established medications; new medications may be inappropriate for the patient's age or renal function. In one study, 95% of patients had a difference between admission and discharge medications (21). Some of these differences were appropriate, such as changes in response to a new diagnosis, or the addition of short-term medications for specific indications (e.g., opioids added for analgesia after surgery or a brief period of anticoagulation started in patients after total knee surgery). Unfortunately, others were inappropriate – nearly 20% of patients in this study were on a dose of medication that was inappropriate for their renal function. Transplant patients will usually require substantial changes in medication regimens. For one thing, the functionality provided by the transplanted organ will obviate the need for many of the prior-to-admission medications or require alterations in their doses. For another, new

medications may be needed, and these may interact with existing medication (e.g., addition of steroids to these patients' regimens may necessitate alterations in their diabetic management) (37). Other admission-to-discharge discrepancies reflect simpler errors, such as when paused medications are inadvertently not restarted (often, anticoagulation or antiplatelet medications) or incorrect doses are prescribed for medications that are continued.

Neglecting to restart suspended medications and to adjust the dosage of those that are restarted is common, particularly for anticoagulation or antiglycemic medications. Diabetic patients may require more insulin at home than in the hospital, where their diet is more tightly controlled, or require more in the hospital, because of the effects of acute surgical stress. They may be discharged home on an insulin regimen based on hospital requirements, which may be either inadequate or too high once they return to their preferred diet. The substantial perturbations in physiology associated with surgery regularly require modification of preexisting medications or expansion of the medication regimen (21). Surgery can exacerbate hypertension (e.g., via pain or fluid overload), requiring alteration or addition of medications that will no longer be needed once the patient has recovered. Alternatively, it can result in hypotension due to fluid shifts or blood loss (and hence anemia in the postoperative period), resulting in suspension of medications that the patient will need to resume once recovery has occurred. It is often difficult to accurately predict the progressive changes in a patient's physiologic state that will occur days or weeks after discharge. This places a greater onus on primary care physicians to monitor and manage medication regimes during this period, but this will be greatly facilitated if the hospital specialists communicate with them clearly about the possible changes that might be anticipated in each particular patient. We believe it is quite unusual for anesthesiologists to engage with primary care physicians in this way. This task often falls to members of the surgical team, but a thoughtful consideration of these nuances may be difficult for a time-pressured surgeon or surgical trainee.

Pediatric patients face many unique risks (38). Dosing should be weight based most of the time, but children are often not weighed. When they are, the weights are not always accurate or may be recorded inaccurately (e.g., weight was performed on kilogram scale, but the notation is for pounds) (39–41). Thus, in one study, pediatric discharge medications were found to have at least one error 80% of the time, but the vast majority of errors simply involved incorrect or missing weights or dates. Although many of these errors may be minor with little potential for harm, a missing or wrong weight makes it difficult for a pharmacist to do a correct double check of the dose, and quite large deviations from appropriate doses might then be missed.

The situation for small children is made even more challenging by the fact that pediatric oral formulations are often unavailable for commonly used medications. This problem is exacerbated by the fact that infants cannot swallow pills. In addition, drug clearance mechanisms are immature at birth and take some years to mature. Clearance has a nonlinear relationship to weight, and there has been insufficient study of pharmacodynamics in children and infants. Thus, simply basing an infant's dose on that of an adult, adjusted for weight alone, may not be accurate, even if the weight itself has been determined precisely (38).

The medications patients actually take after returning home from the hospital may turn out to be different again. Even when every medication prescribed anew or reinitiated at discharge is exactly correct, patients typically receive little education about their new medications or on how to manage other changes in their regimen. In addition, communication with the primary care physician has been shown to be often both inadequate and wrong. Thus, many patients will have a discrepancy between the discharge summary and what patients subsequently report they are actually taking (42,43). In one study where patients were contacted after discharge, all had at least one discrepancy between the discharge summary list of medications and the medications they were actually taking. Many of these discrepancies involved the resumption of normal medications that had not been listed on the discharge summary; other common errors involved patients not being aware that a previously established medication that had been temporarily stopped should have now been resumed. Many others involved incorrect doses (43). Important discrepancies have even been found between the discharge summary medications and the medication list presented to the patient (36). Mixon et al. called patients after discharge and compared the reported medications

being taken with the hospital discharge list. Over 50% of patients had at least one discordant medication, and 59% had a misunderstanding about indication, dose, or frequency of cardiac medications (42). In a study of patients older than 64 years of age, 22% of medications taken prior to admission were restarted with either an altered dose or a within-class substitution (e.g., captopril instead of lisinopril) or were stopped altogether at discharge. The vast majority of patients (70%–80%) had no or only partial understanding of these changes (44). Not surprisingly, patients with lower health literacy or lower subjective numeracy are at increased risk for misunderstandings of this sort (42). To add further risk to this discharge process, almost half of patients investigated by Cornu et al. received a medication list at discharge that was different from the list sent to their primary care provider in the discharge summary. In this study, when there were more than five medications in the patient's discharge medication list, there was a threefold increase in the likelihood of a discrepancy (36).

Most surgical patients leave the hospital with a follow-up surgical visit scheduled. Given the complexities of medication reconciliation at discharge, they should also have a scheduled visit to their primary care physician within 5–7 days, focused on assuring appropriate return-to-home medications.

2.3 Failures in Medication Safety in the Operating Room

Surgical patients who receive either sedation or general anesthesia will be given a variable number of medications during their procedure. In a study of nearly 75,000 anesthetics, the number of intravenous boluses per case ranged from 0 to 39 (the mean was 9.9) although the number of *different types* of medication administered by these boluses was not evaluated (45). In addition, these medications can include inhaled gases or vapors; intravenous infusions given over minutes to hours; and subcutaneous, intramuscular, intraspinal, epidural, and sublingual injections. Medications may also be used for nerve blocks in some patients.

The medication process has sometimes been described as having four steps: "prescribing, dispensing, administering, and monitoring." In fact, this is a substantial oversimplification (see Table 6.1). For clinicians directly caring for patients, the process includes (1) making a diagnosis that

Table 2.1 Some reported rates of medication error during anesthesia, with percentages for common categories of error. All studies are in the context of clinical anesthesia except the 2017 study by Merry et al. in a high-fidelity simulation setting. Note that differences in rate largely reflect differences in methodology. The most reliable estimates are those from the observational studies.

First author and date	Country	Type of study	Rate as the number of anesthetics per error	Most common categories of error[a]
Nanji et al. 2016 (46)	United States	Observational	2	Labeling error (24.2%) Wrong medication (22.9%) Omitted medication (17.6%) Documentation error (17%)
Merry et al. 2011 (47)	New Zealand	Observational RCT (data taken from control group)	1	Wrong dose (61.3%)[b] Recording error (35.6%) Substitution (1.5%) Omission (1.2%) Labeling error (0.3%)
Merry et al. 2017 (48)	New Zealand	Observational RCT (simulated cases: data taken from control group)	1	Wrong dose (47.8%)[b] Recording error (41.8%) Substitution (5.1%) Omission (4.3%) Labeling error (0.9%)
Bowdle et al. 2018 (57)	United States	Facilitated incident reporting (data taken from baseline group 2002–3)[c]	161	Wrong dose (37%) Substitution (26%) Insertion (6.8%) Omission (6.8%) Labeling error (6.8%) Repetition (5.5%) Incorrect route (4.1%)
Zhang et al. 2013 (53)	China	Facilitated medication incident reporting	137	Omission (27%) Wrong dose (23%) Substitution (20%)
Cooper et al. 2012 (58)	United States	Facilitated medication incident reporting	203	Wrong dose (36%) Substitution (25%) Omission (19%)

Table 2.1 (cont.)

Study	Country	Method	N	Findings
Llewellyn et al. 2009 (54)	South Africa	Facilitated medication incident reporting	274	Substitution (60%) Wrong dose (23%)
Webster et al. 2001 (51)	New Zealand	Facilitated medication incident reporting	133	Incorrect dose (32%) Substitution (27%) Omission (18%)
Amor et al. 2012 (56)	Morocco	Facilitated medication incident reporting with denominator data	575	Labeling mistakes (44%)
Abeysekera et al. 2005 (59)	Australia	Voluntary general incident reporting	NA	Wrong medication (34.6%) Overdose (24%) Omission (16.3%) Wrong patient (16.3%)
James 2003 (60)	United Kingdom	Voluntary general incident reporting	NA	Wrong medication (22.7%) Wrong dose (12.9%) Wrong route (11.3%)
Yamamoto et al. 2008 (61)	Japan	Voluntary general incident reporting	NA	Wrong dose (29%) Substitution (23%) Omission (21%) Incorrect route (10%)
Khan and Hoda 2005 (52)	Pakistan	Voluntary general incident reporting	272	Wrong dose (33.3%) Adverse effect/ineffective (33%) Syringe swap (17.6%)
Orser et al. 2001 (50)	Canada	Survey	NA	Syringe swap (70%)

Abbreviation: RCT, randomized controlled trial.
[a] Terminology differs a little between studies.
[b] This was a discrepancy between the recorded dose and the administered dose.
[c] The percentages apply to baseline data collected from 2002 to 2003.

requires a medication, (2) prescribing or selecting the appropriate medication (or medications), (3) dispensing and preparing this medication, (4) administering it, (5) recording its administration, and (6) monitoring its effect. Clearly, the wrong diagnosis can lead to patients receiving inappropriate medications. Unfortunately, much of the literature on medication errors during anesthesia does not appear to include errors in diagnosis within its scope or even errors in the choice of medication for a given diagnosis. A notable exception is the recent study by Nanji et al. (46). Similarly, errors in the recording or documentation of administered medications have seldom been considered in general studies of medication error other than in the observational studies of Nanji et al. and Merry et al. (47,48). We discuss documentation errors in greater detail later in this chapter.

For virtually every medication administered in the hospital other than during anesthesia, a physician writes an order, a pharmacist reviews the order and then dispenses the medication, and a nurse then double-checks and administers this medication and also records what has been given. At each point, there is an opportunity for a "fresh set of eyes" to capture an error. In some institutions, robotic and computerized systems add to the safety of this process. Unlike this robust system of double checks, during anesthesia all of these steps are typically carried out by one individual who makes a diagnosis, selects the medication, draws it up if necessary, administers it without writing a prescription, records the process, and monitors its results. Thus, despite the powerful and inherently dangerous effects associated with many of the agents used for anesthesia, the traditional double checks or forcing functions that are normal for medication safety during the rest of each surgical patient's journey through the hospital are simply missing from this part of patient care.

2.3.1 Rate of Medication Errors and Other Failures in Medication Safety during Anesthesia

As discussed in Chapter 1, measuring medication errors during anesthesia or in the operating room has been done primarily through various forms of voluntary incident reporting. In one of the earliest studies of error in anesthesia, Cooper et al. invited anesthesia providers to provide voluntary reports and take part in interviews to identify errors or equipment failures that they had experienced at any point in their career. The most common type of error reported involved "drug administration" (49). In a different study using a mail survey, over 2000 Canadian anesthesiologists were asked, "Have you ever administered the wrong drug during an anesthetic?" There was a 30% response rate; 85% of these respondents reported at least one error or near miss, with four respondents reporting a death due to the error (50).

Webster et al. used voluntary, ongoing, facilitated reporting in which anesthesiologists in New Zealand were asked to complete a form after *every* anesthetic, not simply those on which they chose to report a medication error (or an incident more generally). The first question on the form asked whether or not a medication error had occurred. More information was required only if the answer was in the affirmative. This approach substantially improved the response rate of the study. These investigators received 7794 study forms from 10,806 anesthetics; the rate of medication administration error per anesthetic was 0.0075, or 1 error per 133 anesthetics (51). This approach has now been used in several countries (see Table 2.1), and a remarkably consistent rate of reported errors has been found – in the region of 1 per 200 anesthetics, which translates approximately to 1 per 2000 medication administrations (52–56). The proportions of types of errors were quite similar as well, with substitution or wrong dose constituting the majority of reported errors in all the studies.

The most reliable method of estimating the rate of medication error is by direct observation. Three such studies have been published in the context of anesthesia, one of which involved high-fidelity simulation. In these observational studies, the rate of medication errors in anesthesia was found to be much higher than any previous estimates (Table 2.1). In two observational studies undertaken by Merry et al. in New Zealand (one in a clinical setting and the other in simulated cases), a rate of approximately one error in medication administration or recording was found per nine medication administrations (47,48). This rate would equate to approximately one error per anesthetic. In the United States, Nanji and colleagues observed 3671 medication administrations in 277 operations and found a rate of medication error of 1 per

2.2 operations, and 1 per 19 administrations (49). This study extended beyond errors of administration and included such things as untreated hypotension. Nevertheless, the results are remarkably similar between the three observational studies.

2.3.2 Documentation Errors and Medication Safety

Errors in documentation were included in the studies of both Merry and Nanji but have not typically been included in incident reporting studies. Accurate recording of administered medications is important for the ongoing management of patients. Although incomplete or omitted documentation may be viewed by some anesthesiologists as trivial infractions rather than clinically important errors (especially for little "bumps" of vasopressors), inaccuracies in the recording of administered medications can lead to subsequent errors, such as overdosing of muscle relaxants, opioids, or antibiotics when a relieving anesthesia provider or a PACU nurse misinterprets the amount that has been given and gives unnecessary additional doses or perhaps has difficulty understanding signs of residual neuromuscular blockade. Accurate documentation is also important for audit, for research, and for medicolegal purposes, and there is a strong argument for including documentation in the list of "rights" of safe medication management, during anesthesia and more generally (Box 2.2).

Inaccuracies in the documentation of anesthetic medications have been specifically studied. Avidan et al. compared direct observation of medication administration to the record made with an anesthesia information system. No documentation was done in 15% of administrations. When it was, there were errors in the recorded medication (17%), dose (8%), and time of administration (4%) (62). The most commonly omitted documentation involved vasoactive medications. Wax and Feit audited used syringes of vasopressors at the end of 100 cases and found complete documentation only 26% of the time. In 36% of the occasions where a syringe clearly had been used (because of the volume remaining in the syringe), there was no documentation of this. In the remaining 62% in which volume was missing from the syringe, only 50% of the doses were charted (63). In a study that compared anesthesia records made manually with records made using an automated anesthesia recording system (AIMS), the AIMS records were more complete than the handwritten records, but there was no significant difference between the recorded number of medication administrations. This likely reflects the fact that entry of medication information into an AIMS is still largely manual, unlike physiological data that can be collected entirely automatically (64).

2.3.3 The "True" Rate of Medication Error during Anesthesia

It is worth commenting further on the difference between the relatively consistent rates identified in the facilitated incident reporting studies and the similarly consistent but much higher rates reported in the observational studies. In essence, incident reporting requires that the reporter knows he or she has made an error or committed a violation. Many errors are not appreciated by the person making them. Many mistakes in diagnosis or choice of medication would be in this category: If the person realized a mistake was being made, he or she would presumably not make it, although the mistake might occasionally be identified later. Similarly, many medication administration errors are made completely unconsciously and are only detected if some obvious physiological response occurs.

Box 2.2 The 10 "rights" of safe medication administration

The *right medication** should be administered to the *right patient** for the *right reason* (or *diagnosis*) in the *right dose** at the *right time** by the *right route* in the *right formulation* with the *right technique* and the *right documentation*, and the *right response* should be confirmed (by monitoring).

Various lists exist, and this one is somewhat longer than many others. In this list, the "right reason" may be taken to include a patient-centered view that not only should the choice of medication be appropriate for the (correctly made) diagnosis but also that it should meet the needs and preferences of the individual patient. Various versions of this list of "rights" have been published since four corresponding wrongs (identified with an asterisk) were identified by Schlossberg in 1958 (see Chapter 3) (67).

These errors can of course be detected in observational studies, directly and through reconciliation of retained empty vials and ampules (47,48). The technique of retaining empty vials and ampules has also been advocated as a part of safe medication management during anesthesia (see Chapter 9) (65). Documentation errors, discussed in the previous section, if identified, would likely be corrected rather than reported. Furthermore, in the studies by Merry et al., one of the methods of identifying errors was reconciling the information documented in the anesthesia record with that obtained by observation and reconciliation of used and unused vials and ampules (47). The results raised questions about the intended medication or dose. It was sometimes unclear whether this was the dose actually given, the one recorded as having been given, or the one on the label of the syringe (there were times when all three were discrepant.) This matter could only really be resolved by interviewing the anesthesiologist concerned, which was not part of the study design and might arguably have influenced its outcome.

There is still some debate over what constitutes a clinically important failure in medication safety during anesthesia. It is relevant to patient safety that some failures are more dangerous than others. Injecting the completely wrong substance into the epidural space is likely to have worse consequences for the patient than a failure to record every last "bump" of ephedrine, for example. One might assume that the rates from facilitated incident reporting reflect failures that participating anesthesiologists thought sufficiently important to report. However, an omitted dose of prophylactic antibiotic is exactly the sort of error that might be overlooked in these studies, and this would obviously be of importance. As discussed in Chapter 1, clear definitions are needed to allow studies to be compared with each other or, at the least, to allow differences in results to be understood. From a clinical perspective, it is hard to discount the argument that medication management is a core role for anesthesia providers and that every effort should be made by them to comply with the list of medication safety "rights" outlined in Box 2.2. From a patient's perspective, the rate that matters will be closer to that seen in observational studies than that seen in studies using facilitated incident reporting.

As a final reflection, an anesthesia provider who gave 20 anesthetics a week, each requiring an average of 10 medication administrations, for 42 weeks a year over a career of 30 years would give a total of just over 25,000 anesthetics involving a quarter of a million medication administrations. He or she would make over 100 medication errors on the basis of the facilitated incident reporting studies, and over 10,000 errors on the basis of the observational studies. It is perhaps surprising that only 1 in 8 respondents to a survey by Merry et al. admitted harming a patient through medication error in anesthesia (66) and that only 4 of the 687 anesthesiologists who responded to a survey in the study by Orser et al., noted in Table 2.1, reported patient deaths from this cause (50). However one looks at the available data, the rate of failures in medication management during anesthesia is clearly far, far too high.

2.3.4 The "Rights" of Safe Medication Management and Classifications of Failures to Achieve These

The classification of failures in medication safety in the overall context of healthcare is discussed in detail in Chapter 7. Some approaches are based on the psychological processes underpinning the errors or violations that lead to these failures. However, these processes can be difficult to evaluate. Phenomenological categorizations in which failures in medication safety are described by their observable characteristics circumvent the need to establish what the practitioner concerned in the particular failure was thinking at the time it occurred and are much more commonly used in reports of such events. In such classifications, errors are often classified in relation to a list of so-called "rights" of safe medication administration (see Box 2.2). However, the safe management of medications involves more than their administration, so reference should also be made to part of the process in which they occurred (see Table 6.1). There is considerable variation in how classification is done in different contexts and studies (see Table 2.2).

As discussed later, medication errors in the hospital but outside the operating room occur most often during the prescribing and administering steps, while the majority of studies of medication

Table 2.2 Examples of different phenomenological approaches to categorizing failures in safe medication management. In this book, we usually adopted the categories in the second column, which have been modified with some additions. An "Other" category is often included in anesthesia publications. Various cognitive processes may underlie examples in any of these categories (see Chapter 7).

"Rights" of medication safety	Category as defined in anesthesia literature	Category as defined by national agencies (NLRS, MEDMARX)	Examples (A = anesthesia example, N = national agency example)
Right medication	**Substitution** – incorrect medication given	Unauthorized drug	A – Syringe or vial swap
			N – Medication not prescribed
	Repetition – extra dose of intended medication given	Extra dose	A/N – Extra dose given
	Insertion – medication given that was not intended at that time or any stage	Not defined	
	Wrong medication – medication given that was not fit for purpose	(Unauthorized)	A/N – Drug given despite allergy or drug/drug interaction
		Deteriorated or expired product	A/N – Expired medication
		Faulty product through failure in manufacture	A/N – Not refrigerated
	Omission – medication not given	Omission error	A/N – Missed dose such as antibiotic
Right patient	**Wrong patient** – medication intended for one patient given to another	Wrong patient	A – Reused syringe from prior case
			A – Syringe prepared in advance for next patient given to current patient
			A/N – Blood given to wrong patient
			N – Medication prescribed to one patient given to a different one
Right reason	**Wrong choice or selection** – wrong medication for correctly diagnosed situation	Prescribing error	A/N – Wrong medication chosen to treat the condition
	Wrong diagnosis – leading to wrong medication for the situation		A/N – Wrong diagnosis
Right dose	**Wrong dose** – desired medication given in the wrong dose	Improper dose/quantity	A/N – Erroneous dilution
			A/N – Infusion pump error
			A/N – Wrong weight used for dose
			A/N – Wrong dose of the right drug for the condition (e.g., epinephrine for hypotension versus anaphylaxis)

(continued)

Table 2.2 (cont.)

"Rights" of medication safety	Category as defined in anesthesia literature	Category as defined by national agencies (NLRS, MEDMARX)	Examples (A = anesthesia example, N = national agency example)
Right time	**Wrong timing** – correct dose of intended medication given at wrong time	Wrong time	A – Antibiotics delivered more than 60 minutes prior to incision N – Prescribed medication given more or less than 30 minutes from correct time
Right route	**Wrong route** – desired medication given by the wrong route	Wrong route	A/N – intravenous versus neuraxial and vice versa; inadvertent intra-arterial injection
Right technique		Wrong technique	N – Bolus versus infusion
	Contaminated medication – through poor asepsis in handling and administration	Not defined	A – Propofol left in syringe greater than 4 hours
	Wrong labeling of syringe, line, or bag containing medication[a]	NA	A – No label, label missing information, or label with incorrect information
Right preparation	**Wrong preparation**	Wrong preparation	A – Pediatric doses prepared from adult formulations N – Normal saline versus water to dissolve, crushing instead of dissolving
Right documentation	**Wrong documentation** – details incorrectly recorded	Not defined	A/N – Missed or erroneous documentation
Right response	**Monitoring error**	Monitoring error	A/N – Failure to recognize adverse reaction (allergic, hemodynamic)

Source: Categories in the second column have been modified from Bowdle et al. 2018 (57).

Abbreviation: NLRS, United Kingdom's National Reporting and Learning System (see Wahr 2014 [68]).

[a] Failures in labeling may include omitting a label altogether and occur one step earlier in the medication process than most of the other listed categories. When they are identified, it may sometimes be difficult to know whether a failure in medication administration actually occurred or, if so, its exact nature (because the type and concentration of the medication in the syringe or bag may not be clear).

errors in anesthesia (Table 2.1) have focused on the dispensing (drawing up from a vial or ampule, labeling, diluting) and administering (by intravenous, inhalational, or other routes) of medications.

2.3.5 Failures in Aseptic Technique during Anesthesia

An important aspect of medication safety that is often ignored by anesthesia providers relates to aseptic technique employed when intravenous medications are handled and administered via peripheral cannulas or central catheters. Although bloodstream infections (BSIs) are more commonly associated with central catheters, even peripheral catheters carry a risk of BSI (69). However, the importance of asepsis in anesthesia practice has only recently gained attention, and it is likely to take a long time to change the habits of current practitioners. As discussed in Chapter 8, many of these failures of asepsis actually represent violations rather than errors. Asepsis is particularly important in relation to the handling of intravenous medications but applies more generally as well. For example, anesthesiologists should remove or change their gloves immediately after intubation of the trachea, with hand hygiene, as simulations have shown that oral contaminants are widely spread around the operating room within 30 minutes if they fail to do this, as they often do (see Figure 2.2) (70,71).

There is at least some evidence to support several potentially important aseptic practices during anesthesia that also align with first principles

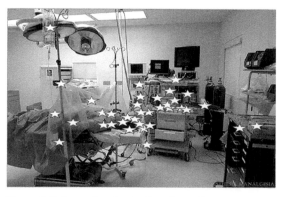

Figure 2.2 Areas of contamination of operating room surfaces from fluorescent dye placed in a simulated patient's mouth within 6 minutes of intubation. Reproduced with permission from Birnbach et al. 2015 (69).

and common sense. For example, the Society for Healthcare Epidemiology of America published expert guidance on infection protection in the anesthesia work area (71), and the U.S. Centers for Disease Control and Prevention published guidelines for placement, maintenance, and accessing of intravenous cannula (72,73). Appropriate hand hygiene (by washing with conventional soap and water or by use of alcohol-based hand rubs) is central to the management of all intravenous cannulas and should be performed prior to placement of a catheter and when accessing the insertion site or an injection port. Skin cleaning with alcohol, povidone-iodine, or chlorhexidine should precede the placement of all intravenous cannulas. In general, insertion of peripheral catheters requires the use of only clean, rather than sterile, gloves, while midline and central venous catheters require full barrier protection for both the patient and the operator (72,74). In addition, any time the intravenous line is accessed for a change of infusion fluids or a port is accessed for addition of an infusion or for a bolus of a medication, aseptic technique should include hand hygiene and a scrub of the port with alcohol.

A common misconception among anesthesia providers is that the rubber stopper of a glass bottle is sterile underneath its metal covering. This is patently not true: These metal covers are meant to serve only as dust covers, they do not protect against microbial contamination, and all rubber stoppers must be scrubbed with alcohol prior to penetration with a needle (75). Multiuse vials should only be used for one patient per vial; syringes for the next case should not be made up during a previous case, particularly with propofol, as any contaminating bacteria can proliferate rapidly in the lipid formulation (76,77). Nevertheless, survey data (78) and anecdotal observation indicate that many practitioners violate these practices routinely. It may be thought that many of these violations are unimportant, but Loftus has led a growing body of research that testifies to the importance of asepsis in anesthetic practice (79–89). A New Zealand team led by one of the authors of this book has added to this evidence by demonstrating that microorganisms are inadvertently injected into some 6% of patients during the process of drawing up and administering intravenous medications during the provision of anesthesia (77,90). A recent report of three cases of sepsis from contaminated propofol (75) is discussed in detail in Chapter 11 (see Box 11.3).

2.3.6 Harm from Failures in Medication Management during Anesthesia

In virtually all studies, the majority of reported medication errors during anesthesia have caused little or no harm. Near misses are common (these have been called pre-errors [51] and, as explained in footnote 5 in Chapter 1, some writers prefer the term "near hits"), but often the number reported seems to be lower than one might expect. An example would be recognizing that an incorrect syringe had been picked up before its contents were administered, and it is possible that many anesthesiologists would see this as too trivial to warrant reporting.

Failures in aseptic technique during the management of intravenous medications during anesthesia are without doubt a potential cause of serious harm and so are erroneous omissions of prophylactic antibiotics. Postoperative infections are recognized as a huge problem worldwide and may manifest as wound infections, pneumonia, or sepsis. However, they typically occur sometime after surgery, and the exact extent to which anesthetic practices contribute to them is currently unknown (see Chapter 12 for a further discussion of this issue).

2.3.7 Closed Claims Databases

Analysis of closed claims databases provides a different perspective on failures in medication safety, as these events have all resulted in sufficient harm that a malpractice suit was brought. In the American Society of Anesthesiologists Closed Claims database, incorrect dose was the most frequent medication error associated with significant harm; syringe or vial swap (substitution) was the second most common (91). In this database, 9% of the medication errors involved the administration of a muscle relaxant to an awake patient, resulting in awareness while paralyzed. This was similar to the National Health Service (NHS) Closed Claims database, where 19 of 93 claims were for awake paralysis (92). In the latter review, virtually all claims were attributed to human error, but less than half would have been prevented using a "double-check" method. In the Danish Closed Claims system, there were 24 deaths attributed to

anesthesia (4.5%), with one-third of these related to a medication error (93).

2.3.8 Medication Errors by and between Different Members of the Operating Room Team

None of the studies listed in Table 2.1 have included medication errors that occurred in the operating room but that were committed by surgeons, nurses, and perfusionists rather than anesthesia providers. Beyea et al. reviewed all operating room medication incidents that were reported to MEDMARX, the voluntary reporting system from the *U.S. Pharmacopeia*, between 1998 and 2003 (94). The majority of the 731 reported incidents involved a surgeon or an operating room nurse. Most were of low harm, but there were several deaths, typically involving dilution errors of epinephrine (e.g., the injection of epinephrine 1:1000 rather than the intended 1:100,000). Non-fatal examples include injecting formaldehyde subcutaneously instead of lidocaine (95) and administering a toxic dose of gentamicin intraocularly (96). These errors led the Association of periOperative Registered Nurses (AORN) to develop evidence-based recommendations for medication management in the operating room (97–100); no follow-up study has been done to determine whether these guidelines have been effective in reducing errors.

Failures in communication in the operating room are common. These include communication to the wrong person (or in which the intended person did not hear the request), at the wrong time, of the wrong information, and with missing or wrong content (101,102). Verbal requests by surgeons for medications to be administered by anesthesia, nursing, or perfusion members of the team may easily be misinterpreted or simply not heard at all. If a request is not explicitly directed to a named person, that person may not know that he or she was the intended audience. One would expect similar failures in communication wherever verbal requests are common, such as in cardiac catheterization laboratories or other procedure rooms, but there are few data on medication errors in these locations.

Two important techniques for ensuring that verbal requests are communicated successfully are "directed communication" (which includes the name of the person for whom the communication is intended) and the "speak back and verify" process, also known as "closing the loop." Closing the loop is routine between surgeons and perfusionists and is improving between surgeons and nurses (as part of the AORN guidelines) but seems to be much less common between surgeons and anesthesiologists (103). A notable exception is in the setting of cardiac surgery where it is well established in at least some units, particularly in respect to administering heparin before going onto cardiopulmonary bypass and protamine after weaning from bypass (103).

2.3.9 Contributory Causes to Failures in Medication Safety in the Operating Room

Reports of medication errors may also include secondary analyses of *contributory or predisposing factors* (see Table 2.3). Frequently cited contributory causes include human factors such as failure to check, distraction, inattention, and haste. Failures in communication, discussed earlier, often feature prominently. Inadequate knowledge or inexperience are uncommonly identified as contributing causes (51,59). This supports a basic premise of human error, namely, that while certain types of

Table 2.3 Contributing factors to failures in the administration of medications during anesthesia; one or more of these factors could be identified as contributing to any of the categories of error listed in Table 7.5.

	Contributing Factor
Provider condition	Distraction, inattention
	Failure to check
	Fatigue
	Inadequate knowledge or experience of the practitioner
Team condition	Failure in communication
	Staff change or use of a relief anesthetist
System condition	Haste or pressure to proceed
	Similarity of ampules
	Unfamiliar workplace or equipment
	Medication label problem[a]

Source: Modified from Webster et al. 2001 (51).
[a] There may be overlap with Table 2.2: Examples could include illegibility or similarity of appearance of otherwise correct labels, misapplied (wrong) labels, and failures to label a medication-containing syringe or bag at all, but the last two examples should more correctly be categorized as errors or violations.

errors may become less frequent with experience (58), errors of one sort or another will occur with practitioners at all levels of experience and expertise (104–106).

As discussed in Chapters 6 and 7, Reason has emphasized the importance of *latent factors* in the system, illustrated as holes in slices of Swiss cheese, which themselves represent layers of defense against accident trajectories (104). Unfortunately, these fundamental vulnerabilities in the wider system are easily overlooked as significant contributing factors. The contribution of complexity, discussed in more detail in Chapter 6, is an ever-present threat to safety in medication management. Other potential vulnerabilities include purchasing look-alike medications in the first place, and then placing them in close proximity to each other, having multiple concentrations of high-risk medications in the anesthesia cart (e.g., for heparin and vasoactive medications), having medications stored in inappropriate locations (e.g., storing hypertonic saline alongside standard infusion fluids), or preparing intravenous chemotherapy agents in the same form (i.e., in similar syringes) as intrathecal agents, with no clear designation of intended route.

Fatigue is often cited as a contributing factor to medication errors. The reasons for fatigue are important, because they can potentially be addressed. They may lie in staffing levels, rosters, and out-of-work activities (including child care). Fatigue overlaps with ill health, and a degree of sophistication is required to deal with both of these factors (107). Fatigue is discussed in considerable detail in Chapter 8.

2.4 Failures in Medication Safety in the Postanesthesia Care Unit

There are very few studies of medication errors in the PACU; one of the first was a review of all incidents reported to the Australian Incident Monitoring Study from its inception (exact dates not given) (108). The authors found that 5% of anesthesia-related incidents reported to this system occurred in the PACU (478/8372), and of these, 11% involved medication errors. The majority of medication errors involved administering an inappropriate medication or an overdose. Hicks and his colleagues analyzed errors reported to MEDMARX. A first study, in 2004 (109), included MEDMARX data from August 1998 through

March 2002, and identified 645 PACU medication errors reported by 189 facilities. The majority of reported errors occurred in the administration phase (59%), and 93% did not result in patient harm. However, 7% did cause at least temporary harm, and several errors were life threatening (e.g., the erroneous administration of neuromuscular blocking agents), although no deaths were reported. The most frequent errors involved wrong doses (24%, primarily involving morphine or heparin) and omitted or extra doses. The latter types of errors were often related to failures in communication between anesthesia staff and PACU nurses (e.g., ketorolac given in the operating room but not reported to the PACU staff, and an additional, improper dose given in PACU).

A follow-up study in 2007 (110) added error reports to those already analyzed, through August 2005. Although there were only 2 years of additional data, the number of facilities reporting had increased to 397, and reports had increased to 3260. The pattern of errors was similar to that in the first report, with only 5.6% of errors associated with harm, and two patient deaths. One death followed a severe overdose of heparin due to confusion of heparin vials (10,000 Units versus the planned 200 Units for an intravenous flush). The authors note that the reported level of harm in the PACU was more than four times that associated with all other medication errors reported to MEDMARX during the same time period, indicating that the PACU may be a particularly high-risk period for patients.

Another review of the MEDMARX data focused on PACU *pediatric* medication errors from September 1, 1998, through August 31, 2004 (111). Of 59 medication errors reported by 42 hospitals, 20% were harmful, a much higher rate than seen in the adult errors reported by Hicks et al. (109). Morphine, acetaminophen, meperidine, and fentanyl accounted for nearly half of the errors, and failures in dose calculation were a common cause of error (including misplacement of the decimal point). The calculation of dose is clearly a source of risk for pediatric patients in general, particularly with certain medications, such as opioids (which are commonly used and potentially very dangerous in overdose). More data on pediatric medication errors are available from the intensive care unit literature and are presented in Chapter 3.

2.5 Conclusions

Failures in medication safety are common in the perioperative period. Patients are at high risk for errors in their medication lists during transitions of care, particularly at admission, and at discharge. Accurate medication history taking is difficult and time consuming, particularly with polypharmacy, increasing age, and decreasing health literacy of the patients. Errors at admission and discharge often involve omission of a medication present prior to admission, but discharge errors also include missed drug-drug interactions, failure to restart a suspended medication, and errors in dosing, particularly when dosing should have been adjusted for age or renal disease. These medication errors place patients at risk of adverse medication events. The management of medications during anesthesia is unique in that a single clinician is responsible for all parts of the process, from diagnosis of the situation and selection of a medication, through its preparation and administration, to recording what has been given and monitoring its effects. Errors and other failures in medication safety are common, but exact rates are difficult to calculate and are likely to vary with context. Communication failures between members of the operating room team contribute to medication errors and, although anesthesia providers administer most medications given in the operating room, other members of the team, notably surgeons, are occasionally responsible for medication errors. The risk of medication errors continues into the PACU. Fortunately, most medication errors cause little or no harm, but some have serious consequences, including fatalities.

Wrong-route medication errors have not been discussed in this chapter. They are less frequent than most other forms of medication error but have a very high potential to cause serious harm. Wrong-route errors can occur in any phase of a patient's care and form a somewhat distinct group, so these are considered in Chapter 10. Medication shortages have been common in anesthesia over recent years and have impacted on medication safety in various ways. These are also addressed more fully in Chapter 10. The advent of the COVID-19 pandemic in December 2019 has thrown a stark new light on the risks of infection to clinical staff, notably anesthesiology providers, and also on the importance of minimizing the risk of transmission of infections from one patient to the next (112).

References

1. Weiser TG, Haynes AB, Molina G, et al. Size and distribution of the global volume of surgery in 2012. *Bull World Health Organ*. 2016;94(3):201–9.

2. Berwick DM. What "patient-centered" should mean: confessions of an extremist. *Health Aff (Millwood)*. 2009;28(4):w555–65.

3. Gray B, Johansen I, Koch S, Bowden T. Electronic health records: an international perspective on "meaningful use." *Commonw Fund Newsletter*. 2011;28:1–18. Accessed January 9, 2020. https://www.commonwealthfund.org/publications/issue-briefs/2011/nov/electronic-health-records-international-perspective-meaningful

4. Cornish PL, Knowles SR, Marchesano R, et al. Unintended medication discrepancies at the time of hospital admission. *Arch Intern Med*. 2005;165(4):424–9.

5. Gleason KM, McDaniel MR, Feinglass J, et al. Results of the Medications at Transitions and Clinical Handoffs (MATCH) study: an analysis of medication reconciliation errors and risk factors at hospital admission. *J Gen Intern Med*. 2010;25(5):441–7.

6. Agrawal A, Wu WY. Reducing medication errors and improving systems reliability using an electronic medication reconciliation system. *Jt Comm J Qual Patient Saf*. 2009;35(2):106–14.

7. Kantelhardt P, Giese A, Kantelhardt SR. Medication reconciliation for patients undergoing spinal surgery. *Eur Spine J*. 2016;25(3):740–7.

8. Fleisher LA, Beckman JA, Brown KA, et al. ACC/AHA 2007 guidelines on perioperative cardiovascular evaluation and care for noncardiac surgery: executive summary: a report of the American College of Cardiology/American Heart Association Task Force on practice guidelines. *Circulation*. 2007;116(17):1971–96.

9. Fleisher LA, Beckman JA, Brown KA, et al. 2009 ACCF/AHA focused update on perioperative beta blockade incorporated into the ACC/AHA 2007 guidelines on perioperative cardiovascular evaluation and care for noncardiac surgery: a report of the American College of Cardiology Foundation/American Heart Association Task Force on practice guidelines. *Circulation*. 2009;120(21):e169–276.

10. Group PS, Devereaux PJ, Yang H, et al. Effects of extended-release metoprolol succinate in patients undergoing non-cardiac surgery (POISE trial): a randomised controlled trial. *Lancet*. 2008;371(9627):1839–47.

11. Fleisher LA, Fleischmann KE, Auerbach AD, et al. 2014 ACC/AHA guideline on perioperative cardiovascular evaluation and management of patients undergoing noncardiac surgery: a report of the American College of Cardiology/American Heart Association Task Force on practice guidelines. *J Am Coll Cardiol*. 2014;64(22):e77–137.

12. Gurses AP, Seidl KL, Vaidya V, et al. Systems ambiguity and guideline compliance: a qualitative study of how intensive care units follow evidence-based guidelines to reduce healthcare-associated infections. *Qual Saf Health Care*. 2008;17(5):351–9.

13. Chrcanovic BR, Albrektsson T, Wennerberg A. Bisphosphonates and dental implants: a meta-analysis. *Quintessence Int*. 2016;47(4):329–42.

14. Foss S, Schmidt JR, Andersen T, et al. Congruence on medication between patients and physicians involved in patient course. *Eur J Clin Pharmacol*. 2004;59(11):841–7.

15. Dexter F, Witkowski TA, Epstein RH. Forecasting preanesthesia clinic appointment duration from the electronic medical record medication list. *Anesth Analg*. 2012;114(3):670–3.

16. Mehta DH, Gardiner PM, Phillips RS, McCarthy EP. Herbal and dietary supplement disclosure to health care providers by individuals with chronic conditions. *J Altern Complement Med*. 2008;14(10):1263–9.

17. Burda SA, Hobson D, Pronovost PJ. What is the patient really taking? Discrepancies between surgery and anesthesiology preoperative medication histories. *Qual Saf Health Care*. 2005;14(6):414–6.

18. Gardella JE, Cardwell TB, Nnadi M. Improving medication safety with accurate preadmission medication lists and postdischarge education. *Jt Comm J Qual Patient Saf*. 2012;38(10):452–8.

19. Curatolo N, Gutermann L, Devaquet N, Roy S, Rieutord A. Reducing medication errors at admission: 3 cycles to implement, improve and sustain medication reconciliation. *Int J Clin Pharm*. 2015;37(1):113–20.

20. Vargas BR, Silveira ED, Peinado II, Vicedo TB. Prevalence and risk factors for medication reconciliation errors during hospital admission in elderly patients. *Int J Clin Pharm*. 2016;38(5):1164–71.

21. von Kluchtzner W, Grandt D. Influence of hospitalization on prescribing safety across the continuum of care: an exploratory study. *BMC Health Serv Res*. 2015;15:197.

22. Lozano-Montoya I, Velez-Diaz-Pallares M, Delgado-Silveira E, Montero-Errasquin B, Cruz Jentoft AJ. Potentially inappropriate prescribing detected by STOPP-START criteria: are they really inappropriate? *Age Ageing*. 2015;44(5):861–6.

23. Boeker EB, Ram K, Klopotowska JE, et al. An individual patient data meta-analysis on factors associated with adverse drug events in surgical and non-surgical inpatients. *Br J Clin Pharmacol.* 2015;79(4):548–57.

24. Unroe KT, Pfeiffenberger T, Riegelhaupt S, et al. Inpatient medication reconciliation at admission and discharge: a retrospective cohort study of age and other risk factors for medication discrepancies. *Am J Geriatr Pharmacother.* 2010;8(2):115–26.

25. Ensing HT, Stuijt CC, van den Bemt BJ, et al. Identifying the optimal role for pharmacists in care transitions: a systematic review. *J Manag Care Spec Pharm.* 2015;21(8):614–36.

26. Eisenhower C. Impact of pharmacist-conducted medication reconciliation at discharge on readmissions of elderly patients with COPD. *Ann Pharmacother.* 2014;48(2):203–8.

27. Cortejoso L, Dietz RA, Hofmann G, Gosch M, Sattler A. Impact of pharmacist interventions in older patients: a prospective study in a tertiary hospital in Germany. *Clin Interv Aging.* 2016;11:1343–50.

28. Charpiat B, Goutelle S, Schoeffler M, et al. Prescriptions analysis by clinical pharmacists in the post-operative period: a 4-year prospective study. *Acta Anaesthesiol Scand.* 2012;56(8):1047–51.

29. Beckett RD, Crank CW, Wehmeyer A. Effectiveness and feasibility of pharmacist-led admission medication reconciliation for geriatric patients. *J Pharm Pract.* 2012;25(2):136–41.

30. Allende Bandres MA, Arenere Mendoza M, Gutierrez Nicolas F, Calleja Hernandez MA, Ruiz La Iglesia F. Pharmacist-led medication reconciliation to reduce discrepancies in transitions of care in Spain. *Int J Clin Pharm.* 2013;35(6):1083–90.

31. Nagpal K, Vats A, Ahmed K, Vincent C, Moorthy K. An evaluation of information transfer through the continuum of surgical care: a feasibility study. *Ann Surg.* 2010;252(2):402–7.

32. ElBardissi AW, Regenbogen SE, Greenberg CC, et al. Communication practices on 4 Harvard surgical services: a surgical safety collaborative. *Ann Surg.* 2009;250(6):861–5.

33. Greenberg CC, Regenbogen SE, Studdert DM, et al. Patterns of communication breakdowns resulting in injury to surgical patients. *J Am Coll Surg.* 2007;204(4):533–40.

34. Salanitro AH, Osborn CY, Schnipper JL, et al. Effect of patient- and medication-related factors on inpatient medication reconciliation errors. *J Gen Intern Med.* 2012;27(8):924–32.

35. Belda-Rustarazo S, Cantero-Hinojosa J, Salmeron-Garcia A, et al. Medication reconciliation at admission and discharge: an analysis of prevalence and associated risk factors. *Int J Clin Pract.* 2015;69(11):1268–74.

36. Cornu P, Steurbaut S, Leysen T, et al. Discrepancies in medication information for the primary care physician and the geriatric patient at discharge. *Ann Pharmacother.* 2012;46(7–8):983–90.

37. Taber DJ, Spivey JR, Tsurutis VM, et al. Clinical and economic outcomes associated with medication errors in kidney transplantation. *Clin J Am Soc Nephrol.* 2014;9(5):960–6.

38. Merry AF, Anderson BJ. Medication errors – new approaches to prevention. *Paediatr Anaesth.* 2011;21(7):743–53.

39. Harris M, Patterson J, Morse J. Doctors, nurses, and parents are equally poor at estimating pediatric weights. *Pediatr Emerg Care.* 1999;15(1):17–8.

40. Black K, Barnett P, Wolfe R, Young S. Are methods used to estimate weight in children accurate? *Emerg Med.* 2002;14(2):160–5.

41. Luscombe MD, Owens BD, Burke D. Weight estimation in paediatrics: a comparison of the APLS formula and the formula "'Weight = 3(age) + 7." *Emerg Med J.* 2011;28(7):590–3.

42. Mixon AS, Myers AP, Leak CL, et al. Characteristics associated with postdischarge medication errors. *Mayo Clin Proc.* 2014;89(8):1042–51.

43. Downes JM, O'Neal KS, Miller MJ, et al. Identifying opportunities to improve medication management in transitions of care. *Am J Health Syst Pharm.* 2015;72(17 suppl 2):S58–69.

44. Ziaeian B, Araujo KL, Van Ness PH, Horwitz LI. Medication reconciliation accuracy and patient understanding of intended medication changes on hospital discharge. *J Gen Intern Med.* 2012;27(11):1513–20.

45. Webster CS, Larsson L, Frampton CM, et al. Clinical assessment of a new anaesthetic drug administration system: a prospective, controlled, longitudinal incident monitoring study. *Anaesthesia.* 2010;65(5):490–9.

46. Nanji KC, Patel A, Shaikh S, Seger DL, Bates DW. Evaluation of perioperative medication errors and adverse drug events. *Anesthesiology.* 2016;124(1):25–34.

47. Merry AF, Webster CS, Hannam J, et al. Multimodal system designed to reduce errors in recording and administration of drugs in

anaesthesia: prospective randomised clinical evaluation. *BMJ*. 2011;343:d5543.

48. Merry AF, Hannam JA, Webster CS, et al. Retesting the hypothesis of a clinical randomized controlled trial in a simulation environment to validate anesthesia simulation in error research (the VASER study). *Anesthesiology*. 2017;126(3):472–81.

49. Cooper JB, Newbower RS, Kitz RJ. An analysis of major errors and equipment failures in anesthesia management: considerations for prevention and detection. *Anesthesiology*. 1984;60(1):34–42.

50. Orser BA, Chen RJB, Yee DA. Medication errors in anesthetic practice: a survey of 687 practitioners. *Can J Anaesth*. 2001;48(2):139–46.

51. Webster CS, Merry AF, Larsson L, McGrath KA, Weller J. The frequency and nature of drug administration error during anaesthesia. *Anaesth Intensive Care*. 2001;29(5):494–500.

52. Khan FA, Hoda MQ. Drug related critical incidents. *Anaesthesia*. 2005;60(1):48–52.

53. Zhang Y, Dong YJ, Webster CS, et al. The frequency and nature of drug administration error during anaesthesia in a Chinese hospital. *Acta Anaesthesiol Scand*. 2013;57(2):158–64.

54. Llewellyn RL, Gordon PC, Wheatcroft D, et al. Drug administration errors: a prospective survey from three South African teaching hospitals. *Anaesth Intensive Care*. 2009;37(1):93–8.

55. Bowdle A, Kruger C, Grieve R, Emmens D, Merry A. Anesthesia drug administration errors in a university hospital. *Anesthesiology Annual Meeting Abstract Archives*. 2003:A-1358. Accessed January 1, 2020. http://www.asaabstracts.com/strands/asaabstracts/abstractArchive.htm

56. Amor M, Bensghir M, Belkhadir Z, et al. [Medication errors in anesthesia: a Moroccan university hospitals survey]. *Ann Fr Anesth Reanim*. 2012;31(11):863–9.

57. Bowdle TA, Jelacic S, Nair B, et al. Facilitated self-reported anaesthetic medication errors before and after implementation of a safety bundle and barcode-based safety system. *Br J Anaesth*. 2018;121(6):1338–45.

58. Cooper L, DiGiovanni N, Schultz L, Taylor AM, Nossaman B. Influences observed on incidence and reporting of medication errors in anesthesia. *Can J Anaesth*. 2012;59(6):562–70.

59. Abeysekera A, Bergman IJ, Kluger MT, Short TG. Drug error in anaesthetic practice: a review of 896 reports from the Australian Incident Monitoring Study database. *Anaesthesia*. 2005;60(3):220–7.

60. James RH. 1000 anaesthetic incidents: experience to date. *Anaesthesia*. 2003;58(9):856–63.

61. Yamamoto M, Ishikawa S, Makita K. Medication errors in anesthesia: an 8-year retrospective analysis at an urban university hospital. *J Anesth*. 2008;22(3):248–52.

62. Avidan A, Dotan K, Weissman C, et al. Accuracy of manual entry of drug administration data into an anesthesia information management system. *Can J Anaesth*. 2014;61(11):979–85.

63. Wax DB, Feit JB. Accuracy of vasopressor documentation in anesthesia records. *J Cardiothorac Vasc Anesth*. 2016;30(3):656–8.

64. Edwards KE, Hagen SM, Hannam J, et al. A randomized comparison between records made with an anesthesia information management system and by hand, and evaluation of the Hawthorne effect. *Can J Anaesth*. 2013;60(10):990–7.

65. Merry AF, Webster CS, Mathew DJ. A new, safety-oriented, integrated drug administration and automated anesthesia record system. *Anesth Analg*. 2001;93(2):385–90.

66. Merry AF, Peck DJ. Anaesthetists, errors in drug administration and the law. *N Z Med J*. 1995;108(1000):185–7.

67. Schlossberg E. 16 Safeguards against medication errors. *Hospitals*. 1958;32(19):62; passim.

68. Wahr JA, Shore AD, Harris LH, et al. Comparison of intensive care unit medication errors reported to the United States' MedMarx and the United Kingdom's National Reporting and Learning System: a cross-sectional study. *Am J Med Qual*. 2014;29(1):61–9.

69. Maki DG, Kluger DM, Crnich CJ. The risk of bloodstream infection in adults with different intravascular devices: a systematic review of 200 published prospective studies. *Mayo Clin Proc*. 2006;81(9):1159–71.

70. Birnbach DJ, Rosen LF, Fitzpatrick M, et al. Double gloves: a randomized trial to evaluate a simple strategy to reduce contamination in the operating room. *Anesth Analg*. 2015;120(4):848–52.

71. Munoz-Price LS, Bowdle A, Johnston BL, et al. Infection prevention in the operating room anesthesia work area. *Infect Control Hosp Epidemiol*. 2019;40(1):1–17.

72. O'Grady NP, Alexander M, Burns LA, et al. Guidelines for the prevention of intravascular catheter-related infections. *Am J Infect Control*. 2011;39(4 suppl 1):S1–34.

73. O'Grady NP, Alexander M, Burns LA, et al. Summary of recommendations: guidelines for the prevention of intravascular catheter-related infections. *Clin Infect Dis*. 2011;52(9):1087–99.

74. Pronovost P, Needham D, Berenholtz S, et al. An intervention to decrease catheter-related bloodstream infections in the ICU. *N Engl J Med.* 2006;355(26):2725–32.

75. Hilliard JG, Cambronne ED, Kirsch JR, Aziz MF. Barrier protection capacity of flip-top pharmaceutical vials. *J Clin Anesth.* 2013;25(3):177–80.

76. Cilli F, Nazli-Zeka A, Arda B, et al. Serratia marcescens sepsis outbreak caused by contaminated propofol. *Am J Infect Control.* 2018(5):582–84.

77. Gargiulo DA, Mitchell SJ, Sheridan J, et al. Microbiological contamination of drugs during their administration for anesthesia in the operating room. *Anesthesiology.* 2016;124(4):785–94.

78. Ryan AJ, Webster CS, Merry AF, Grieve DJ. A national survey of infection control practice by New Zealand anaesthetists. *Anaesth Intensive Care.* 2006;34(1):68–74.

79. Loftus RW, Koff MD, Brown JR, et al. The dynamics of Enterococcus transmission from bacterial reservoirs commonly encountered by anesthesia providers. *Anesth Analg.* 2015;120(4):827–36.

80. Loftus RW, Koff MD, Brown JR, et al. The epidemiology of *Staphylococcus aureus* transmission in the anesthesia work area. *Anesth Analg.* 2015;120(4):807–18.

81. Loftus RW, Koff MD, Birnbach DJ. The dynamics and implications of bacterial transmission events arising from the anesthesia work area. *Anesth Analg.* 2015;120(4):853–60.

82. Loftus RW, Brown JR, Patel HM, et al. Transmission dynamics of gram-negative bacterial pathogens in the anesthesia work area. *Anesth Analg.* 2015;120(4):819–26.

83. Fernandez PG, Loftus RW, Dodds TM, et al. Hand hygiene knowledge and perceptions among anesthesia providers. *Anesth Analg.* 2015;120(4):837–43.

84. Loftus RW, Patel HM, Huysman BC, et al. Prevention of intravenous bacterial injection from health care provider hands: the importance of catheter design and handling. *Anesth Analg.* 2012;115(5):1109–19.

85. Loftus RW, Brown JR, Koff MD, et al. Multiple reservoirs contribute to intraoperative bacterial transmission. *Anesth Analg.* 2012;114(6):1236–48.

86. Loftus RW, Brindeiro BS, Kispert DP, et al. Reduction in intraoperative bacterial contamination of peripheral intravenous tubing through the use of a passive catheter care system. *Anesth Analg.* 2012;115(6):1315–23.

87. Loftus RW, Muffly MK, Brown JR, et al. Hand contamination of anesthesia providers is an important risk factor for intraoperative bacterial transmission. *Anesth Analg.* 2011;112(1):98–105.

88. Koff MD, Loftus RW, Burchman CC, et al. Reduction in intraoperative bacterial contamination of peripheral intravenous tubing through the use of a novel device. *Anesthesiology.* 2009;110(5):978–85.

89. Loftus RW, Koff MD, Burchman CC, et al. Transmission of pathogenic bacterial organisms in the anesthesia work area. *Anesthesiology.* 2008;109(3):399–407.

90. Gargiulo DA, Sheridan J, Webster CS, et al. Anaesthetic drug administration as a potential contributor to healthcare-associated infections: a prospective simulation-based evaluation of aseptic techniques in the administration of anaesthetic drugs. *BMJ Qual Saf.* 2012;21(10):826–34.

91. Bowdle TA. Drug administration errors from the ASA closed claims project. *ASA Newsletter.* 2003;67(6):11–3.

92. Cranshaw J, Gupta KJ, Cook TM. Litigation related to drug errors in anaesthesia: an analysis of claims against the NHS in England 1995–2007. *Anaesthesia.* 2009;64(12):1317–23.

93. Hove LD, Steinmetz J, Christoffersen JK, et al. Analysis of deaths related to anesthesia in the period 1996–2004 from closed claims registered by the Danish Patient Insurance Association. *Anesthesiology.* 2007;106(4):675–80.

94. Beyea SC, Hicks RW, Becker SC. Medication errors in the OR – a secondary analysis of MEDMARX. *AORN J.* 2003;77(1):122, 5–9, 32–4.

95. Putterman AM. Accidental formaldehyde injection in cosmetic blepharoplasty. Case report. *Arch Ophthalmol.* 1990;108(1):19–20.

96. Jalali S, Batra A. Visual recovery following intraocular infiltration of gentamicin. *Eye.* 2001;15(pt 3):338–40.

97. AORN. AORN Guidance Statement: "do-not-use" abbreviations, acronyms, dosage designations, and symbols. *AORN J.* 2006;84(3):489–92.

98. Association of periOperative Registered Nurses. AORN guidance statement: safe medication practices in perioperative settings across the life span. *AORN J.* 2006;84(2):276–83.

99. Brown-Brumfield D, DeLeon A. Adherence to a medication safety protocol: current practice for labeling medications and solutions on the sterile field. *AORN J.* 2010;91(5):610–7.

100. Hicks RW, Wanzer LJ, Denholm B. Implementing AORN recommended practices for medication safety. *AORN J.* 2012;96(6):605–22.

101. Lingard L, Espin S, Whyte S, et al. Communication failures in the operating room: an observational classification of recurrent types and effects. *Qual Saf Health Care.* 2004;13(5):330–4.

102. Weller J, Civil I, Torrie J, et al. Can team training make surgery safer? Lessons for national implementation of a simulation-based programme. *N Z Med J.* 2016;129(1443):9–17.

103. Santos R, Bakero L, Franco P, et al. Characterization of non-technical skills in paediatric cardiac surgery: communication patterns. *Eur J Cardiothorac Surg.* 2012;41(5):1005–12.

104. Reason J. *Human Error.* Cambridge: Cambridge University Press; 1990.

105. Keers RN, Williams SD, Cooke J, Ashcroft DM. Causes of medication administration errors in hospitals: a systematic review of quantitative and qualitative evidence. *Drug Saf.* 2013;36(11):1045–67.

106. Merry AF, Brookbanks W. *Merry and McCall Smith's Errors, Medicine and the Law.* 2nd ed. Cambridge: Cambridge University Press; 2017.

107. Merry AF, Warman GR. Fatigue and the anaesthetist. *Anaesth Intensive Care.* 2006;34(5):577–8.

108. Kluger MT, Bullock MF. Recovery room incidents: a review of 419 reports from the Anaesthetic Incident Monitoring Study (AIMS). *Anaesthesia.* 2002;57(11):1060–6.

109. Hicks RW, Becker SC, Krenzischeck D, Beyea SC. Medication errors in the PACU: a secondary analysis of MEDMARX findings. *J Perianesth Nurs.* 2004;19(1):18–28.

110. Hicks RW, Becker SC, Windle PE, Krenzischek DA. Medication errors in the PACU. *J Perianesth Nurs.* 2007;22(6):413–9.

111. Payne CH, Smith CR, Newkirk LE, Hicks RW. Pediatric medication errors in the postanesthesia care unit: analysis of MEDMARX data. *AORN J.* 2007;85(4):731–40; quiz 41–4.

112. Cook TM, Harrop-Griffiths W. Kicking on while it's still kicking off – getting surgery and anaesthesia restarted after COVID-19. *Anaesthesia.* 2020;19:9.

Failures in Medication Safety in the Intensive Care Unit and Ward

3.1 Introduction

In Chapter 2 we discussed the unique challenges presented by the perioperative period to safe medication management, but this is by no means the only period during which surgical patients are at risk from failures in medication safety. Medication errors have been found, in multiple studies, to be the most common cause of medical errors in hospitals, and lead to death and disability in up to 6.5% of all admissions (1,2). Bond et al. reported a rate of 1.3–3.3 medication errors per occupied bed per year (3). In this study, the average hospital reported 382 medication errors per year, and 5% of these errors harmed patients. On average, hospitals experienced a medication error every 22 hours (3). A study from Denmark of the medication process on a surgical and a medical ward found 1065 errors in 2467 opportunities for error (43%) (4). There was a 39% error rate in the prescription phase, 56% in the transcription phase (there was no computerized order entry system in place), just 4% in the dispensing phase, and 41% in the administration phase. In a detailed study of every admission, van Doormaal et al. found that 60% of all medication orders in the hospital contained an error (5). These rates are supported by a recent meta-analysis: Among 25 publications regarding medication errors in pediatric inpatients, there was a rate of 0.175 for prescribing errors (17.5%), and 0.209 (20.9%) of medication administrations contained an administration error (6).

As we discuss in Chapters 4 and 5, medication errors that result in adverse medication events (AMEs) carry economic, physical, and emotional costs to the patient and their families, and also to the clinician making the error and to the institution. However, it is difficult to establish just how costly medication errors are overall. A single inpatient AME has variously been calculated to cost from $80 to $8000 (7–9). These cost estimates should be viewed cautiously, as most compare the total cost of care of patients with a medication error with the cost of those without an error. Since medication errors increase with increasing severity of illness and with increasing numbers of medications (10,11), patients with medication errors are likely to be sicker and thus naturally incur higher costs during hospitalization. Furthermore, the upper limit of this estimate is clearly too conservative: The true costs of rendering a patient paraplegic through administering tranexamic acid via a neuraxial route, for example, would be much higher than $8000, and so would the cost to the family and community of an avoidable death of a patient, but in the absence of a successful lawsuit, there may be little cost to the hospital in which this occurred. Emotional costs are huge as well, for both the patient and the clinicians involved in the adverse event, with several well-documented suicides of healthcare workers who have made harmful errors. These topics are covered in more detail in Chapters 4 and 5.

Despite a large number of publications regarding medication errors in the intensive care unit (ICU) or on the ward, it is very difficult to make any sense of what their actual rate is. For a start, there are undoubtedly real differences in the rates of medication error that grow out of the variable work processes that exist in different institutions and countries, between rural and urban hospitals, and among different cultures. A study that compared ICU medication errors reported to MEDMARX (United States) and those reported to the National Reporting and Learning System (NRLS, United Kingdom) found that gentamicin was the most commonly reported medication involved in an error in the United Kingdom, accounting for 7.4% of all reported errors, but it was involved in only 0.74% of the errors reported in the United States (12). This difference was postulated to be due to the process in place at the time in the United Kingdom, where, once a gentamicin prescription was written, a nurse would immediately take a vial of gentamicin from the unit's medicine cabinet and prepare and administer it. An intervening pharmacist review, particularly for dose corrections needed for renal function, was customary in the United States but was not usual in the United Kingdom at the time of this review.

There are also substantial differences in the medication processes that are used in different institutions. For example, the prescription process can range from the manual writing of scripts to electronic order entry with manual transcription in the pharmacy, to comprehensive electronic systems. In these comprehensive systems, all orders are entered electronically and flow immediately into the pharmacy work queues, where they are reviewed electronically and dispensed by pharmacists using barcode technology to be administered on the wards using electronic checks tied to the pharmacy record. There is variability in the degree of decision support (e.g., allowing for only certain doses, prespecifying the frequency for a given medication, alerting to allergies or medication-medication interactions) and the type of dispensing process (e.g., from pharmacy, by nurses from medication cabinets on the ward or using unit-based dosing with pharmacy-stocked carts or automated dispensing units on the ward) (13). Studies are not always sufficiently explicit about the details of the processes they have evaluated.

Finally, as discussed in Chapter 1, different studies have used various definitions of error, reported various metrics, focused on various phases of the medication process, and employed various methods (e.g., observational data collection versus voluntary reporting). Table 3.1 (14–26) provides a snapshot of information from some of the studies of medication error in the ICU or ward, and it will be quickly apparent how varied they have been.

Thus, it is very difficult to obtain a clear picture from the various reports of medication errors in the ICU and on the ward; in the overview that follows, the emphasis should be on the main messages that emerge from the literature rather than on any apparent precision in numbers.

3.2 Intensive Care Unit versus Ward Errors

The rate of medication errors reported in ICUs varies substantially among published reports (see Table 3.1), with rates as low as 1.2% of administrations in

hospitals with both computerized physician order entry (CPOE) and automated dispensing cabinets (ADCs) (21), 9.8% of prescriptions without such sophisticated technology (17), to as high as 52% of prescriptions (26). Some of this variability can be ascribed to the differences already enumerated, but some is attributable to differences in the type of unit, with neonatal and pediatric ICUs (NICUs and PICUs) tending to have higher rates of prescribing errors (predominantly in dosage errors) than adult units. Dosage error rates from two NICUs using a mixed manual and CPOE system were 3.8% and 3.1% of prescriptions; overdosing was as common as underdosing (23). Rothschild et al. reported 127.8 medication errors per 1000 patient days in an ICU, and 131.5 medication errors per 1000 patient days in a coronary care unit; the most common errors were dose related (27). An intensive study to determine the point prevalence of sentinel events included 250 ICUs in 29 countries over a single 24-hour period (28): medication errors had a point prevalence of 10.5 per 100 patient days, with similar percentages of prescription and administration errors (54% and 46%, respectively). Using variable logistic regression, the authors found that organ failure, number of medications, and patient-to-nurse ratio were independent risk factors for any sentinel event (28).

Cullen et al. conducted a prospective, observational study of the medication process in five ICUs and six general surgery wards (29). The rate of medication error was higher in ICUs than in general wards (19 versus 10 per 1000 patient days), but this difference disappeared when adjusted for number of medications administered (1.27 versus 1.07 per 1000 patient days per medication). In this study, errors occurred predominantly in the administration and prescription phases (44% and 38%, respectively) (29). In a study of 839,554 inpatient medication errors reported to MEDMARX, only 6.6% were from ICUs, while 93.4% were from non-ICUs (30). The greater number of ward errors is to be expected, given the distribution of inpatients between wards and ICU. However, the authors found that errors in the ICU were more likely to be associated with harm (odds ratio [OR] 1.89) and death (OR 2.48) than non-ICU errors. Administration errors were the most common type of error in both locations (ICU 44%, non-ICU 33%) (30). A recent systematic review of the rate of prescribing errors with high-risk medications highlights the difficulty of defining

Table 3.1 Some studies on the nature and rate of medication error in the intensive care unit

Author, year	Unit	Study type	Comments
Venkataraman et al. 2016 (14)	Pediatric ICU, UK	Prospective, observational	132 handwritten scripts for infusions, 32.6% had an error 119 using infusion calculator, less than 1% error rate
Hirata et al. 2019 (15)	Pediatric ED, US	Retrospective chart review	Errors in recording weight – 0.63%, but when weight was wrong, 34% led to dosing error
Terkola et al. 2017 (16)	Pediatric oncology, Europe	Prospective observational	Gravimetric system demonstrated that 7.89% of 759,060 prepared doses of antineoplastic medications had deviation of greater than 10% from that ordered (dispensing error)
Khoo et al. 2017 (17)	PICU, NICU, pediatric wards, Malaysia	Chart review	17 hospitals, 17,889 prescriptions, 9.2% error rate: CPOE worse than manual (16.9% versus 8.2%); 1.7% judged to be serious, 0.1% were potentially fatal
Ewig et al. 2017 (18)	PICU, Hong Kong	Prospective observational chart review	46% of patients had at least one potential AME; prescribing error rate of 6.8 errors per patient, 3.1 errors per ICU patient. Incorrect dose calculation most common type of error (48%). Majority were potentially serious or harmful, 98% intercepted before reaching patient
Gokhul et al. 2016 (19)	PICU, South Africa	Observational, plus chart review	76% of staff made errors in calculation of doses/infusions (rate of infusion and conversion of mL to mEq/mg). 94.9% of patients exposed to at least one medication error
Pawluk et al. 2017 (20)	NICU, Qatar	Voluntary electronic reporting system	201 errors reported over 15 months; none reached the patient, 98% in prescription phase, 58.7% calculation errors
Cochran et al. 2016 (21)	Ward, US	Observational	12 hospitals. 6497 medication administrations observed; error rate 1.2% per administration; fewer errors if pharmacy department dispensed, decreased errors for single cell medication drawer (0.19%) versus multicell drawer (0.45%) or cabinet (0.77%); barcode administration had higher rate of error interceptions prior to patient (66.7%) versus manual double checks (10%) or no check (30.4%)
Shehata et al. 2016 (22)	Ward (66%), ICU (23%), outpatient (11%), Egypt	Voluntary online pharmacist reported errors	12,000 reports included. Phases of care involved: 54% prescription; 25% monitoring; 16% administration. Errors: wrong dose (20%), drug-drug interaction, wrong medication, wrong frequency. 51% harmless, 25% potential, 11% prevented, 13% with patient harm
Horri et al. 2014 (23)	NICU, France	Retrospective review of manual prescriptions	Error rate 3.8% with manual prescriptions ($n = 676$); over- and underdosing equally common; 47% of manual prescriptions were for off-label or unlicensed medications
Vazin and Delfani 2012 (24)	ICU, Iran	Prospective observational (manual scripts)	7.6% error rate (442/5785); 6.8% in prescription phase, 3.3% in transcription, 2.3% in dispensing, 9.8% in administration
Kane-Gill et al. 2010 (25)	Adult ICU and ward; university hospital, US	Voluntary reporting	3252 medication error reports in 4.5 years; primary type of error was prescribing in ICU and omission in general care units. Associated with harm in 12% in ICU and 6% in general care
Agalu et al. 2011 (26)	Adult ICU, Ethiopia	Retrospective review of all prescriptions	52.2% of medication prescriptions contained an error: wrong combinations of medicines (25.7%), wrong frequency (15.5%), and wrong dose (15.1%)

Abbreviations: AME, adverse medication event; CPOE, computerized physician order entry; ED, emergency department; ICU, intensive care unit; NICU, neonatal intensive care unit; PICU, pediatric intensive care unit; UK, United Kingdom; US, United States.

a precise rate. The definition of prescribing errors in one study was based on whether or not an error-prone abbreviation was used, and whether the local pharmacy guidelines for "good prescribing" were followed. The authors of this review found that the denominator used to determine incidence varied and included the number of medication orders, patient admissions, and prescriptions. The error rate ranged from 0.24 to 89.6 per 100 orders of high-risk medications (31).

Table 3.2 Risk factors for medication error in critical care units

Patient risk factors	• Severity of illness (organ failure and high intensity of care increase risk) • Poor medication reconciliation • Sedation and mechanical ventilation • Extremes of age
Provider risk factors	• Inexperience (junior doctors and nurses make more errors) • Lack of medication knowledge • Physiologic and physical state (e.g., fatigue, stress, sleep deprivation)
ICU environment	• Number of medications • Frequent changes in medications and doses • Type of ICU (e.g., error rate is higher in medical and pediatric units) • Initiation of temporary therapies • Lack of communication • Number and complexities of interventions • Use of novel technologies and treatments
Type of medication	• High-risk medications more commonly involved: cardiovascular, sedatives, analgesics, anticoagulants, and anti-infectives
Organizational factors	• Patient-to-nurse ratio • Frequent change in personnel • Frequent handover of care • Difficult working conditions • Inadequate supervision • Premature or nighttime discharge

Source: From Camire et al. 2009 (32) and Valentine et al. 2006 (28).

A detailed review of medication errors in critical care that included 17 articles identified the potential risk factors for error: their findings are summarized in Table 3.2 (32). The authors also collated potential strategies for preventing error, which are largely consistent with those discussed in Chapter 9. The reviewing authors echo our difficulty in understanding the literature when they write that "medication error rates vary widely among clinical settings, patient populations, and studies; the lack of standard definitions and reporting techniques make comparisons across organizations, regions or countries difficult."

3.3 Prescribing Errors

Prescribing is part of the wider process by which medications are manufactured, delivered to hospitals, selected by practitioners, and administered to patients (see Table 6.1). It begins with diagnosing the disease state correctly. From this diagnosis, the correct medication for the disease state is then chosen. These two cognitive steps open the door widely for mistakes to occur (see Chapters 6 and 7) (33). These mistakes can be subtle and even debatable, and estimation of the rate of diagnostic errors is particularly difficult (34). Of course, if the diagnosis is wrong, it is nearly inevitable that the prescribed medication(s) will be wrong as well. The third step is usually writing the prescription, and the fourth involves transcribing this from one location (physician orders) to another (pharmacy log or medication records), but prescriptions can sometimes be written in ward charts, in which case this transcribing may not occur. These last two processes may be manual or electronic, and electronic aids may support the first two.

Prescribing error is the rate of choosing 1) the wrong or inappropriate medication or 2) the wrong dose, formulation, frequency, or route of the right medication. An extensive systematic review of prescribing error in 2009 included 65 publications (35). Most of the studies came from high-income countries (the United States and United Kingdom accounted for 47/65 studies), so their broader applicability is uncertain. As with all other reviews, this one found extensive variability in the rate of prescription errors, from 0.4 errors per 100 admissions to 323 errors per 100 admissions. The median rate was 52 (interquartile range [IQR] 8–227) errors per 100 admissions. The authors conclude, "Prescribing errors are common, affecting a median of 7% of medication orders, 2% of patient days and 50% of hospital admissions" (35).

In an investigation of patients with acute coronary syndrome and chronic kidney disease, Milani et al. found that 17% were prescribed anticoagulation medications that are contraindicated in patients with renal failure (36). Medications that are contraindicated in older adults nevertheless get prescribed to them with great frequency, so much so that multiple methods have been developed to identify medications that are inappropriate, such as the Beers Criteria (see https://dcri.org/beers-criteria-medication-list/, accessed 6 September 2020) and Screening Tool of Older People's Prescriptions (STOPP)/Screening Tool to Alert to Right Treatment (START) criteria (37). A meta-analysis of studies examining application of the STOPP/START criteria found efficacy in reducing falls, dementia, and length of stay but not in reducing overall mortality (38).

The difficulty in keeping up with advances in pharmacology and the tremendous proliferation of new medications was discussed in Chapter 2. In addition, as discussed in Chapter 10, seemingly endless and constantly fluctuating medication shortages mean that physicians must often switch from a familiar medication to one they know less about. This lack of knowledge may extend to the medication's dose, frequency of administration, interactions, and potential side effects and may make prescription errors more likely (39). Virtually all medication classes have been affected as well as all disciplines; cancer treatment has been delayed by such shortages. Surveys done by the Institute for Safe Medication Practices in 2010–2012 uncovered at least 17 deaths attributable to medication shortages. These have reflected physicians' unfamiliarity with substitute medications, risks created by the need to purchase look-alike medications, or confusion around potency or formulation (40).

Although computerized order entry systems are increasingly present, handwritten prescriptions continue to predominate in many countries, including many high-income countries. Reports of errors with handwritten prescriptions come from around the world with error rates that vary from 3.8% to 56% of prescriptions (41–45). Researchers at a major academic hospital in the United States in 2003 found that they could not verify the prescriber 34% of the time because of illegibility (46). Omission of key data (e.g., prescriber name, route, frequency) was also common in handwritten prescriptions (44, 47). In nearly all studies, dangerous abbreviations and potentially misleading numerical notations (notably the use of a trailing zero, with the risk that the decimal point might be omitted or overlooked) were common: in one study, 27% of all prescriptions contained one or more of these abbreviations (46). The large number of errors related to the use of abbreviations, trailing zeros, and symbols led to a sentinel alert published by the Joint Commission (JC) in 2001. The JC (www.jointcommission.org/facts_about_do_not_use_list/, accessed January 20, 2020) and Institute for Safe Medication Practices (www.ismp.org/recommendations/error-prone-abbreviations-list, accessed January 20, 2020) have published lists of "do not use" or dangerous abbreviations and symbols.

In most studies, wrong dose is the most common form of prescription error, particularly in pediatric patients (35,48,49), where weight-based dosing predominates, and where errors can occur due to the wrong dose chosen for the correct weight or due to a wrong weight in the record. In three studies using voluntary medication error reporting, errors at the prescription phase predominated (54%–98% of all errors) with wrong dose or wrong calculation responsible for 20%–30% of prescription errors (20,22,50). Many studies, both in real life and in simulations, have shown that many providers simply cannot perform calculations accurately, whether at the prescribing phase or at the preparation and administration phases (51–54).

3.3.1 Contributing Causes and Factors for Prescription Errors

One highly publicized event that sparked intense scrutiny of medication errors was the death of Libby Zion (Box 3.1: this case is discussed further in Chapter 8). A junior doctor's excessive workload and consequent fatigue, her lack of supervision, and her unfamiliarity with both the medications involved in Libby's treatment and her diagnosis were factors that may have contributed to both the diagnostic error and the prescribing error in this case.

Unfortunately, causes of and factors associated with prescribing errors are infrequently studied. A systematic review in 2009 found only 16 such studies (55). Of these 16, only 7 specifically reported causes of prescribing errors. When interviewed about an error, individuals most often cited a lack of knowledge as the primary cause of the error, whether about the medication itself (including

---

Box 3.1 The death of Libby Zion

Libby Zion was an 18-year-old college freshman with a history of depression, taking phenelzine. Late one evening in 1984, she presented to the emergency room at New York Hospital with fever, agitation, and seemingly uncontrolled jerking. She was admitted for hydration, but without a definitive diagnosis, and sent to a ward staffed by a first-year resident who had 40 other patients under her care. This junior doctor, together with her supervising resident (a second-year resident), ordered meperidine (Demerol) to control Libby's shaking. Instead, Libby became more agitated. She was given haloperidol and physically restrained. At 6 a.m., Libby was found to have a temperature of over 41°C, suffered a cardiac arrest, and died. Although the initial diagnosis and cause of death was judged to be a high fever due to an unknown infection, anesthesiologists will recognize this as serotonin syndrome. Libby's presenting signs were quite typical for this syndrome and were likely due to her prescribed phenelzine; her condition would then have been exacerbated by meperidine.

Libby's father, a prominent lawyer and journalist, used his daughter's death to highlight the inhumane levels of stress and responsibility placed on very junior doctors – 36 hours without sleep, little to no supervision or backup from senior physicians, workloads that boggle the mind (e.g., 40 patients for a single intern/resident team). Ultimately Mr. Zion's efforts led to reform of intern and resident on-duty hours, both in the United States and around the world.

---

appropriate dosing), about a patient's condition, or about side effects or interactions associated with the medication. A survey of 185 physicians found that medication incidents were associated with a higher perceived workload, higher inpatient caseloads, and higher emotional stress scores (56). Other commonly cited causes or contributing factors include the following:

- Excessive workload, long working hours, fatigue
- Inadequate supervision or access to expertise
- Poor access to information about a medication or the patient
- Unwillingness to challenge authority (e.g., when having been instructed to write a prescription by senior staff)
- Low importance attached to prescribing

- Communication failures

Ashcroft et al. more recently performed an extensive study of the level of experience on prescribing errors. Pharmacists in 20 hospitals collected data over 7 days on the total number of medications written and checked, the details of any prescribing errors, and the level of training of the prescriber (57). First- and second-year trainees were twice as likely to make prescribing errors as senior physicians, and errors were 70% more likely to occur during the admission process than during the later hospital stay. Nearly one-third of errors were omissions on admission or discharge, and 10% involved underdosing. Electronic prescriptions were less likely to be associated with errors than handwritten ones.

Contributing causes for errors are explored in more detail in Chapter 7.

The Ashcroft study included a substudy of the causes underlying 85 of the prescription errors. Of the 85 errors, 34 were felt to be rule based, 18 were knowledge based, with the remainder slips and lapses. Although many errors were due to simple lack of knowledge about a medication (including its dose, interactions, contraindications, etc.), many were incorrect application of a good rule (i.e., poor framing of the current clinical situation). These authors also uncovered error-producing conditions, such as workload and stress due to busyness, and fatigue. They also identified serious cultural issues, including a steep hierarchical structure that prevented junior doctors seeking help or receiving adequate supervision. Junior doctors described not seeking advice for fear of looking incompetent or being afraid of "annoying" the senior physicians (Box 3.2) (58).

3.4 Dispensing Errors

Dispensing errors tend to be relatively uncommon in most modern studies of medication error, typically accounting for 6.5%–10% of all errors (6,59,60). Differences between studies are likely based at least in part on how medications are dispensed. As noted earlier, on some units, a nurse receives a manual prescription from a provider, retrieves the appropriate medication vial from a local cabinet, and administers the medication. In others, centralized pharmacies provide unit-based dosing: Individual doses of patient medications to be administered by the nurses on an ordered schedule are prepared by the pharmacy and placed in labeled packets or in individual medication drawers in a cart delivered daily to the patient's unit. Dispensing errors with this system would occur by improper preparation of the packets or medication carts and should be infrequent, given the standardized processes and double-checking prevalent in most pharmacies. The latest evolution of dispensing involves ADCs, where each unit has a locked, computer-controlled cabinet that allows for local storage and retrieval of medications. ADC systems decrease the time from prescription to administration, but unless electronically linked to the CPOE, they can increase dispensing errors (61). Errors can occur both when the wrong medication is retrieved (e.g., because the drop-down menu has diazepam listed directly above diltiazem) or when the wrong dose is retrieved (e.g., when a nurse read 1.0 mg of colchicine as 10 mg; had the medication been dispensed by a pharmacist, this error would have been less likely) (61). As discussed in Chapter 9, ADC systems provide additional safety when they are linked to the central pharmacy record.

Errors can occur when stocking these cabinets (although the risk is reduced by the use of barcoding or automated restocking). In a widely publicized case from Pennsylvania, 10,000 units/mL heparin had been loaded into the ADC drawer that usually held 10 units/mL; three infants died, and three were injured when nurses used these vials to prepare intravenous flushes (62). Although the root cause of this tragedy was a dispensing error, there was also administration error, in that nurses failed to accurately read the vials or to use a second nurse to double check.

3.5 Administration Errors

One of the earliest studies of medication error, published in 1958, focused on voluntarily reported preparation and administration errors. Of 360 medication errors reported by nurses, 12% involved the wrong patient, 16% a wrong dosage, 26% a wrong medication, and 46% a wrong time. From this study, Eli Schlossberg made recommendations to prevent medication administration errors, most of which will be familiar to any student of these errors (Table 3.3) (63). Two years later, Safren and Chapanis reported on another critical incident study using voluntary reports by nurses (64,65). This two-part study also focused on administration errors and ignored all other phases of the medication process. These investigators analyzed 178 errors reported over 7 months in a 1100-bed hospital and expanded on the 4 wrongs identified by Schlossberg (Box 2.2): they noted that the errors identified belonged to seven categories: (1) wrong patient, (2) wrong dose, (3) wrong time, (4) omitted medication, (5) wrong medication, (6) extra dose, and (7) wrong route or preparation. These three reports published 60 years ago clearly identified key types of medication errors and many best practices to prevent them (see Table 3.3); distressingly, our current error landscape continues to look much the same as in 1958.

In many studies of medication errors, administration errors account for a large percentage (often more than half) of all errors, whether observed or voluntarily reported. This is unlikely to change in the near future, as administration is the phase of the process most vulnerable to human error and the least amenable to technology improvements. Administration of medication is truly the "sharp-end of the stick," where a clinician reads the prescription, obtains the prescribed medication and dose, and then physically walks it to the patient and delivers it. Production pressure, workload, task complexity, poor lighting, noise, and interruptions all conspire to distract and confuse an all-too-human operator.

An exhaustive review of the literature on administration errors was published in 2013 by Keers et al. (66), who analyzed 91 direct observa-

Table 3.3 Measures to prevent medication administration errors

Labeling	• Clearly label every vial, ampule, and bag (with indelible ink) with name and potency of the medication, expiration date, and if appropriate, patient's name • Use standard nomenclature for medication name
General measures	• Establish written rules and procedures to govern use of medications • Establish role responsibility (i.e., for pharmacists, physicians, nurses) so that medications are always under strict control and correctly labeled • Ensure that all nurses receive orientation to medication policies and procedures, including correct administration techniques • Set responsibility for preparing medication (i.e., for nurse versus pharmacy) • Use single-dose forms of injectable medications • Use the metric system • Standardize medicine cabinets on all wards • Inspect medicine cabinets monthly (a nurse and pharmacist should do this together) • Ban all unidentified and unlabeled medications from nursing stations • Provide a location for medication preparation that is well lighted, quiet, and free of traffic • Communicate information about new medicines, especially indications, dosage, side effects, and storage • Review procedures for identification of patients prior to medication administration • Review medicine card information for abbreviations, new medicines, or discontinuation of old orders • Institute a system for reporting of medication errors • Establish a committee on patient safety, with representatives from pharmacy, nursing, and medical staff to review and analyze reported medication errors and to establish means to assure patient safety

Source: Adapted from Schlossberg 1958 (63).

tional studies of medication administration carried out between 1985 and May 2012 in long-term care settings or inpatient settings. Their overarching definition of medication error was "a deviation from the prescriber's medication order as written on the patient's chart, manufacturers' preparation/administration instructions, or relevant institutional policies." These authors reported a median error rate (IQR) of 19.6% (8.6%–28.3%) of total opportunities for error when timing errors were included, and 8.0% (5.1%–10.9%) when timing errors were excluded (66). Intravenous medications were associated with a high median adverse event rate (53.3% versus 20.1% for nonintravenous); wrong time, omission, and wrong dosage were the three most common medication administration error subtypes. The rate of error was depressingly consistent across the three decades of studies included in the review. For example, one of the most recent studies, which involved four units and 24 days of observation, reported rates of 27.6% with timing errors and 7.5% without timing errors (66).

In an even more recent observational study on medical wards, al Tehewy et al. reported that among 2090 medication administrations, 5531 errors were observed, with an average of 2.7 errors per administration (67). The overall error rate was 37.8 errors per 100 opportunities, and over 85% of observations had at least 1 error. Fortunately, only 0.8% of errors involved patient harm. The majority of administrations (91%) involved an error in documentation, 78% involved an error in technique and a third of all administrations involved either a wrong time or a wrong dose (67).

3.5.1 Preparation

Errors in the preparation of medications form a subcategory of administration errors. These are more likely to occur in the ICU, where medications are often provided in a concentrated form or in a powder needing preparation with a diluent and then diluted in a syringe for continuous infusion. Certain high-risk medications may be provided in multiple concentrations (e.g., heparin, insulin), predictably leading to confusion and harm (we have already mentioned the well-known case of the harm associated with mistaken heparin concentrations in infants [62]). Although infusions are increasingly prepared in a central or decentralized (i.e., on the ward) pharmacy, local preparation of medications by nurses is still common. As noted earlier, multiple studies have shown that many providers simply cannot perform calculations and dilutions accurately (51–54). Labeling is also problematic – in a study of hospitals in the United Kingdom, Germany, and France, prepared medications were not labeled or were incorrectly labeled 43%, 99%, or 20% of the time. The wrong diluent was used 1%, 49%, and 18% of the time (68).

3.5.2 Factors Contributing to Administration Errors

In addition to their systematic review of the *rate* of errors, Keers et al. performed a systematic review of 54 studies that reported on *causes* of medication administration errors (69). Unlike prescribing errors, where mistakes predominate, administration errors tended more commonly to be skill-based errors (slips and lapses), with misidentification of either medication or patient frequently reported slips, and wrong time or omitted doses common lapses. Misreading a medication label, forgetting to sign a medication record, and confusing look-a-like or sound-a-like medications were also common.

Despite the predominance of skill-based errors, nurses report mistakes in the administration of medications arising from deficiencies in their personal knowledge about the relevant medications, patient, or equipment (69). Interestingly, 14 studies in the systematic review by Keers included reports of violations, such as not adhering to protocols (Box 3.3; violations are discussed in detail in Chapter 8). Reasons for these protocol violations included poorly designed protocols, trusting one's senior colleagues, poor supervision, and lack of staff (which led to intentionally giving medications too early or too late) (69).

Latent or personal conditions contribute to administration errors, with workload cited frequently as a contributing factor (70–72). As noted, administrations at the wrong time or missed doses are common errors. Over time, the definitions of a correct time to administer medications have become increasingly restrictive, and in many hospitals, a medication that is given more than 20–30 minutes after the prescribed time is now considered a "wrong-time" error. This definition is based on a completely false construct. Although there are a few classes of medications where the specific time of administration does have physiologic consequences (e.g., medications for Parkinson disease), the majority of medications that we administer are equally effective when given across a range of times. Pharmacokinetics would dictate that twice a day dosing should be given every 12 hours, but virtually no patients or hospitals administer medications this way. Instead most choose a convenient time such as 8 a.m. and 5 p.m. for this task. In many hospitals, "three times a day" defaults to a standardized dosing schedule, such as 9 a.m., 1 p.m., and 5 p.m. (this may be automatically assigned by computer), but there is little or no physiologic consequence if the medication is given an hour earlier or later, for example. These automatic defaults can reduce confusion about when medications should be given, because every single "three times a day" medication defaults to the same administration time in that institution. However, the result is a variable workload, where suddenly at 9 a.m., there are a host of medications to be given, while at 10 a.m., there may be none. This artificial construct places unnecessary pressure on the administering nurses, who must rush to get all the medications given within 30 minutes of the computer assigned dosing time or face being chastised for "wrong-time administrations." It seems only reasonable that some nurses might choose to administer medications a little early in order to complete the myriad of tasks assigned to them. Similarly, a patient scheduled for magnetic resonance imaging (MRI) at 9 a.m. may have her 9 a.m. medications given at 8 a.m. to prevent a "too late" dose on return from having the MRI.

Nurses also have continually changing work shifts and frequently work multiple long shifts with minimal breaks between them. In Chapter 10, we discuss the widely publicized death of a young parturient due to intravenous administration of bupivacaine that had been intended for the epidural route; the nurse who made that error had worked back-to-back 8-hour shifts that ended at midnight, had slept

---

Box 3.3 Causes of medication administration errors

"[Y]ou'd be thinking, I need to get these medicines finished, because in an hour and a half's time, I've got my lunch time drugs to get out. So, that would have been a factor [in not clarifying an illegible prescription]."

"[W]ith the nature of the ward and it being so busy, I think it's becoming just a bit of a habit to people to just check the expire date, check it's the right drug and then, yeah, it's fine … up until this incident I'd still say that if a sister asked me to check something, I would check it by the look of it […] she'll have done it right."

Source: Taken from Keers et al. 2015 (71).

a few hours at the hospital, and was back on duty at 7 a.m. (73). Number of hours worked and amount of voluntary overtime are both independent risks associated with increased rates of error (74,75). Olds et al. analyzed 11,516 responses to a nursing survey and found that working more than 40 hours in a week or working more than 4 hours of voluntary paid overtime were both independently associated with medication administration errors and also with work injuries and needlestick injuries to the nurse (75). A federal law specifically limits the number of hours a nuclear power operator or railroad engineer may be at work, and the Federal Aviation Administration, Navy, and Army strictly limit duty hours of their pilots. By contrast, in the United States, only Maine, Oregon, and California have rules about nurse shift hours. In addition to their long hours, nurses will often "stick around" to help colleagues for an hour or two when the wards are busy or staffing is low. We discuss the relationship between fatigue and error in more detail in Chapter 8.

3.6 Conclusions

Although it is impossible to precisely define the rate of various types of medication errors on the wards and in the ICUs, it is clear that:

- Nearly every patient in the ICU or on the wards will experience at least one medication error.
- Many medication errors are intercepted by a pharmacist or nurse, but serious harm and fatalities are reported in virtually every study, even for errors deemed to be entirely preventable.
- Prescribing errors are common in the ICU: physicians commonly fail to recognize medication-medication interactions and often prescribe the wrong dose or wrong frequency.
- Pediatric patients and neonates have a much higher rate of dosing errors than adult patients, with both erroneous weights (resulting in the correct dose being given for a wrong weight) and erroneous calculations (resulting in the wrong dose for a correct weight) contributing to these.
- Administration errors are common on general care wards, particularly omissions of a prescribed dose.
- The likelihood of medication errors in intensive care units is increased with patients

who are sicker (i.e., have more failing organs), those receiving an increased number of infusions, more patients per nurse, and more patients on the unit (76).

- Many clinicians have difficulty in calculating doses or infusion rates.
- The presence of CPOE and computer prompts does not obviate prescribing error, as orders are often written for medications that are inappropriate for the patient's condition.
- Certain groups of patients are at particularly high risk for error, including those needing psychotropic agents (77) and antiviral agents (78–80).
- High-risk medications, such as opioids, insulin, and antibiotics, are the most common classes of medications involved in reported errors, particularly harmful errors; anticoagulant medications, vasoactive infusions, and potassium administration are close behind.

At the heart of this problem lies the enormous system vulnerabilities harbored by most hospitals. Heavy and variable workloads (for all team members), distractions, interruptions, and variable penetration of technologies that could reduce errors all conspire to allow human errors to undermine the safety of medication management. In the next two chapters, we reflect on the harm these errors can cause to patients and clinicians.

References

1. Leape LL, Brennan TA, Laird N, et al. The nature of adverse events in hospitalized patients. Results of the Harvard Medical Practice Study II. *N Engl J Med.* 1991;324(6):377–84.

2. Thomas EJ, Studdert DM, Burstin HR, et al. Incidence and types of adverse events and negligent care in Utah and Colorado. *Med Care.* 2000;38(3):261–71.

3. Bond CA, Raehl CL, Franke T. Medication errors in United States hospitals. *Pharmacotherapy.* 2001;21(9):1023–36.

4. Lisby M, Nielsen LP, Mainz J. Errors in the medication process: frequency, type, and potential clinical consequences. *Int J Qual Health Care.* 2005;17(1):15–22.

5. van Doormaal JE, van den Bemt PM, Mol PG, et al. Medication errors: the impact of prescribing and transcribing errors on preventable harm in hospitalised patients. *Qual Saf Health Care.* 2009;18(1):22–7.

6. Koumpagioti D, Varounis C, Kletsiou E, Nteli C, Matziou V. Evaluation of the medication process in pediatric patients: a meta-analysis. *J Pediatr (Rio J)*. 2014;90(4):344–55.

7. Choi I, Lee SM, Flynn L, et al. Incidence and treatment costs attributable to medication errors in hospitalized patients. *Res Social Adm Pharm*. 2016;12(3):428–37.

8. Nuckols TK, Paddock SM, Bower AG, et al. Costs of intravenous adverse drug events in academic and nonacademic intensive care units. *Med Care*. 2008;46(1):17–24.

9. Bates DW, Spell N, Cullen DJ, et al. The costs of adverse drug events in hospitalized patients. Adverse Drug Events Prevention Study Group. *JAMA*. 1997;277(4):307–11.

10. Alhawassi TM, Krass I, Bajorek BV, Pont LG. A systematic review of the prevalence and risk factors for adverse drug reactions in the elderly in the acute care setting. *Clin Interv Aging*. 2014;9:2079–86.

11. Saedder EA, Lisby M, Nielsen LP, Bonnerup DK, Brock B. Number of drugs most frequently found to be independent risk factors for serious adverse reactions: a systematic literature review. *Br J Clin Pharmacol*. 2015;80(4):808–17.

12. Wahr JA, Shore AD, Harris LH, et al. Comparison of intensive care unit medication errors reported to the United States' MedMarx and the United Kingdom's National Reporting and Learning System: a cross-sectional study. *Am J Med Qual*. 2014;29(1):61–9.

13. Chapuis C, Roustit M, Bal G, et al. Automated drug dispensing system reduces medication errors in an intensive care setting. *Crit Care Med*. 2010;38(12):2275–81.

14. Venkataraman A, Siu E, Sadasivam K. Paediatric electronic infusion calculator: an intervention to eliminate infusion errors in paediatric critical care. *J Intensive Care Soc*. 2016;17(4):290–4.

15. Hirata KM, Kang AH, Ramirez GV, Kimata C, Yamamoto LG. Pediatric weight errors and resultant medication dosing errors in the emergency department. *Pediatr Emerg Care*. 2019;35(9):637–42.

16. Terkola R, Czejka M, Berube J. Evaluation of real-time data obtained from gravimetric preparation of antineoplastic agents shows medication errors with possible critical therapeutic impact: results of a large-scale, multicentre, multinational, retrospective study. *J Clin Pharm Ther*. 2017;42(4):446–53.

17. Khoo TB, Tan JW, Ng HP, et al. Paediatric in-patient prescribing errors in Malaysia: a cross-sectional multicentre study. *Int J Clin Pharm*. 2017;39(3):551–9.

18. Ewig CLY, Cheung HM, Kam KH, Wong HL, Knoderer CA. Occurrence of potential adverse drug events from prescribing errors in a pediatric intensive and high dependency unit in Hong Kong: an observational study. *Paediatr Drugs*. 2017;19(4):347–55.

19. Gokhul A, Jeena PM, Gray A. Iatrogenic medication errors in a paediatric intensive care unit in Durban, South Africa. *S Afr Med J*. 2016;106(12):1222–9.

20. Pawluk S, Jaam M, Hazi F, et al. A description of medication errors reported by pharmacists in a neonatal intensive care unit. *Int J Clin Pharm*. 2017;39(1):88–94.

21. Cochran GL, Barrett RS, Horn SD. Comparison of medication safety systems in critical access hospitals: combined analysis of two studies. *Am J Health Syst Pharm*. 2016;73(15):1167–73.

22. Shehata ZH, Sabri NA, Elmelegy AA. Descriptive analysis of medication errors reported to the Egyptian national online reporting system during six months. *J Am Med Inform Assoc*. 2016;23(2):366–74.

23. Horri J, Cransac A, Quantin C, et al. Frequency of dosage prescribing medication errors associated with manual prescriptions for very preterm infants. *J Clin Pharm Ther*. 2014;39(6):637–41.

24. Vazin A, Delfani S. Medication errors in an internal intensive care unit of a large teaching hospital: a direct observation study. *Acta Med Iran*. 2012;50(6):425–32.

25. Kane-Gill SL, Kowiatek JG, Weber RJ. A comparison of voluntarily reported medication errors in intensive care and general care units. *Qual Saf Health Care*. 2010;19(1):55–9.

26. Agalu A, Ayele Y, Bedada W, Woldie M. Medication prescribing errors in the intensive care unit of Jimma University Specialized Hospital, Southwest Ethiopia. *J Multidiscip Healthc*. 2011;4:377–82.

27. Rothschild JM, Landrigan CP, Cronin JW, et al. The Critical Care Safety Study: The incidence and nature of adverse events and serious medical errors in intensive care. *Crit Care Med*. 2005;33(8):1694–700.

28. Valentin A, Capuzzo M, Guidet B, et al. Patient safety in intensive care: results from the multinational Sentinel Events Evaluation (SEE) study. *Intensive Care Med*. 2006;32(10):1591–8.

29. Cullen DJ, Sweitzer BJ, Bates DW, et al. Preventable adverse drug events in hospitalized patients: a comparative study of intensive care and general care units. *Crit Care Med*. 1997;25(8):1289–97.

30. Latif A, Rawat N, Pustavoitau A, Pronovost PJ, Pham JC. National study on the distribution,

causes, and consequences of voluntarily reported medication errors between the ICU and non-ICU settings. *Crit Care Med.* 2013;41(2):389–98.

31. Alanazi MA, Tully MP, Lewis PJ. A systematic review of the prevalence and incidence of prescribing errors with high-risk medicines in hospitals. *J Clin Pharm Ther.* 2016;41(3):239–45.

32. Camire E, Moyen E, Stelfox HT. Medication errors in critical care: risk factors, prevention and disclosure. *CMAJ.* 2009;180(9):936–43.

33. Groopman J. *How Doctors Think.* Boston, MA: Houghton Mifflin Harcourt; 2007.

34. Singh H, Graber ML, Hofer TP. Measures to improve diagnostic safety in clinical practice. *J Patient Saf.* 2019;15(4):311–16.

35. Lewis PJ, Dornan T, Taylor D, et al. Prevalence, incidence and nature of prescribing errors in hospital inpatients: a systematic review. *Drug Saf.* 2009;32(5):379–89.

36. Milani RV, Oleck SA, Lavie CJ. Medication errors in patients with severe chronic kidney disease and acute coronary syndrome: the impact of computer-assisted decision support. *Mayo Clin Proc.* 2011;86(12):1161–4.

37. Hill-Taylor B, Sketris I, Hayden J, et al. Application of the STOPP/START criteria: a systematic review of the prevalence of potentially inappropriate prescribing in older adults, and evidence of clinical, humanistic and economic impact. *J Clin Pharm Ther.* 2013;38(5):360–72.

38. Hill-Taylor B, Walsh KA, Stewart S, et al. Effectiveness of the STOPP/START (Screening Tool of Older Persons' potentially inappropriate Prescriptions/Screening Tool to Alert doctors to the Right Treatment) criteria: systematic review and meta-analysis of randomized controlled studies. *J Clin Pharm Ther.* 2016;41(2): 158–69.

39. Rinaldi F, de Denus S, Nguyen A, Nattel S, Bussieres JF. Drug shortages: patients and health care providers are all drawing the short straw. *Can J Cardiol.* 2017;33(2):283–6.

40. Fox ER, Sweet BV, Jensen V. Drug shortages: a complex health care crisis. *Mayo Clin Proc.* 2014;89(3):361–73.

41. Al-Jeraisy MI, Alanazi MQ, Abolfotouh MA. Medication prescribing errors in a pediatric inpatient tertiary care setting in Saudi Arabia. *BMC Res Notes.* 2011;4:294.

42. Bates K, Beddy D, Whirisky C, et al. Determining the frequency of prescription errors in an Irish hospital. *Ir J Med Sci.* 2010;179(2):183–6.

43. Martinez-Anton A, Sanchez JI, Casanueva L. Impact of an intervention to reduce prescribing errors in a pediatric intensive care unit. *Intensive Care Med.* 2012;38(9):1532–8.

44. Sada O, Melkie A, Shibeshi W. Medication prescribing errors in the medical intensive care unit of Tikur Anbessa Specialized Hospital, Addis Ababa, Ethiopia. *BMC Res Notes.* 2015; 8:448.

45. Khammarni M, Sharifian R, Keshtkaran A, et al. Prescribing errors in two ICU wards in a large teaching hospital in Iran. *Int J Risk Saf Med.* 2015;27(4):169–75.

46. Garbutt J, Milligan PE, McNaughton C, et al. Reducing medication prescribing errors in a teaching hospital. *Jt Comm J Qual Patient Saf.* 2008;34(9):528–36.

47. Belela AS, Peterlini MA, Pedreira ML. Medication errors reported in a pediatric intensive care unit for oncologic patients. *Cancer Nurs.* 2011;34(5):393–400.

48. Glanzmann C, Frey B, Meier CR, Vonbach P. Analysis of medication prescribing errors in critically ill children. *Eur J Pediatr.* 2015;174(10):1347–55.

49. Bolt R, Yates JM, Mahon J, Bakri I. Evidence of frequent dosing errors in paediatrics and intervention to reduce such prescribing errors. *J Clin Pharm Ther.* 2014;39(1):78–83.

50. Samsiah A, Othman N, Jamshed S, Hassali MA, Wan-Mohaina WM. Medication errors reported to the National Medication Error Reporting System in Malaysia: a 4-year retrospective review (2009 to 2012). *Eur J Clin Pharmacol.* 2016;72(12):1515–24.

51. Avidan A, Levin PD, Weissman C, Gozal Y. Anesthesiologists' ability in calculating weight-based concentrations for pediatric drug infusions: an observational study. *J Clin Anesth.* 2014;26(4):276–80.

52. Simpson CM, Keijzers GB, Lind JF. A survey of drug-dose calculation skills of Australian tertiary hospital doctors. *Med J Aust.* 2009;190(3):117–20.

53. Wheeler DW, Remoundos DD, Whittlestone KD, House TP, Menon DK. Calculation of doses of drugs in solution: are medical students confused by different means of expressing drug concentrations? *Drug Saf.* 2004;27(10):729–34.

54. Parshuram CS, To T, Seto W, et al. Systematic evaluation of errors occurring during the preparation of intravenous medication. *CMAJ.* 2008;178(1):42–8.

55. Tully MP, Ashcroft DM, Dornan T, et al. The causes of and factors associated with prescribing errors in hospital inpatients: a systematic review. *Drug Saf.* 2009;32(10):819–36.

56. Dollarhide AW, Rutledge T, Weinger MB, et al. A real-time assessment of factors influencing medication events. *J Healthc Qual.* 2014;36(5):5–12.

57. Ashcroft DM, Lewis PJ, Tully MP, et al. Prevalence, nature, severity and risk factors for prescribing errors in hospital inpatients: prospective study in 20 UK hospitals. *Drug Saf.* 2015;38(9):833–43.

58. Lewis PJ, Ashcroft DM, Dornan T, et al. Exploring the causes of junior doctors' prescribing mistakes: a qualitative study. *Br J Clin Pharmacol.* 2014;78(2):310–19.

59. Karthikeyan M, Lalitha D. A prospective observational study of medication errors in general medicine department in a tertiary care hospital. *Drug Metabol Drug Interact.* 2013;28(1):13–21.

60. Kuo GM, Touchette DR, Marinac JS. Drug errors and related interventions reported by United States clinical pharmacists: the American College of Clinical Pharmacy practice-based research network medication error detection, amelioration and prevention study. *Pharmacotherapy.* 2013;33(3):253–65.

61. Grissinger M. Safeguards for using and designing automated dispensing cabinets. *P T.* 2012;37(9): 490–530.

62. Arimura J, Poole RL, Jeng M, Rhine W, Sharek P. Neonatal heparin overdose – a multidisciplinary team approach to medication error prevention. *J Pediatr Pharmacol Ther.* 2008;13(2):96–8.

63. Schlossberg E. Sixteen safeguards against medication errors. *JAHA.* 1958;32:62.

64. Safren MA, Chapanis A. A critical incident study of hospital medication errors. Part 2. *JAHA.* 1960;34:53.

65. Safren MA, Chapanis A. A critical incident study of hospital medication errors. *JAHA.* 1960;34:32–4.

66. Keers RN, Williams SD, Cooke J, Ashcroft DM. Prevalence and nature of medication administration errors in health care settings: a systematic review of direct observational evidence. *Ann Pharmacother.* 2013;47(2):237–56.

67. al Tehewy M, Fahim H, Gad NI, El Gafary M, Rahman SA. Medication administration errors in a university hospital. *J Patient Saf.* 2016;12(1):34–9.

68. Cousins DH, Sabatier B, Begue D, Schmitt C, Hoppe-Tichy T. Medication errors in intravenous drug preparation and administration: a multicentre audit in the UK, Germany and France. *Qual Saf Health Care.* 2005;14(3):190–5.

69. Keers RN, Williams SD, Cooke J, Ashcroft DM. Causes of medication administration errors in hospitals: a systematic review of quantitative and qualitative evidence. *Drug Saf.* 2013;36(11): 1045–67.

70. Keers RN, Williams SD, Cooke J, Ashcroft DM. Understanding the causes of intravenous medication administration errors in hospitals: a qualitative critical incident study. *BMJ Open.* 2015;5(3):e005948.

71. Berdot S, Roudot M, Schramm C, et al. Interventions to reduce nurses' medication administration errors in inpatient settings: a systematic review and meta-analysis. *Int J Nurs Stud.* 2016;53:342–50.

72. Cottney A, Innes J. Medication-administration errors in an urban mental health hospital: a direct observation study. *Int J Ment Health Nurs.* 2015;24(1):65–74.

73. Smetzer J, Baker C, Byrne FD, Cohen MR. Shaping systems for better behavioral choices: lessons learned from a fatal medication error. *Jt Comm J Qual Patient Saf.* 2010;36(4):152–63.

74. Saleh A, Awadalla N, El-masri Y, Sleem W. Impacts of nurses' circadian rhythm sleep disorders, fatigue, and depression on medication administration errors. *Egypt J Chest Dis Tuberc.* 2014;63:145–53.

75. Olds DM, Clarke SP. The effect of work hours on adverse events and errors in health care. *J Safety Res.* 2010;41(2):153–62.

76. Valentin A, Capuzzo M, Guidet B, et al. Errors in administration of parenteral drugs in intensive care units: multinational prospective study. *BMJ.* 2009;338:b814.

77. Wolf C, Pauly A, Mayr A, et al. Pharmacist-led medication reviews to identify and collaboratively resolve drug-related problems in psychiatry – a controlled, clinical trial. *PLoS One.* 2015;10(11):e0142011.

78. Guo Y, Chung P, Weiss C, Veltri K, Minamoto GY. Customized order-entry sets can prevent antiretroviral prescribing errors: a novel opportunity for antimicrobial stewardship. *P T.* 2015;40(5):353–60.

79. Chiampas TD, Kim H, Badowski M. Evaluation of the occurrence and type of antiretroviral and opportunistic infection medication errors within the inpatient setting. *Pharm Pract.* 2015;13(1):512.

80. Jen SP, Zucker J, Buczynski P, et al. Medication errors with antituberculosis therapy in an inpatient, academic setting: forgotten but not gone. *J Clin Pharm Ther.* 2016;41(1):54–8

4 Impact of Medication Errors on the Patient and Family
Managing the Aftermath

4.1 Introduction

It would seem that this should be the shortest chapter of all time in a medical textbook and consist of only the words spoken by Sorrel King, "our lives were shattered and changed forever" (see www.youtube.com/watch?v=b2DQg7JNwKI&list=PLMdfxb3KK n3op6y3JdgjvmG-jwuAOSRaw, accessed January 20, 2020), but we cannot turn our eyes away so quickly or save ourselves from hearing and feeling the impact medication errors have on patients and their family. All healthcare providers should listen again to Sorrel King describe her frantic attempts to prevent her daughter's death, and hear her desperate words when Josie lay dying: "You did this to her and now you have to fix her." All healthcare providers should also hear her comments about those who had participated, wittingly or unwittingly, "No one in the room could look at me." Human error in medication administration can and has caused enormous pain and loss. We would be negligent and callous if we were to simply look away, so we will undertake this journey to experience what our errors actually do to the patients whom we only intended to protect and to heal. As indicated in Chapter 1, we consider not only patients and their immediate families, but also their extended families.[1]

In Chapter 10 we discuss the horrors of the intrathecal vincristine catastrophes (1). The agonizing, painful, and excruciatingly slow progression from paralysis to death in these cases has been well documented. To make matters worse, the patients involved in these errors have sometimes been young, and at least one was in remission from the cancer for which these medications were being administered (2). Here, we consider examples from a comparable series of medication disasters that has involved young, healthy pregnant women (3).

In 2001, Angelique Sutcliff presented to her local hospital in England in early labor (3,4). She went on to have a caesarean section under a spinal anesthetic with hyperbaric bupivacaine 0.5%. Postdelivery, she developed severe back pain and urinary retention. Two weeks later she required an intracranial shunt for raised intracranial pressure. She continued to deteriorate, becoming progressively paraplegic. Magnetic resonance imaging demonstrated a severely damaged spinal cord with multiple adhesions.

In some countries, epidural trays come with a self-contained swabstick (press the barrel, and the solution is delivered to the sponge at the tip of the device) of the antiseptic chlorhexidine and separate vials or syringes of saline. In other health systems, epidural trays are locally prepared, and the assisting nurse pours a saline solution into one sterile bowl, usually unlabeled, and the skin antiseptic (chlorhexidine) into another. Both these solutions may be clear unless a coloring agent has been added to the chlorhexidine. However, even if colored chlorhexidine solution is used, a potential trap may be set if a bloody tap occurs and the saline (flushed back into the container) becomes slightly blood stained (3).

In Angelique's case, the anesthesia provider appropriately prepped the skin with chlorhexidine 0.5% in alcohol 70%. Although the point is controversial and has never been definitively proven, the judge of the High Court in the civil case that considered this event concluded that the injectate had become contaminated with "a measurable quantity" of chlorhexidine. Chlorhexidine seems to be the most effective product for sterilizing the skin in this context, but it is a denaturing agent and disrupts cell membranes. How much chlorhexidine would be needed to cause such an event, and under what circumstances, is not clear (3).

The case of Grace Wang, 10 years after Angelique's (5), was much clearer (Box 4.1). In her case,

---

[1] Whānau," an inclusive Māori term for all those who care for and support one another, captures this concept of an extended family perfectly.

Box 4.1 Grace Wang: "My epidural hell"

"We try to get our normal life back as much as we can," says Jason. "But with people here all the time and Grace's physical condition, we have lost the emotion and spontaneity and the passion that most married couples share.

"We want to have our life back as a normal couple. A stupid mistake permanently deprived us of all our rights as a normal husband and wife, as normal parents to enjoy our life with our son.

"My son will never know the feeling like the other kids when his mother cuddles him. I miss the feeling we shared when we held each other and the passionate hugs we had before. I am afraid that I might lose that feeling forever. I wish God would give us our other life back."

Source: From Sheather 2012 (5).

---

the anesthesiologist apparently drew up some 8 mL of chlorhexidine from the wrong bowl and injected this into Grace's epidural space (3). The consequences were similar to those suffered by Angelique but were much more immediate. Both of these women had been perfectly healthy pregnant women, happily anticipating seeing and holding their babies for the first time.

Grace was quadriplegic before her son Alex was born a few hours later. She has never held her child, walked, or been able to feed herself since this event. As with the vincristine disasters, the knowledge gained from these terrible errors has not been able to prevent subsequent events. Tragically, despite these two events as warning, another such event happened in Australia in 2010 (6), and yet another in Malmo, Sweden, in 2014 (7), each with the same sickeningly common theme: a healthy pregnant woman anticipating her baby's arrival needs an epidural and is inadvertently injected with a potent neurotoxin. In addition, there have been multiple case reports of tranexamic acid given intrathecally, including some involving obstetrical patients; consequences typically included ventricular arrhythmias and myoclonic seizures, with both fatal and nonfatal outcomes (8,9). Most involved vials or ampules where the tranexamic acid and heavy bupivacaine were remarkably similar in appearance (see Figure 7.2).

In Chapters 6 and 7 we explore in depth how both human and system vulnerabilities open the door to these tragedies. None of the previous events were malicious; every provider intended to deliver excellent care. These events occurred in the normal, busy, hectic flow of an anesthesiologist's life, and likely occurred in the same flow (e.g., with look-alike unlabeled bowls on a sterile field) that the provider had accomplished without error many times previously. We already acknowledged that the vast majority of medication errors either do not reach the patient or are of minor consequence. Similarly, error-prone processes are accomplished flawlessly many times without error. The rarity of these devastating harm events can lead us to a dangerous sense of complacency, or a misplaced confidence that such an event would never occur with us. But, as James Reason has put it, "What we have here is not an error-prone individual. What we have here is an error-prone situation, an error trap" (10). Without appropriate process and system changes, these error traps will continue to ensnare well-meaning and highly trained professionals and to destroy patient lives. Furthermore, even significant system changes are not entirely effective. Certainly, vincristine should always be provided to end users in a minibag rather than a syringe, and swab sticks would seem to be much safer than the use of bowls containing chlorhexidine. However, merely changing to swab sticks might ignore important steps such as allowing the solution to dry before performing the epidural (3). Unfortunately, the potential for other errors in the intraspinal administration of medications is not eliminated by focusing on just those known to have occurred but requires both system changes and heightened vigilance.

In Chapter 8 we explore how normalized deviance can creep into our everyday lives, where harmless medication errors (or error-prone processes such as unlabeled bowls of toxic substances on a sterile field, or look-alike vials of tranexamic acid and bupivacaine) are accepted as of no importance. The events presented earlier demonstrate in stark reality the ever-present potential to harm patients, and underpin our view that normalized deviance is not acceptable and that no medication error should be dismissed as minor.

4.2 Long-Term Impact

Our stories have focused on the immediate physical impact of particular medication errors.

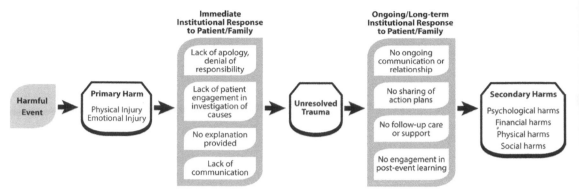

Figure 4.1 Conceptual model of potential secondary harms to patients and their families after medical error. Reprinted with permission from Ottosen et al. 2018 (12).

Unfortunately, physicians and institutions have long compounded iatrogenic injury by abandoning injured patients and their families, by refusing to acknowledge errors, and by failing to communicate or to provide adequate explanations for what has gone wrong. For all of us, acknowledging an error is an admission of fallibility in a setting that deserves infallibility and perfection. We feel shame and are terrified of losing the respect of our colleagues. We are suddenly face-to-face with our inadequacy (11). It is not difficult to understand why our primary response has often been to "deny and defend," to refuse to provide financial compensation, to board up all lines of communication, and even seek to blame the patient for the adverse outcome (11). But this cruel abandonment of patients and their families adds unresolved psychological and emotional trauma and other forms of secondary harm to the primary physical harm that has been suffered (Figure 4.1) (12).

Harmed patients and their families experience a myriad psychological, emotional, and financial hardships over their lifetime. Ottosen et al. (12) conducted 32 interviews with 72 patients who had suffered harmful healthcare events and their family members, at a minimum of 5 years after the event. Of these events, 56% had caused permanent harm, and 31% had been fatal. Medication errors accounted for 16%. Virtually all those interviewed (94%) reported experiencing long-term impact: 59% had "dramatic changes in their lives and their view of themselves," with loss of career and of their ability to enjoy life. Despite counseling, most continued to see themselves as victims, not survivors. Comments quoted in the paper from patients who suffered harm in various ways are very moving (see Table 4.1) (12). Many voiced a complete lack of trust in healthcare and would not seek further treatment. This distrust had as much or more to do with the way the hospital and staff dealt with them after the event, ignoring their requests, and refusing to apologize or even acknowledge the event. Continuing anger was mentioned by many of the respondents (50%) and may increase as they are denied access to hospital records and are simply ignored or even lied to. Some reported being blamed for the event. Patients and families, naturally, have vivid memories of that time, using words such as "horrifying" and "terrifying." They are beset with self-doubt or even self-anger, that they ignored their gut sense that something was wrong, that they trusted the system, that they did not speak up or challenge authority. In addition to physical defects and disabilities (64%), patients and families suffer psychological scars, including depression, grief, sadness, and even suicidal thoughts.

As we bear witness to our patients' and their families' anguished "what ifs" and desperate accounting of their loss, we know that we cannot truly understand or fathom their distress. We cannot assuage it, we cannot "fix her" as Josie's mother implored. But when these events happen and we cannot fix what we have just done, what then? Knowing that abandonment will further injure our patients, what can we do, what should we do, to rectify these wrongs? As it turns out, there are specific steps that we as providers should and must take, steps that the victims of preventable adverse medication events and their families tell us that they want us to do (13).

Table 4.1 Selected quotes from patients regarding long-term impact of adverse events during healthcare

Social and behavioral impacts	Altered life view of self	"I'm an educational researcher. I was. Now I can't do very much about anything. I have a lot of very nonfunctional days. I'm classified as permanently disabled. … It has limited my life."
	Altered healthcare-seeking behaviors	"And when you're very sick in the hospital, you're afraid to speak up initially. I'm not anymore, because I've been through so much that I certainly will tell them everything I need to say, and they better do it as long as I'm conscious and aware of what's going on."
Psychological impacts	Anger	"But what turns you into the bitter, angry patient is the fact that you can't get answers … or there are key pieces missing out of your medical record … or things are incorrect … or the hospital won't talk to you. Or you start to uncover lies that have been told to you."
		"That sends a very bad message to the people who are now having their lives crucified because of this guy's arrogance. They all put their lives and their careers on the line to cover up for this guy's arrogance because he wouldn't dare admit he had made a mistake."
	Vivid memories	"It was almost like this bad movie. They surrounded me in the entryway, in the lobby there, and started arguing with me about why I shouldn't want the records, which is my right as a consumer to see the records."
		"As I said, I was in intractable pain that was not dealt with. They forced a breathing tube down my throat while I was wide awake. And I actually thought it was going to kill me. … I can't forget everything that happened to me there."
	Loss of trust in healthcare	"It's left a lasting impact on me because I used to have a lot of confidence in our healthcare and now I don't have much at all. … I'm even afraid if I ever have to go to a hospital, I'm going to be terrified. Because I used to think hospitals were a place that you went to get adequate care and you got better and you came home. I didn't realize you could go in with one thing, and then wind up dead from another and it terrifies me."
		"When we went in, things were just one after another … afterward we learned there was deception, their arrogance, they were [not] communicative. It shattered my confidence and the image about the medical profession."
	Grief	"The traumas that I've been through are really sad [crying]. If you stop and look at everything that happened to me over these years. … I lost everything. I lost a career, a salary. Like I said I could have lost my kid."
	Self-blame	"And I wish I had listened to my inner voice. My inner voice was trying to tell me something wasn't right, but I silenced it because I had trusted this guy for 20 years. So, and he was a doctor. You know? He was the authority."
	Psychological scars	"The minute I walk into that door and say, 'You hurt me and let me just talk about it.' … they would not talk to me … they didn't care that they had hurt me. Nobody did. The thing is I am one of the luckier ones … I'm able to at least still have a life. I wasn't paralyzed. I wasn't maimed. I wasn't, you know, physical injured. But I think we all … all of us who have been a victim or a survivor of patient harm, all share the same psychological scars. This has been about, I don't know, 5 years ago, I guess. I mean I've been suicidal over this."
Physical impacts		"As an outcome of that [surgical error]. … I was totally and irreversibly blind very early into the first recovery period after the first morning surgery. And to date, I am 100% blind in both eyes … I have no light perception."
Financial impacts		"I was disabled from the beginning. I went back to work. I tried for the first 6 months, because I was being promoted to vice president. And I didn't want to lose my job. So I really tried hard to go back to work. But I just was too sick … And then within 4 years or so, I ended up in a wheelchair … I lost everything. I lost a six-figure job."

Source: From Ottosen et al. 2018 (12).

4.3 Our Sacred Promise Is "First, Do Not Harm" but When We Do, What Is the Next Promise?

The Hippocratic oath has, arguably, set the medical profession an impossible (albeit worthy) aspiration. If an entire professional ethos is invested in the idea that harming a patient should never happen, it is not surprising that the importance of responding to harm when, inevitably, it does occur has been overlooked. Responses to harm have traditionally often varied from inadequate to positively harmful in their own right.

Over the nearly 20 years since the Institute of Medicine published its seminal analysis of human error in medicine, "To Err Is Human" (14), we have developed a much deeper appreciation and understanding of how to manage the aftermath of an adverse medical event. When asked, patients and their families clearly want timely and full disclosure of errors, acknowledgment of responsibility, description of how and why the error occurred, what the physician or hospital will do to mitigate the consequences, and when error is involved, what steps will be taken to prevent a recurrence of the same error (13,15). They may also need and want medical care directed at treating the harm that has occurred and compensation for the losses they have experienced consequent to that harm. Finally, they might reasonably expect accountability for the failures in care that they have experienced. Instead of these things, attempts to find out what happened have often been met with a stony silence devoid of any sense of empathy. They have had to go to the courts to get the information that should be theirs by right. Similarly, accountability and compensation have often only been available through prolonged, expensive, and adversarial legal processes. At the very time when they most need the ongoing support and care of their hospital and its physicians, nurses, and other staff, they end up rejected.

Today, it is increasingly recognized that harm does occur and that the "next promise" should be to continue to care compassionately for one's patients when it does. In Chapters 11 and 12, we discuss the legal and regulatory aspects of responding to those who have been harmed by healthcare. In the rest of this chapter, we consider the role of disclosure and compassion in mitigating the secondary harm that so often follows the primary harm that only too frequently arises directly from failures in healthcare.

4.4 Disclosure and Compassion

One of the most eloquent responses to preventable adverse harm came from George Dover, the director of the Johns Hopkins Children's Center, Baltimore, Maryland, who went to the home of Tony and Sorrel King in the days after Josie's death, to apologize to the grieving parents (Box 4.2). In a striking departure from what commonly occurs after a medical error (i.e., silence), the top leadership of the system that had failed Josie King went personally to her grieving family, stood on the doorstep, pledged to delve deeply into what happened,

---

Box 4.2 No room for error – but room for compassion

On March 4, 2001, George Dover stood outside a Baltimore home, rang the doorbell, and changed the future of Johns Hopkins Medicine.

The director of the Johns Hopkins Children's Center had come to the home of Tony and Sorrel King to apologize to the grieving parents.

Six weeks earlier, the Kings' 18-month-old daughter Josie had wandered into an upstairs bathroom, turned on the hot water, and climbed into the tub. By the time her screams brought her mother, Josie had second-degree burns on more than half of her body. The toddler was rushed by ambulance to the Johns Hopkins Hospital, where she received skin grafts and healed. Within weeks, she was acting like her old self. Then her condition deteriorated. Josie grew pale and unresponsive. She died February 22 of what was ultimately identified as septic shock, compounded by an erroneous narcotic injection, just days before she was scheduled to return home.

"The first thing I said to the Kings was that I was terribly sorry," says Dover. "In those days, that was not fashionable. We told Tony and Sorrel we would find out exactly what had happened, we would communicate what we found, and we would do our best to make sure it never happened again."

The transparency and compassion allowed Tony and Sorrel to move past their natural anger and devastation and embark on a remarkable partnership with Dr. Peter Pronovost and Johns Hopkins Hospital to effectively change the face of patient safety at Hopkins (see http://josieking. org/programs/josie-king-patient-safety-program/, accessed January 20, 2020).

Source: Excerpted, verbatim except for the last paragraph, from Nitkin et al. 2016 (16).

promised that their health system would do their very best to make sure that this would never happen again, and *promised to return frequently to update the family* on what was learned about how and why these errors had happened. This commitment to improving patient safety was remarkable, but the more remarkable aspect of this story is the deep compassion shown by Dover to the parents of the little girl who had died in his institution. Of course, nothing can make up for the loss of a child, but the common failure to engage with those who have been harmed in responding to that harm, both practically and emotionally, can certainly add to the pain and anger that follow such an event.

Disclosing errors and apologizing for them is a recent change in physician and institutional behavior. Of 114 house officers completing a questionnaire in 1991 about their most recent error, only 24% had informed the patient of the error, despite serious adverse outcomes in 90% of the incidents (17). Although medical errors have been presented and discussed for hundreds of years at departmental morbidity and mortality (M&M) conferences, the prevailing view was that medical errors were due to the negligence of individual physicians, due to malpractice, which translates literally to to "bad practice." The concept of "error traps" (10) was not yet on the horizon. These M&M sessions were held behind closed doors, and there was little or no public recognition or discussion of medical errors. The tort system for settling negligence cases served to enhance this secrecy, by heightening the fear that discussion of an error would lead to a lawsuit. To complete the circle, the tort system was traditionally viewed as a way to "deter negligent action by physicians, hospitals and others," despite no evidence that this was so (18) (see also Chapters 11 and 12). Although Safren and Chapanis in 1960 (19) and Cooper et al. in 1984 (20) used the critical incident approach to analyze preventable adverse events, the emphasis was on the "detection and prevention" of errors (20), and there was no discussion of disclosure of these errors to patients.

In 1984, David Hilfiker wrote a moving essay for the *New England Journal of Medicine* titled "Facing Our Mistakes" (21). In it he describes his own errors in his rural Minnesota practice. He actually practiced full disclosure with his patients, but he expressed his frustration and loneliness in the process:

Somehow, I felt, it was my responsibility to deal with my guilt alone. … Everyone of course, makes mistakes, and no one enjoys the consequences. But the potential consequences of our medical mistakes are so overwhelming that it is almost impossible for practicing physicians to deal with their errors in a psychologically healthy fashion. Most people – doctors and patients alike – harbor deep within themselves the expectation that the physician will be perfect. … The climate of medical school and residency training … is an environment in which precision seems to predominate … and when a doctor does make an error it is first whispered about in the halls, as if it were a sin. … Indeed, errors are rarely admitted or discussed. … The medical profession simply seems to have no place for its mistakes. There is no permission given to talk about errors, no way of venting emotional responses. Indeed, one would almost think that mistakes are in the same category as sins: it is permissible to talk about them only when they happen to other people.

One resident used the analogy of error as a sin and confessing to one's peers in the M&M conference: "You are supposed to give full disclosure. Don't hold anything back. And it is almost a religious experience. You get up, you confess your sins. They assign a punishment to you. You sit back down, and you are forgiven for your sins" (13).

Within the traditional atmosphere of secrecy and concealment, it is clear that full disclosure of errors not only did not happen between peers, it also did not often occur between a physician or institution and the patient. The failure to include the patient in the process of confession and forgiveness noted in the previous paragraph about the M&M process is striking. David Hilfiker was an outlier. The patient and families were left alone, without answers or empathy at a time when those were most needed. Today there is a much greater recognition of the fact that, when an unanticipated outcome occurs, patients want and deserve to know what happened and whether an error has been made. In 1999, the widespread approach was "deny and defend." Fortunately, the public accounting of medical errors has allowed many clinicians to embrace the fact that all of us make mistakes, that our mistakes do not indicate we are bad doctors, nurses, or pharmacists, and that reporting and disclosing our errors is not only ethical and appropriate but also critical to the psychological health of our patients and (as we discuss in Chapter 5) ourselves. There is still much work to be done on this front, but progress is being made.

In 2006, Boyle et al. proposed a medical error disclosure framework in which providers should apologize, empathize, engage in corrective action, and provide compensation (22). Implicit in this framework is that there be full disclosure of what happened, to the extent that answers are known at the time. Disclosure of the facts should happen as quickly as possible but with adequate time for the team to understand the basic elements of what went wrong (23). There should be a standard process in an institution of how to disclose. Preparation for disclosure should include emotional preparation that allows the clinician involved to make sense of the event. Time should be allowed for information seeking and consideration given to who should be present (23). Disclosure should be viewed as a process, with a clear indication that the patient and family will be continually updated and informed as the institution works through the process of understanding what happened. Although beyond the scope of this chapter, formal communication management strategies are available to guide both physicians and institutions through the intricate process of full disclosure (23).

Disclosing an error to patients or their families is still difficult, especially as many of us continue to hold ourselves to an unrealistic ideal. For example, in a study of prescribing errors among trainee doctors, Duncan et al. found that many held the view that *they were capable of prescribing without error.* Disconcertingly, many also thought that *prescribing errors were unlikely to have consequences* for patients (24). Of course, as we have repeatedly noted, many medication errors are of minor consequence. In Chapter 11 we consider the controversial question of the threshold at which disclosure should occur. Nevertheless, if an adverse outcome occurs or an error is potentially material to the patient for any other reason, then full disclosure is imperative. Rosner et al. (25) state: "Errors do not necessarily constitute improper, negligent, or unethical behavior, but failure to disclose them may." Disclosure preserves trust between patients and their providers, especially when the patient is already suspicious that an error has occurred (25). Disclosure recognizes the ethical aspect of patient autonomy, that patients have the right to know exactly what has transpired, and that this knowledge is necessary for patients to make informed decisions about subsequent care (26,27). Residents who score the

highest on ethical reasoning tests were those most likely to both provide full disclosure and take personal responsibility (27). Clearly, disclosure is necessary to prevent the secondary harms that follow the primary injury (12).

Although agreement in theory that all harmful errors should be disclosed is increasingly widespread, we often fail to practice what we preach. We are still a long way from the 100% disclosure that patients want (13,28), that medical societies recommend (15), and that regulatory bodies are beginning to mandate (29). In a study of iatrogenic medical events including medication errors, Lehmann found that only 5% of charts had any documentation of disclosure to patients or their families (30). An interview study conducted in 2005 found that only 26% of patients who believed they had experienced a medical error had received disclosure (31). A study of physicians found that 100% of them would want full disclosure if they were the patient, but only 50% reported that they had ever provided disclosure after an error (28). Barriers to reporting and to disclosure include the psychosocial profile of physicians, the often poor communication between physician and patient, the common institutional culture of blame and shame, and the medicolegal environment (Table 4.2) (11,32).

In addition to a clear explanation of what happened, patients very much want those involved to acknowledge that they were harmed, and this acknowledgment should include a direct apology (13). Physicians, institutions, and risk management entities have understandably been concerned that explicitly stating "I am sorry that we did not provide appropriate care" or "I am sorry that this error happened," will serve as a confession of guilt and have legal ramifications. There is evidence that this is not the case (see the VA and University of Michigan data, later; also see the discussion of this issue in Chapter 11). Furthermore, many states specifically preclude apologies from being entered into evidence during a malpractice lawsuit. Nevertheless, these fears still constrain many clinicians from simply saying sorry. Everyday human experience tells us how distressing a lack of apology can be when a mistake has clearly been made. Petronio et al. capture this point in an approach where the goal of a full apology includes a desire to provide emotional support and an explanation of what the physician and institution have learned from the error (23). If

Table 4.2 Barriers to error reporting and disclosure

Intra- and interpersonal barriers	Psychosocial profile of physicians	• Inadequate education regarding moral character or professionalism in medical school • Unwillingness to report or disclose peers' errors (to preserve friendships) • Infrequent discussion or education around ethics of medicine • Inadequate empathy development • Medical profession's ethos of perfectionism: errors constitute personal failure, erode respect among one's peers, threaten one's identity as a healer, lead to loss of self-esteem
	Physician-patient communication	• Insensitivity in managing disclosure, poor communication skills regarding disclosure • Patients sense that facts are concealed • Unrealistic expectations of patients for outcome of treatment; expectation of error-free practice • Lack of frank discussion of expectations prior to treatment
Institutional barriers	Healthcare culture and policies	• Climate that perpetuates blame, secrecy, fear • Punitive response from institution (for one's own errors) • Retaliation from peers or superiors (for disclosing a peer's or superior's errors) • Uncertainty about how to report or disclose errors • Lack of safe, nonjudgmental environment in which to discuss medical errors • Inherent resistance to change • Hierarchical structure that inhibits junior staff from speaking up; deference to authority by those lower in hierarchy • Historical lack of response to reported errors or concerns • Disregard of leadership of frontline workers' opinions
Societal barriers	Medicolegal environment	• Threat of legal punishment and financial losses • Mandatory reporting is limited only to serious errors, thus missed opportunities to correct vulnerabilities identified via near misses

Source: From Perez et al. 2014 (11) and Etchegaray et al. 2017 (32).

inappropriate conduct or behavior was involved in the mistake, there should also be a promise to correct that behavior and provide compensation when appropriate (see Chapters 11 and 12) (23).

Perhaps more than an explicit "mea culpa," patients want empathy (33). They want to be heard, sometimes at great length. They want time to tell those involved what impact the error has had on their life; they want to know that their suffering and distress are recognized (12). Unfortunately, because disclosure and apology are difficult, they often fail to receive these important things. Our natural tendency is to "hit and run," to rapidly state the error, briefly express sympathy, and leave. This abrupt approach can actually shock the patient, who may not even be aware an error has led to the adverse outcome. It leads to a perception of the physician as cold and uncaring, just when the patient most needs empathy and emotional support. Unfortunately, many of us clinicians are unprepared to offer either, especially when we ourselves are expe-

riencing very natural guilt, shame, and emotional trauma (see Chapter 5). The fact is that many physicians find that they have to subconsciously detach from the emotional intensities of caring for patients and thus do become depersonalized and appear to be cold and uncaring (Box 5.2). Several studies in the early 2000s found a significant decline in medical student empathy levels across the curriculum, particularly in the clinical years (34). A systematic review in 2011 found that of 11 studies among medical students, 9 described declines in empathy (35).

Fortunately, a more recent scoping review included 20 studies, 12 of which reported either empathy gains or nonstatistically significant changes (36). Over the past 20 years, there have been sweeping changes to the medical school curriculum to include professionalism, nontechnical skills, ethics, and empathy. These changes may be contributing to a healthier view of our imperfect human natures and increasing the willingness of interns and residents to disclose errors (37). Attitudes are changing, largely through education of those in training. Surveys of interns in 1999–2001 and again in 2008–9 found that the percentage of interns who were willing to fully disclose an error that resulted in an adverse outcome increased from 29% among the earlier cohort to 55% in the later group (37). Coexistent with this change, the percentage of interns who felt that errors could be prevented with adequate education decreased from 49% to 31% (37).

It is important to recognize that physicians are not the only clinicians involved in the care of patients harmed by medication errors. The importance of pharmacists and nurses in improving medication safety has been emphasized in Chapters 2 and 3 and is discussed again in Chapter 9. Furthermore, these clinicians, particularly nurses, often spend more time with patients than physicians do and often have a strong rapport with them. They should be seen as an essential part of the team not only in delivering safe care but also in responding appropriately, compassionately, and effectively when things go wrong (Box 4.3).

Box 4.3 An example of interprofessional training of health professionals about adverse medication events

The University of Auckland's Faculty of Medical and Health Sciences runs an annual 2-day quality and safety intensive for third-year medical, nursing, pharmacy, and optometry students (38). These students work in small interprofessional groups to undertake root-cause analyses of real adverse medication events. This group work is interspersed with didactic lectures from a similarly interprofessional faculty, supported by guest lectures from people such as New Zealand's Health and Disability Commissioner and the chief medical officer of its Health Quality and Safety Commission. The first day starts with the true story of a teenage patient who died following an anesthetic for appendicitis. This story is told, on video, by this patient's mother, and the long-lasting secondary impacts of the adverse event are strongly conveyed. Other key themes of the "intensive" are those outlined in this chapter, including disclosure and apology. One of the exercises carried out by the students involves composing a letter to go to the patient or family explaining what happened and what is going to be done to prevent a similar thing happening again.

In recognition of the difficulties that many physicians and providers have with disclosure, many healthcare organizations are developing formal communication and resolution programs (CRPs) to better interact with patients and families after medical error. Moore et al. (39) conducted semi-structured interviews with patients, family members, and staff who had experienced an error and subsequently partook in a CRP. The majority, but not all (18/30 patients/family) reported a positive experience, and 18/30 continued to receive their care at that institution. Patients expressed a strong desire to be listened to without interruption and to receive updates on efforts to prevent a recurrence. The promise to provide ongoing updates is critical: Since full disclosure needs to happen rather quickly after an error has occurred, the incident and the antecedents will not yet be fully understood or appreciated. A full root-cause analysis may take weeks, and design and implementation of interventions to prevent similar events in the future even longer. Patients should receive the bare-bones information up front and then be provided additional information as it emerges. Unfortunately, in the study by Moore et al., 24/30 respondents reported receiving no such updates, despite the fact that these institutions were clearly devoted to that ideal.

In these interviews, patient and family comments were informative, speaking to the need for the physical space to provide privacy, the right people (the treating and lead physician should both be present), a liaison person (someone not involved in the error but who represents the institution), good communication practices (listening for as long as it takes, sitting calmly with the family, allowing all family members to speak), giving updates regarding patient safety improvements, and asking for feedback about the CRP (39). One interesting approach included patients and families in the adverse event reviews and asking them for their views about what factors might have contributed to the adverse event and for recommendations to address these factors (40). Each participant identified at least one contributing factor with an average of 3.67 (40). Clearly, involving patients and families in a review of the adverse event they experienced not only provides emotional support, but it also strongly validates any institutional and provider statements about transparency and about efforts to improve safety

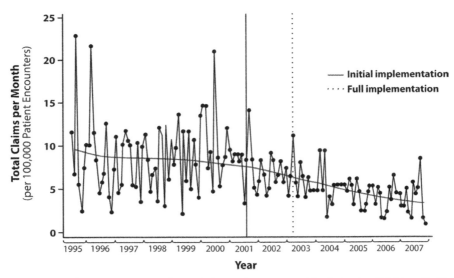

Figure 4.2 Monthly rates of total liability costs before and after implementation of the University of Michigan Health System disclosure-with-offer program. Reprinted with permission from Kachalia et al. 2010 (42).

and prevent a recurrence of the event in question. In some cases, this may also allow patients to gain insight into how difficult the latter objective can sometimes be. Conversely, in other cases, the involvement of patients in this way may help the institution to identify improvements that are clearly, needed, affordable, and practicable and ensure that these are actually implemented. Most importantly, this approach is the antithesis of rejection.

As noted earlier, one of the greatest fears about disclosure of errors has been increased exposure to litigation. We return to this issue in Chapter 11, but on balance, the result seems to be quite the opposite. One of the earliest institutions to embrace full disclosure, the Veterans Affairs Medical Center in Lexington reported that, 10 years after instituting full disclosure, the median liability payment for their facility was one-fifth of that for the private sector. Another of the first to lead the way to full disclosure was the University of Michigan, who in 2001 made a strong commitment to "openness and honesty with regard to the investigation, defense, and settlement of potential malpractice claims" (41). Richard Boothman, lead counsel, envisioned a world of full disclosure with compensation, where patients who were injured would receive quick and fair compensation, where patients would have the complete picture of what happened, including any mistakes that had been made and how these experiences would be used to improve a system's learn-

ing. Applying this model in 2001 led to a significant reduction in total liability costs over the next 6 years (Figure 4.2) (42). Unfortunately, despite clear evidence that patients have been harmed by medication error in the Swiss medical system (43), a recent series of structured interviews with Swiss medicolegal stakeholders found that at least some liability insurance companies still inhibit communication with harmed patients after errors (44). Developing appropriate disclosure policies and practices will require coordinated efforts at all levels of the healthcare industry.

4.5 Conclusions

The proportion of patients harmed by medication errors is small, but when harm does occur it can be very serious. Furthermore, this primary harm is only the tip of the iceberg. Patients and their families also have long-term psychological, emotional, and financial impacts added to physical injury. These secondary effects are aggravated by failures to respond to adverse events in a caring, compassionate, and transparent manner, fulfilling what we have called "the next promise." The approach of the clinicians and institution involved in a harmful medication error is critical to recovery and requires 1) full and transparent disclosure of all known causes for the error; 2) an apology that includes empathy and emotional support, listening at length to the patients and their families without any attempt to deflect blame or downplay the impact; 3) appropriate and rapid compensation; 4) accountability; and 5) regular feedback to all regarding ongoing investigations into the event and interventions that have been made to prevent this event from happening to another patient. There is an excellent body of knowledge to guide institutions and their interprofessional clinical teams about how to design and implement a communication and resolution program that is ethical, patient centered, and provides emotional support not only to patients and their families but also to staff involved in the error.

References

1. Noble DJ, Donaldson LJ. The quest to eliminate intrathecal vincristine errors: a 40-year journey. *Qual Saf Health Care*. 2010;19(4):323–6.

2. Merry AF, Brookbanks W. *Merry and McCall Smith's Errors, Medicine and the Law*. 2nd ed. Cambridge, UK: Cambridge University Press; 2017.

3. Bogod D. The sting in the tail: antiseptics and the neuraxis revisited. *Anaesthesia*. 2012;1(12):1305–9.

4. Nathanson MH. Guidelines on skin antisepsis before central neuraxial blockade. *Anaesthesia*. 2014;1(11):1193–6.

5. Sheather M. Grace Wang: my epidural hell. *Australian Women's Weekly*. 2012. Accessed January 9, 2020. https://www.nowtolove.com.au/celebrity/celeb-news/epidural-victim-grace-wang-im-terrified-my-husband-will-leave-me-9747

6. Clinical Safety Quality and Governance Branch. Safety Notice 010/10. Correct identification of medication and solutions for epidural anaesthesia and analgesia. NSW Department of Health; 2010. Accessed January 9, 2020. https://www.health.nsw.gov.au/sabs/Documents/2010-sn-010.pdf

7. Swede asks for epidural and gets disinfectant. *The Local*. 2014. Accessed December 5, 2019. https://www.thelocal.se/20140813/pregnant-woman-treated-with-disinfectant-for-pains

8. Patel S, Loveridge R. Obstetric neuraxial drug administration errors: a quantitative and qualitative analytical review. *Anesth Analg*. 2015;121(6):1570–7.

9. Hatch DM, Atito-Narh E, Herschmiller EJ, Olufolabi AJ, Owen MD. Refractory status epilepticus after inadvertent intrathecal injection of tranexamic acid treated by magnesium sulfate. *Int J Obstet Anesth*. 2016;26:71–5.

10. Reason J. *The Human Contribution: Unsafe Acts, Accidents and Heroic Recoveries*. Burlington, VT: Ashgate Publishing; 2008.

11. Perez B, Knych SA, Weaver SJ, et al. Understanding the barriers to physician error reporting and disclosure: a systemic approach to a systemic problem. *J Patient Saf*. 2014;10(1):45–51.

12. Ottosen MJ, Sedlock EW, Aigbe AO, et al. Long-term impacts faced by patients and families after harmful healthcare events. *J Patient Saf*. Published online January 17, 2018. doi:10.1097/PTS.0000000000000451

13. Gallagher TH, Waterman AD, Ebers AG, Fraser VJ, Levinson W. Patients' and physicians' attitudes regarding the disclosure of medical errors. *JAMA*. 2003;289(8):1001–7.

14. Kohn LT, Corrigan JM, Donaldson MS, eds. *To Err Is Human: Building a Safer Health System*. Washington, DC: National Academy Press, Institute of Medicine; 1999.

15. Committee Opinion No. 681 Summary: disclosure and discussion of adverse events. *Obstet Gynecol*. 2016;128(6):1461.

16. Nitkin K, Broadhead L, Smith L, Smith P. No room for error. *The Johns Hopkins Newsletter*. January/February 2016. Accessed January 20, 2020. https://www.hopkinsmedicine.org/news/articles/no-room-for-error

17. Wu AW, Folkman S, McPhee SJ, Lo B. Do house officers learn from their mistakes? *JAMA*. 1991;265(16):2089–94.

18. Hiatt HH, Barnes BA, Brennan TA, et al. A study of medical injury and medical malpractice. *N Engl J Med*. 1989;321(7):480–4.

19. Safren MA, Chapanis A. A critical incident study of hospital medication errors. *Hospitals*. 1960;34:32–4.

20. Cooper JB, Newbower RS, Kitz RJ. An analysis of major errors and equipment failures in anesthesia management: considerations for prevention and detection. *Anesthesiology*. 1984;60(1):34–42.

21. Hilfiker D. Facing our mistakes. *N Engl J Med*. 1984;310(2):118–22.

22. Boyle D, O'Connell D, Platt FW, Albert RK. Disclosing errors and adverse events in the intensive care unit. *Crit Care Med*. 2006;34(5):1532–7.

23. Petronio S, Torke A, Bosslet G, et al. Disclosing medical mistakes: a communication management plan for physicians. *Perm J*. 2013;17(2):73–9.

24. Duncan EM, Francis JJ, Johnston M, et al. Learning curves, taking instructions, and patient safety: using a theoretical domains framework in an interview study to investigate prescribing errors among trainee doctors. *Implement Sci*. 2012;7:86.

25. Rosner F, Berger JT, Kark P, Potash J, Bennett AJ. Disclosure and prevention of medical errors. Committee on Bioethical Issues of the Medical

Society of the State of New York. *Arch Intern Med.* 2000;160(14):2089–92.

26. Lipira LE, Gallagher TH. Disclosure of adverse events and errors in surgical care: challenges and strategies for improvement. *World J Surg.* 2014;38(7):1614–21.

27. Cole AP, Block L, Wu AW. On higher ground: ethical reasoning and its relationship with error disclosure. *BMJ Qual Saf.* 2013;22(7):580–5.

28. D'Errico S, Pennelli S, Colasurdo AP, et al. The right to be informed and fear of disclosure: sustainability of a full error disclosure policy at an Italian cancer centre/clinic. *BMC Health Serv Res.* 2015;15(1):130.

29. Eadie A. Medical error reporting should it be mandatory in Scotland? *J Forensic Leg Med.* 2012;19(7):437–41.

30. Lehmann LS, Puopolo AL, Shaykevich S, Brennan TA. Iatrogenic events resulting in intensive care admission: frequency, cause, and disclosure to patients and institutions. *Am J Med.* 2005;118(4):409–13.

31. Schoen C, Osborn R, Huynh PT, et al. Taking the pulse of health care systems: experiences of patients with health problems in six countries. *Health Aff (Millwood).* 2005;(suppl; web exclusives):W5-509-25.

32. Etchegaray JM, Ottosen MJ, Dancsak T, Thomas EJ. Barriers to speaking up about patient safety concerns. *J Patient Saf.* Published online November 4, 2017. doi:10.1097/PTS.0000000000000334

33. Nazione S, Pace K. An experimental study of medical error explanations: do apology, empathy, corrective action, and compensation alter intentions and attitudes? *J Health Commun.* 2015;20(12):1422–32

34. Hojat M, Vergare MJ, Maxwell K, et al. The devil is in the third year: a longitudinal study of erosion of empathy in medical school. *Acad Med.* 2009;84(9):1182–91.

35. Neumann M, Edelhauser F, Tauschel D, et al. Empathy decline and its reasons: a systematic review of studies with medical students and residents. *Acad Med.* 2011;86(8):996–1009.

36. Ferreira-Valente A, Monteiro JS, Barbosa RM, et al. Clarifying changes in student empathy throughout medical school: a scoping review. *Adv Health Sci Educ Theory Pract.* 2017;22(5):1293–313.

37. Varjavand N, Bachegowda LS, Gracely E, Novack DH. Changes in intern attitudes toward medical error and disclosure. *Med Educ.* 2012;46(7):668–77.

38. Horsburgh M, Merry A, Seddon M, et al. Educating for healthcare quality improvement in an interprofessional learning environment: a New Zealand initiative. *J Interprof Care.* 2006;20(5):555–7.

39. Moore J, Bismark M, Mello MM. Patients' experiences with communication-and-resolution programs after medical injury. *JAMA Intern Med.* 2017;177(11):1595–603.

40. Etchegaray JM, Ottosen MJ, Aigbe A, et al. Patients as partners in learning from unexpected events. *Health Serv Res.* 2016;51(suppl 3):2600–14.

41. Biermann JS, Boothman R. There is another approach to medical malpractice disputes. *J Oncol Pract.* 2006;2(4):148.

42. Kachalia A, Kaufman SR, Boothman R, et al. Liability claims and costs before and after implementation of a medical error disclosure program. *Ann Intern Med.* 2010;153(4):213–21.

43. Schwappach DL. Frequency of and predictors for patient-reported medical and medication errors in Switzerland. *Swiss Med Wkly.* 2011;141:w13262.

44. McLennan S, Shaw D, Leu A, Elger B. Professional liability insurance and medical error disclosure. *Swiss Med Wkly.* 2015;145:w14164.

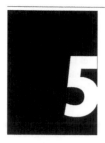

Consequences for the Practitioner

5.1 Introduction

In Chapter 4, we discussed the impact of avoidable adverse medication events on patients. This is variable but may include psychological, emotional, physical, financial, and other forms of harm, and sometimes death. Those close to the patient, family, and friends are also affected. A strong theme in this book is that too many avoidable adverse medication events occur in healthcare, and the response to them should include caring for the harmed patients and seeking ways to reduce the occurrence of similar events in the future. It is with some reticence that we now raise the matter of whether this response should also address the effects of these events on the practitioners who have been involved with them and perhaps also on others associated with the event and on the

institution in which it occurs. As an illustrative case, we turn to that of Dr. Bawa-Garba (Box 5.1) and her patient, Jack Adcock (1): her case is explored in further detail in Chapter 12. It is certainly illustrative of how serious the consequences of an adverse event in healthcare can be on the practitioner involved in its generation.

5.2 The Concept of the "Second Victim"

In 2000, the *British Medical Journal* (*BMJ*) devoted an entire edition to medical errors (2). In an editorial in this edition (3), Wu discussed the impact of such errors on the doctors, nurses, pharmacists, and other practitioners who have made them. He acknowledged "a norm of not criticizing" but

---

Box 5.1 Jack Adcock and Dr. Hadiza Bawa-Garba (see also Chapter 12)

Jack Adcock presented to the Leicester Royal Infirmary in February 2011. He was 6 years old and had been unwell the previous night, with vomiting and diarrhea. Dr. Hadiza Bawa-Garba had recently returned to work after 13 months of maternity leave. Before her leave, she had been managing children with nonacute conditions in a community setting. There were shortages of both medical and nursing staff, so she agreed to cover the hospital's acute pediatric services. She saw Jack at 10:30 a.m. and diagnosed dehydration and viral gastroenteritis. She administered fluids but not antibiotics, despite a lactate of 11 mmol/L and a pH of 7.0. Jack improved with fluids, and on a second measurement, pH was 7.24 (this sample was insufficient for a lactate measurement). Around 3 p.m., Jack was sitting up and taking fluids, but a chest radiograph showed infection, and antibiotics were started. At around 8 p.m., he collapsed and died: At postmortem, it was concluded that death had been due to streptococcal infection and sepsis. Dr. Bawa-Garba received very little direct supervision during this day – her first

ward round with her consultant (i.e., attending) was in the late afternoon, and he did not see and assess Jack himself (1).

The people who have suffered most from this case are without question Jack and his family, particularly his mother. Nevertheless, Dr. Bawa-Garba has suffered too. There seems to be little doubt that she, like any doctor, would have experienced strong emotional regret over the death of a child in her care. In addition, over the subsequent 7 years, she was charged twice with manslaughter, was convicted once, and was struck off the medical register and was then reinstated – all at an immense emotional and financial cost.

One's view of all this will depend on the degree of culpability one sees in the events leading to Jack's death. This aspect of the case is discussed in detail in Chapter 12. What matters for this chapter is the stark illustration provided by this case of the potential consequences for a practitioner when something goes wrong while trying to do the right thing with very sick patients in difficult circumstances with inadequate support.

---

suggested that unconditional sympathy and support from colleagues are rare. He cited the seminal account in 1984, mentioned in Chapter 4, in which Hilfiker, a primary healthcare physician, discussed several errors that he had made personally. Hilfiker's central point was that it is inevitable that all doctors will make errors at some stage of their careers, and he expressed a need for confession, restitution, and absolution when these occur. He called for more honesty about mistakes, both with patients and with colleagues, and also more understanding of them. He argued that these two things would advance both patient safety and the well-being of physicians. More recently, Gawande has made similar points (4,5). Wu expanded on these themes and coined the term "second victim" to capture the idea that the impact of errors on the clinicians who make them is often substantial (3).

This term has gained considerable traction: Gomez-Duran et al. were recently able to find more than 100 articles in PubMed with this phrase in the title (6). The idea of subsidiary "victims" has been extended to include a potential "third victim." This term has been applied to the "collective harm in self-esteem and confidence" experienced by an institution as a "social organism" (7,8) after an adverse event. It has also been applied, more poignantly, to a subsequent patient cared for by the same clinician who also suffers avoidable harm. The idea here is that the emotional impact on a clinician who has inadvertently injured one patient might impair that clinician's ability to practice safely, at least temporarily, and thereby make a subsequent error more likely (9).

Some commentators have expressed reservations about this terminology. Notably, Clarkson et al., in a recent editorial subtitled "An appeal from families and patients harmed by medical errors" argued that the term should be abandoned, for reasons that we find cogent (10). These authors argue that the term "victim" implies that the healthcare professionals and institutions bear no responsibility for causing the harm in question. In Chapters 6, 7, and 8, we discuss how things go wrong in healthcare, and in Chapters 11 and 12, we explore this question of responsibility for adverse events in healthcare in considerable depth. Chance does play an important role in the genesis of iatrogenic harm. Nevertheless, it is not by any means the only factor, and in the context of this book, we agree with Clarkson et al. that there is a tendency to dismiss preventable adverse medication errors too lightly as inevitable and simply the result of "bad luck." They argue that this subtle implication "is a threat to enacting the deep cultural changes needed to achieve a patient centered environment focused on patient safety." Tumelty reported results of qualitative research in Ireland showing dissatisfaction with the term among healthcare providers and argued that use of the word "victim" is "insensitive to the patient, as well as dissipating the professional identity of the healthcare provider" (11). None of these authors questions the idea that the impact of an avoidable adverse event on the involved practitioners is often substantial. This is primarily a debate about framing and terminology. In one view, the term "second victim" has the advantage of being dramatic enough to capture the attention of managers and policymakers (12). In an alternative view, which we tend to share, this importance can be conveyed more effectively by retaining sensitivity to the primary victims. Furthermore, we agree that the connotations of being a "victim" do tend to reflect an underlying fatalism about the high rate of avoidable adverse events in healthcare – in effect, the implication is that these adverse events are beyond the control of healthcare practitioners and managers and therefore preventing them is not really their responsibility. At the very least, we think the term "second victim" should be reserved for those cases where the punishment visited on a practitioner who has demonstrably been trying to do the right thing is clearly disproportionate to any failure in the standard of care. It does seem to us that at least some practitioners have been the victims of an overzealous legal system that does not grasp the nature of human error.

In Chapters 6, 7, and 8, we argue that errors are not in themselves culpable, in contrast to violations, which may be, to a varying degree. Thus, the term "second victim" might more justly be reserved for only those practitioners who are subjected to prosecution, litigation, complaints, or other formal responses after simply making an error. This has not always been the case. Furthermore, the central idea behind the use of this term is that simply harming a patient is in itself enough to precipitate substantial feelings of stress, shame, remorse, and sorrow in the practitioner who has done this. This was the point made by Hilfiker (13) – he referred to the possibility of being sued, but this was not by any means the most important issue for him. His article paints a very clear picture of his emotional response to having inadvertently harmed some of the patients whom he was actually trying to help. Our personal experience confirms that remorse over even the possibility of having caused harm to a patient may be substantial, and our observation of colleagues confirms that remorse for this reason may exceed any emotional response to the secondary legal consequences of having done this.

Nevertheless, the legal and regulatory responses to an adverse event may add considerably to this emotional response. It might be thought that this is reasonable given that there has been a failure in the care provided to a patient. However, as we have noted, such failures are not *necessarily* blameworthy. In Chapters 11 and 12, we discuss the tendency to punish the *consequences* of an error rather than its *moral culpability*. Notably, only those medication errors that cause serious harm tend to be punished in any way, yet their moral blameworthiness is typically no greater than that associated with the myriad medication errors that cause little or no harm. The example concerning dopamine discussed in Chapters 7 and 11 is a case in point. Many examples can be found in which the consequences to the practitioner (in this anesthesiologist's case, conviction for manslaughter) are so far out of proportion with the moral blameworthiness of the underlying failures in care (a medication error made while trying to manage an emergency) that the term "second victim" may well be justifiable. Nevertheless, our sense is that this term has been overused.

It has been observed that no better term has so far been found (12), but perhaps no term is needed: perhaps it is enough to simply refer to the effect of avoidable adverse events on the practitioners who inadvertently caused them. The idea that practitioners involved with patients who have suffered serious adverse events should not adopt the passive role of a "victim" does not necessarily discount the potential value of proactive and well-construed support for practitioners under these circumstances. The challenge lies in doing this while keeping the main focus on the need to acknowledge and support the harmed patient and their loved ones.

We have gone to some lengths to discuss this important matter of terminology and perspective before turning to the empirical evidence on the nature and extent of the effects of adverse events on practitioners and a consideration of how best to mitigate these effects. We have done so because of our conviction that the primary and undisputed victims of avoidable adverse events in healthcare, including adverse medication events, are the harmed patients and their families and other people close to them. In no small part, the argument for a more supportive approach to the clinicians in whose hands the care of these patients has failed lies in the belief that this will contribute to making patient care safer.

5.3 The Emotional Aftermath of Adverse Events

Before delving further into the question of the stress faced by practitioners when a patient suffers avoidable harm, it is worth considering the wider context of the human condition in today's world.

5.3.1 Traumatic Events in Everyday Life

We live in a world where violence, injury, and unexpected death are common and reported in varying degrees of explicitness. The terrorist attack on March 15, 2019, on two mosques in Christchurch, New Zealand, that killed 51 people and seriously injured many more provides one recent example. As is often the case, the number of people directly impacted by this attack was substantial and included families, rescuers, the police, eyewitnesses, and many others. In addition, the attack was livestreamed on Facebook. The video was spread widely across the Internet for almost half an hour before being taken down (14). One can only guess how many people have seen this material. In fact, there is no shortage of emotionally traumatic events in the lives of ordinary people, or of horrific material available on both social and conventional media. The attacks in the United States on September 11, 2001, provide a second obvious example. The direct impact of these attacks was huge, and the visual images of the burning Twin Towers and of people jumping from them to their deaths were seen around the world. Earthquakes, bushfires, floods, epidemics of infectious diseases, wars, and many other disasters regularly devastate many lives and are shown graphically in both the formal and informal media on a daily basis. It turns out that exposure to traumatic events should be considered as being within the normal range of human experience. Benjet et al. undertook general population surveys of 24 countries, with 68,894 adult respondents (15). Over 70% of respondents reported having experienced a traumatic event, and many had been exposed to several. Half the reports dealt with five types of events: witnessing a death or serious injury, the unexpected death of a loved one, being mugged, being in a life-threatening automobile accident, and experiencing a life-threatening illness or injury.

Turning more specifically to the workplace, healthcare is not the only stressful profession known to man. Many occupations are arguably much more challenging than being a doctor, a nurse, or a pharmacist in a modern civilian healthcare facility. For example, active service in the military involves exposure to people killed and injured during war, often in very distressing ways. Rescue and ambulance services, firefighting, policing, and many other activities also frequently expose workers to emotionally traumatic situations. As with healthcare, people continue to enter these fields of employment, and most seem to cope with the stress. Indeed, the prevailing expectation both in healthcare and in other fields is that people who take up these occupations should accept the stress that goes with them (Box 5.2). It is relevant to ask whether the emotional challenges of these stressful events result in difficulties in employing people within particular fields. In most cases, including healthcare, this does not seem to be the case. As a general matter, any negative impact

---

Box 5.2 "If you can't stand the heat …"

Internationally, routine cardiac surgery is associated with a mortality rate of over 1%, depending on case mix. Every surgeon and anesthesiologist with a reasonable caseload can therefore expect to be confronted with at least one or two deaths a year, possibly more, particularly if the acute case load is substantial. The physicians and nurses who work in postcardiac surgical intensive care units would deal with most of these deaths and thus face this sort of event much more frequently than that.

The loss of any patient undergoing elective surgery is likely to be emotionally stressful for any caring practitioner. These deaths require very personal interactions with the patient's family and other loved ones, who have to be told bad news, often over time as the clinical condition deteriorates, and then finally after the event. Subsequently, deaths of this sort are typically presented and reviewed at multidisciplinary meetings where the discussion is often robust but somewhat coldly clinical rather than emotionally empathic. It is common for areas to be identified where the clinical management of the case could have been better. The issues canvassed are wide ranging and may well include the management of medications – in the context of supporting a failing heart, for example. Thus, the anesthesiologist and others involved in the case may be subject to criticism as well as the surgeon. Criticism may not imply that serious errors necessarily occurred in most of these cases, instead it may simply reflect the pursuit of perfection with the benefit of hindsight in the context of complex and high-risk surgery. Nevertheless, an analysis of this sort can readily come over as being critical of an individual clinician's performance and hence may add to the emotional stress for that person. If a formal complaint or a lawsuit follows the death, the emotional impact is likely to become even greater and much more prolonged.

Recently, one of the authors of this book had reason to meet with a senior cardiac surgeon to discuss certain challenges faced by a particular surgical unit. The Resilience in Stressful Events (RISE) program at Johns Hopkins Hospital (discussed later in this chapter) was mentioned. The cardiac surgeon had not heard of this program, nor of anything like it. He was polite about the idea that emotional support may be needed for clinicians involved with adverse events, but his body language suggested that it did not resonate with him. Although not explicitly articulated, the message was clear: He believed that people who want to do this kind of work need to accept the associated emotional challenges. Language resonant of heroic stereotypes of film and television could provide some color to this view. In essence, though, his point was that stress is simply a fact of life in cardiac surgery and anesthesia.

As noted elsewhere in this chapter, occupational stress is not confined to physicians. The saying "If you can't stand the heat, you better get out of the kitchen" was apparently used by Harry S. Truman from time to time, notably in a speech in Washington, DC, on December 17, 1952. He is quoted as saying, "The President gets a lot of hot potatoes from every direction anyhow, and a man [sic] who can't handle them has no business in that job" (16).

of these adverse events seems to be offset by the many positive aspects of these occupations. However, when one looks at individuals, a different picture emerges. It has long been known that even if some people do cope well with stressful events, others sometimes experience serious psychological consequences, sometimes with serious impact on their work and personal life. In the context of healthcare, it is a long and expensive process to train doctors, nurses, and pharmacists, so the loss of even a few of these valuable professionals is important. Also, as noted in relation to the concept of the "third victim," the consequences of underperformance in the aftermath of a stressful adverse event may be very serious. In particular, it is not difficult to imagine that a practitioner's ability to manage medications safely may be impacted for some considerable period of time after being involved in an event of this type. Thus, the real question is not whether there is a problem, but rather, what is the extent of the problem and how best can it be ameliorated? In the next section, we review some of the key concepts of managing the aftermath of being involved in a traumatic event of any type. We then turn specifically to what techniques may be available to return a professional involved in a serious adverse medication event to a high performing level.

5.3.2 Post-traumatic Stress Disorder and Psychological First Aid

The stress that may follow exposure to a traumatic event may, in its more extreme manifestations, lead to post-traumatic stress disorder (PTSD; Box 5.3). PTSD is just one of the "trauma and stress-related disorders" listed in the American Psychiatric Association's *Diagnostic and Statistical Manual of Mental Disorders* (17). Its lifetime prevalence varies between countries, from 1.3% to 12.2%. Among others, its features include avoidance of reminders of the triggering event, disturbed sleep, alteration of mood and cognition, a pervasive sense of imminent threat, and hypervigilance. There is a strong consensus that PTSD is a serious problem and worthy of proactive initiatives to reduce its occurrence and to provide treatment when it occurs (18). To this end, it is useful to be able to predict which people are at particular risk for developing PTSD and to make a clear diagnosis in those suspected of having developed PTSD. Validated screening instruments suitable for

> **Box 5.3 Key points about post-traumatic stress disorder**
>
> - Highly traumatic events are experienced by people from all walks of life, surprisingly frequently.
> - Stress-related disorders, including PTSD, may follow such events.
> - Screening for PTSD is feasible and may be warranted.
> - Various therapeutic options are available for PTSD and may be effective in some patients.
> - However, effect size tends to be small, many patients do not respond, and overmedication may occur.
> - Early intervention to prevent or mitigate the effects of stressful events is logical, but evidence to inform and support initiatives to provide this is limited.

use by primary healthcare physicians are available for this purpose (19).

Treatment options for PTSD have been summarized in a recent review article by Shalev et al. (20). Mainstream approaches include psychological interventions and pharmaceutical therapies. Of the former, cognitive behavioral therapy appears to have the best supporting evidence, but there are many variations on the details of how this is provided, and not all approaches are equal. Antidepressants, anxiolytics, and antipsychotics are all used to treat PTSD, but although symptoms may be alleviated, remission is less commonly achieved.

Given the challenges of treating PTSD, early intervention to reduce the immediate aftermath of any traumatic event is an obvious priority, and efforts have been made in recent decades to offer early psychosocial support to people who have experienced such an event. Dieltjens et al. recently undertook a systematic review of the literature for the Belgian Red Cross-Flanders (BRC) on one of the more popular strategies for doing this, called psychological first aid (PFA) (18).

PFA has been defined by the World Health Organization as "a humane, supportive response to a fellow human being who is suffering and who may need support." These authors explain that PFA includes listening, comforting people, helping them to connect to others, and providing information and practical support to address their basic needs. PFA can be delivered by laypeople. The BRC offers a 3-hour basic course to laypeople and a more comprehensive 28-hour course to health professionals. Unfortunately, the conclusion of their literature search was that "there is a complete lack of high-quality experimental and observational studies on the effectiveness of PFA in the immediate aftermath of a disaster." They discuss possible reasons for this, including the variety of definitions and frameworks that underpin PFA. In this context, debriefing is also commonly recommended for PTSD and may be an element of PFA. However, a Cochrane review found no evidence demonstrating that a single debriefing session can reduce the likelihood of PTSD, and some of the studies reviewed suggest that debriefing may actually make PTSD and depression more likely (21). A lack of evidence of effect does not equate with evidence of no effect, but as Dieltjens et al. further conclude, more research is needed "before evidence-based PFA guidelines on how to train laypeople and professionals can be developed."

A fundamental point about PTSD is that this is not a simple and homogenous condition. There is considerable variation in the precipitating events and in the responses of the individuals exposed to these. It is not surprising that its effective management requires expertise and time. Notwithstanding the uncertainties that characterize approaches to treating or preventing PTSD, there are many practical reasons for early intervention after people have been exposed to a stressful event. We agree with Shalev et al. that each person's individual priorities should be identified and that stabilizing their lives after the traumatic event should be given priority. Attention should also focus on reducing the risk of self-destructive behavior and addressing the potential for loneliness and despair (20). In the context of a clinician with PTSD, reducing the risk of harm to patients should be added to this list of priorities.

5.3.3 Harming Instead of Helping

For the most part, when people experience emotionally traumatic situations through their work or during their daily lives outside of work, they will not have contributed to causing the stressful situations that confront them or had a preexisting professional relationship with the harmed person. The military should be viewed as a special case in this regard: The emotional implications of an explicit expectation to kill

people officially designated as "the enemy" as part of one's job is beyond the scope of this chapter.

Health professionals are in the position of having to undertake dangerous things for individuals who have come to them seeking help. This is expressed in the following observation that can be found on page 55 of the recent "Independent Review of Gross Negligence Manslaughter and Culpable Homicide" by the General Medical Council (GMC) (22):

Although no one is above the law, the nature of our profession, where every act from a prescription to a diagnosis or mis- diagnosis, to a minor or major invasive procedure inflicts actual or potential harm to an individual is very different. We are tasked with doing potentially dangerous and fatal things to members of the public on a daily basis, as an integral part of our professional roles unlike any other profession and this must be legally recognised. We incise, operate, insert and inject but then suddenly we are deemed to be assaulting and inflicting grievous harm – but only when it suits…

Health professionals may experience emotionally traumatic situations of two types during their work: those in which they have had no role in causing the situation and those in which they were its cause.

Like those who work in various other fields, clinicians are exposed to many distressing circumstances that are not of their making but rather the results of illnesses and accidents. It can be very distressing to see patients suffering or dying from these causes, perhaps more particularly with certain categories of patient, such as children. The COVID-19 pandemic provides a striking example of this, which extends to the loss of colleagues who die as a consequence of their commitment to caring for patients. There is usually little need for a clinician to feel any personal guilt over the position these patients find themselves in, and there may even be emotional gain in working to ameliorate the situation. However, we would be poorer as physicians if we relentlessly simply "moved on" and were not in any way impacted by our patients' suffering. Ameliorating suffering is, after all, why many people enter these professions in the first place.

Unfortunately, despite their best efforts, practitioners sometimes fail to help these sick and traumatized patients. Sometimes they even cause new harm in a way that should have been completely avoidable. Some failures are understandable but still disappointing (e.g., failing to save the life of a patient undergoing high-risk emergency surgery for a dissection of the aorta). Others are much more confronting (e.g., having a patient with a known allergy die from anaphylaxis from a contraindicated medication inadvertently administered during a routine, low-risk operation such as a tonsillectomy).

The phenomenon of inadvertently causing harm while trying to alleviate a difficult situation is not confined to health professionals. For example, a high-speed police-car chase might end up in the death of a pursued person whose crime was relatively trivial. Even in this example, however, the person harmed would not usually be in an explicit and dependent prior relationship with the police officer who has caused that harm in the way that a patient is with a physician or other healthcare practitioner. Patients harmed by avoidable medication events are not bystanders, nor are they offenders who need to be arrested. They are innocent victims in the true sense of the word.

For a clinician whose responsibility is to help a patient to instead actually cause harm to the patient is a failure so fundamental that it is not surprising that the emotional response to such an event is often profound and may include feelings of shame, guilt, remorse, and self-anger (23,24). In the end, the comparative frequency and severity of post-traumatic psychological consequences between occupations is not the point of greatest relevance – the point here is rather that there is every reason to believe that this problem is likely to be of considerable importance in healthcare. Given the frequency of adverse medication events, it is, furthermore, highly relevant to safe medication management.

5.4 Blame and the Question of Negligence

A fundamental assumption that underpins advocacy for the emotional support of practitioners involved in inadvertently harming patients is that they are blameless. For example, Wu et al. wrote: "The blame they often apportion to themselves may not be deserved. In some cases, patient harm may be unavoidable. In addition, many patients have bad outcomes that occur despite the best of care" (12). As stated, this is clearly correct. What is not always acknowledged, however, is that this assumption is *not always* correct.

As explained in Chapters 6 and 7, many avoidable adverse medication events are indeed the result of blameless errors for which the primary causes lie in the complexity of healthcare and the imperfections of the system. Unfortunately, as we discuss in Chapter 8, it is also true that violations are too common in healthcare and often contribute to medication errors by making them more likely or making the consequences more severe if an error occurs. Although many of these violations may arguably be minor, they are avoidable, and they reflect at least some degree of negligence. We expand on this difficult theme of blameworthiness in Chapters 11 and 12, but these issues lie at the heart of the argument of Clarkson et al. (10), and Tumelty (11). We would agree with these authors that it is not good enough to passively accept all adverse events in healthcare as both inevitable and completely blame free.

This is important, because if one attributes avoidable adverse medication events to negligence, then one might well argue that feelings of shame, distress, and remorse are entirely appropriate. Furthermore, if a patient suffers harm in a manner that is clearly outside the normal progress of disease and treatment, it seems reasonable from the perspective of a patient to ask that someone look into the question of whether negligence was involved, even if doing so adds to the stress of the practitioner in question.

An inquiry would be common if someone was inadvertently harmed in other occupations – notably in our example involving a police officer. In healthcare, such an inquiry will seldom follow an adverse medication event. The likelihood of this will depend on how visible the harm from the event is and how clearly it is coupled with an identifiable failure in care. A considerable element of luck may also be involved, manifesting through the complex interactions of the system, the prevailing culture, and the context of the event. Put more simply, the same medication error may be accepted with minimal response in one institution given an uncomplaining patient, become the subject of a root-cause analysis in another institution with a similarly uncomplaining patient, and precipitate a lawsuit in either of these institutions if the patient happens to be litigious. The relationship between an action for malpractice and the degree of negligence associated with iatrogenic harm of all types is quite variable (25), and the data on adverse medication events suggest that they are no exception to this: only a small minority are investigated, but when they are, the subsequent actions may occasionally be very harsh and even extend to loss of licensure and criminal prosecution (26). When this happens, as in the example of Dr. Bawa-Garba, there is often tension between the medical professionals who may see the severity of punishment as disproportionate to the level of blameworthiness involved in the failures of care and the family of the harmed patient who may see it as disproportionately lenient given the severity of the harm (in this case, death). On one side there have been many calls for a blame-free culture in which the focus is entirely on improving the system, and on the other many calls for greater accountability on the part of health professionals.

In summary, then, there is an increasing understanding that harming patients is to some extent unavoidable and an inherent part of healthcare. At the same time, there is an increasing sense that some of this harm could be avoided by greater engagement in patient safety, both at the institutional level and at the level of individual practitioners. On balance, though, it seems that very few of these events involve "bad" people. Mostly, health professionals have actually been trying to do their jobs properly, often under difficult situations and usually to very much the same standards as those of their colleagues. An investigation to identify negligence is likely to add considerably to the stress that is already being experienced by these practitioners, even if it finds the practitioners to have been completely blameless. On one hand, it seems undesirable to respond to adverse events in ways that needlessly or unjustly result in demoralizing a substantially innocent workforce. On the other, it seems equally problematic to adopt a priori an entirely blame free approach, whether in healthcare, the police force, or any other occupation. The notion that the public should simply trust health professionals because they are health professionals is particularly unsupportable.

An underlying theme in this book is that of a just culture. Within a just culture, it seems appropriate to investigate any serious adverse medication event that might potentially have been avoidable, and an investigation should address the care and attention to safety displayed by the involved practitioners. Even from the perspective of improving the system, it is important to acknowledge that humans are part of the system and that appropriate accountability for their actions is reasonable.

The point here is not *whether* such investigations should be conducted, but *how*. It is very important that they are conducted by expert people. The investigators should have an adequate appreciation of the science underlying success and failure in a complex system and the nature of human error. They should also be trained in the sensitive conduct of such an inquiry, with the aim of minimizing stress for both the patient and family and the practitioners. Actually, there is ample evidence that inquiries are often very stressful for patients and families as well as for clinicians. An approach that includes stress reduction for one group will very likely reduce stress for everyone. This is only one of many reasons why such investigations should be carried out in a well-founded, careful, and consistent manner by suitably trained and qualified people.

Given this view, it is particularly disconcerting to read in a recent report of a lack of consistency in the way investigations are carried out in the British National Health Service. The GMC's "Independent Review of Gross Negligence Manslaughter and Culpable Homicide" notes that "some organisations have 'dedicated investigators but too often, investigators are clinicians or managers (with other 'day jobs') and who have had limited training in the science and art of investigation' and 'limited time to spend on this task'" and that "the investigation function usually needs to be re-built every time" (22).

There is no particular reason to believe that other countries would be very different in this regard, although there will be variation, and some institutions are likely to be better than others in the way investigations into adverse events are conducted. Our points so far add weight to our observation that practitioners may have to learn to cope with *some* emotional stress when they inadvertently harm patients, and it seems that many do. At the same time, there should be reasonable limits to this. If at all avoidable, practitioners who are well motivated and competent should not end up as casualties themselves simply because they make an error while trying their best to care for patients. Even where some blame may be appropriate, the aim of investigation should surely be remedial where possible. This brings us back from theory to the empirical data on the nature and extent of the impact of adverse events on involved practitioners in healthcare systems as they actually function today.

5.5 The Impact of Avoidable Adverse Medication Events on Practitioners

A practitioner involved with any adverse medication event is likely to experience some combination of consequences over a variable period of time (Box 5.4). The various processes that follow such an event may take years, will consume time, and may be emotionally and financially challenging. The impact of a serious adverse event will not usually be confined to the practitioner alone – it will typically extend to the practitioner's colleagues, family, and friends, and perhaps to the institution as a whole.

5.5.1 Emotional Impact

There does not appear to have been much research focused specifically on the emotional impact of adverse medication events during anesthesia and the perioperative period on the practitioners, but Busch et al.[1] published a careful systematic review and meta-analysis of the psychological and psychosomatic symptoms of the "second victims" (as they call them) of adverse events in healthcare in general (24). Among a final selection of 18 studies encompassing 11,649 participants from various countries published between 1991 and 2016, this review included a survey of 5000 anesthesiologists to assess the proportion who had experienced catastrophic events (85% – at least some were adverse medication events) and their responses to such events (27). It also included a study of emergency medicine residents' responses to errors (28), a study of errors made by house surgeons in the United States (29), a survey exploring the emotional responses and coping strategies of family physicians and their office staff following "patient safety incidents" (30), and a study of changes in practice following errors made by nurses in Greece (31). All of these included at least some medication errors, and the authors also included one study of medication errors in particular, made by nursing students in Turkey (32). Thus, although the results apply to all types of adverse events, it is reasonable to assume that they can be extrapolated to adverse medication events as well as the various

> **Box 5.4 The costs of an adverse event to a practitioner involved in its causation; included are emotional costs, time, financial costs, and reputational costs, among others**
>
> - The emotional response to the immediate situation
> - The impact on routine work of attending to the immediate needs of the patient (e.g., the next case may need to be cancelled or an alternative practitioner found to continue the scheduled work)
> - The time required to document the event and file an incident report and other notifications
> - The costs of participating in an inquiry, root-cause analysis, or other internal investigation
> - The costs of participating in a coroner's inquest
> - The costs of defending a civil lawsuit
> - The costs of defending a criminal prosecution

other types of adverse events included in these 18 studies.

The primary outcome measure of this review was the prevalence of psychological and psychosomatic symptoms among healthcare providers involved in an adverse event. They included any healthcare professional of any age or sex, in both inpatient and outpatient settings. The authors did not seek to determine whether the adverse events were avoidable or not. The principal findings of their meta-analysis are reproduced in Table 5.1. In summary, "more than two-thirds of providers reported troubling memories, anxiety, anger,[2] remorse, and distress. More than half reported fear of future errors, embarrassment, and guilt. A third reported difficulty sleeping." Respondents seemed to be more concerned about the reactions of their colleagues than about those of their patients: 39% expressed concern about colleagues' reactions, while only 8% expressed concern about patients' reactions, although these estimates come from only three and two studies, respectively. In discussion, these authors comment on what they see as the need to shift away from an approach of blame and judgment to one of a just culture. They concluded that the summarized data provided evidence of a severe psychological burden on practitioners involved with adverse events, with potentially

---

[1] Dr. A. W. Wu who first introduced the term "second victim" is one of the authors.

[2] The reported anger involved the practitioners being angry with themselves.

Table 5.1 Overall prevalence rates of psychological and psychosomatic symptoms experienced by healthcare professionals involved in an adverse event

Symptom	Overall prevalence rate (%)	95% Confidence interval	I^2 [a] Studies	n
Troubling memories	81	46–95	27.8	3
Anxiety/concern	76	33–95	46.1	3
Anger toward oneself	75	59–86	4.8	5
Regret/remorse	72	62–81	0	3
Distress	70	60–79	0	2
Fear of future errors	56	34–75	0	5
Embarrassment	52	31–72	13.6	4
Guilt	51	41–62	53.1	12
Frustration	49	43–55	0	2
Anger	44	6–91	0	3
Fear	43	32–54	0	3
Feelings of inadequacy	42	27–59	0	7
Reduced job satisfaction	41	36–47	52.2	3
Concern regarding colleagues' reactions	39	14–71	0	3
Symptoms of depression	36	20–56	48.6	9
Fears of repercussions/official consequences	36	21–54	0	6
Sleeping difficulties	35	22–51	5.0	5
Anger toward others	33	18–52	0	4
Loss of confidence	27	18–38	6.5	10
Concern regarding patients' reactions	8	0–70	0	2
Self-doubts	6	2–14	0	2

Source: Reproduced (with slight modification) with permission from Busch et al. 2019 (24).
[a] The I^2 statistic provides an estimate of heterogeneity, with 30% to 60% being moderate and 50% to 90% substantial.

serious repercussions for the healthcare workforce. They suggest that programs to support practitioners in this sort of situation would have the potential to increase patient safety and the quality of care.

Busch et al. did not quantify the severity or duration of the emotional responses to adverse events, but some of the studies included in their review indicate a considerable range for both. For example, in the study of anesthesiologists in the United States mentioned earlier, recovery took a few days for some respondents and more than a year for others (27).

5.5.2 The Risk of Suicide

The possibility that such an event might precipitate suicide is mentioned by several authors cited in this chapter (6,9) but not by Busch et al., and it is difficult to find strong evidence of a clear relationship between involvement in an adverse event and a subsequent decision to commit suicide. The following comment about the stress of investigations is to be found on page 42 of the GMC's "Independent Review of Gross Negligence Manslaughter and Culpable Homicide" in the United Kingdom (22): "We heard frequent reference to the phenomenon of the 'second victim' and the perceived lack of support for staff involved in investigations. We heard of instances where this has led to mental breakdown and even the suicide of individuals under investigation."

Grissinger reported the specific example of Kimberly Hiatt, a nurse who committed suicide 7 months after making a fatal error in the calculation of the dose of a medication for a child (33). Kimberly lost her job after 27 years of employment with the same institution. To satisfy state licensing requirements, she paid a fine and accepted a 4-year period of supervision of medication administration in any future nursing position. It appears that she was, in general, a competent nurse. She was well liked by her patients, many of whom attended her funeral. However, she was unable to find new employment, and one might expect that this would have contributed to her ultimate despair. No doubt there have been other individual cases of this type, but there is no obvious way to identify them if they have not been reported. Furthermore, such reports will always represent a small proportion of the total number of suicides to which a sense of failure arising from one or more adverse medication events was a contributing factor. The decision to take one's own life typically reflects a complex set of interacting factors, and it would be difficult to know in any individual case exactly how much the experience of an adverse event and its aftermath had contributed to this. Prospective studies of larger groups of clinicians typically measure risk factors for suicide rather than the incidence of suicide. For example, in a study of surgeons in the United States, there was a threefold increase in the risk of suicide ideation within 3 months of having made a major medical error (the base rate of suicide ideation being 5.4%) (34). Anesthesiologists are widely believed to have an increased risk of suicide regardless of whether or not they have recently been involved with an adverse event (35). In fact, the absolute rate is still quite low compared with other causes of death (such as coronary artery disease), and it is quite difficult to be certain that this perception is correct (although it probably is). There is at least one possible reason for this increase, if it is real. Suicide attempts in general are often not fatal. Once the impulse has passed, survivors of these attempts often continue their lives without further attempts to kill themselves. Thus, ready access to highly effective means of suicide (which anesthesia providers certainly have) does increase the likelihood that acting on impulse will be successful. The despair associated with having harmed a patient could plausibly precipitate such an impulse, particularly in a person in whom other risk factors are already present.

Thus, although the data are sparse, it seems likely that a serious adverse medication event in the background of other risk factors would increase the chance of a practitioner committing suicide.

5.5.3 The Impact of Conversations or Writing about an Adverse Event

There is evidence that emotional release through conversations may have benefit for physical and psychological health in general, and conversations are an important part of dealing with any traumatic event in life.

In Chapter 11, we discuss the practical importance of talking with colleagues in the management of the immediate consequences of an adverse medication event, with the aim of ameliorating its effects on the patient. This may well imply disclosure of errors to colleagues, and this information may result in criticism or even notification of the event by these colleagues to the authorities, which might add to the stress of the overall situation. Conversely, and very importantly, successful mitigation of harm is probably the most important single thing that can be done to reduce the emotional consequences of an error both in the short term and in the long term through reducing the likelihood of potential complaints, lawsuits, and prosecutions. It is also the right thing to do, and we suggest that a sense of having done the right thing is in itself likely to increase emotional resilience.

However, the actual impact of a particular conversation on a practitioner who has experienced an adverse medication event depends substantially on the nature of that conversation. Some conversations may be therapeutic, while others may be unhelpful. Silence can be particularly difficult to cope with. A narrative review by Coughlan et al. confirmed that talking with colleagues is often found to be an important mechanism for coping with an adverse event in healthcare (36). May and Plews-Ogan undertook in-depth interviews of 61 physicians about their experience of coping with a serious medical error (37). They found that some physicians remained silent about the events they had been involved in, on the advice of their lawyers, to mitigate risk more generally or out of a sense of shame. Such silence was described as "terribly isolating." Silence from others, notably colleagues and supervisors, was also distressing and created a sense of having been abandoned. Some participants were lied to by colleagues who were trying to absolve themselves of responsibility, and this was clearly unhelpful. Some of the people these participants talked with were found to be insensitive and even cruel, while others tended to minimize the event. By contrast, honest conversations with patients, families, colleagues, and mentors were considered helpful. Disclosure and apology to patient and families were reported as making a particularly important contribution to healing. The ongoing relationship with the patient was emphasized as was the responsibility to continue providing care. Various other conversations were reported, including with spouses, priests, and God, sometimes seeking forgiveness.

There may be differences between disciplines in the extent to which practitioners engage with patients and families after an adverse event. It would be almost universal for the patient's attending surgeon to be involved in discussions of this sort, even in the context of an adverse medication event during surgery and the perioperative period, notwithstanding the fact that the attending surgeon may not have had any part in the generation of the event. If a nurse was involved in the failure of medication safety, it is not at all certain that the nurse would personally be included in such a conversation, particularly at the early stages of managing the situation. One might speculate that the same would often be true for a pharmacist who contributed materially to a medication error, but we know of no data on this. In their study of catastrophic events in the perioperative setting, Dhillon et al. found that anesthesiologists only participated in disclosing information to the family in about half the cases reviewed. We find this quite worrying: Dhillon et al. comment that an anesthesiologist can be an asset to an honest discussion with the family, and also that participation in a team-based approach to interacting with the family can reduce the sense of isolation and engender mutual trust (27). We strongly endorse these points and agree entirely that any clinician directly involved with an adverse event should normally participate actively in communicating with the family from the outset. It is very important that a harmed patient and the patient's loved ones see that the person responsible for the event cares. It is also important that the practitioner is seen to be a human being, rather than be allowed to grow in the injured people's imagination into some demonized manifestation of callousness. From the practitioner's perspective, a difficult discussion with the patient or family is not likely to become easier by being postponed. The response of any particular individual is of course unpredictable, and we discuss the management of meeting with patients or families to discuss an adverse medication event in Chapter 11. Nevertheless, personal contact is likely, in most cases, to be directly therapeutic to both the patient and the practitioner and, in the case of physicians, can also be seen as integral to the ongoing patient-doctor relationship.

Writing can also be a means of emotional expression and can be therapeutic (38,39). In 1986, Pennebaker and Beall undertook experiments with psychology students that showed that writing about earlier traumatic events in their lives was associated with long-term decreases in health problems (40). Subsequent work by various investigators has confirmed this general point (38,39), but it is difficult to know how to translate findings under experimental conditions to the context of this chapter, or whether the positive impact relates to events for which one is responsible rather than for events where one was the actual victim.

Documentation is obviously important at every step of managing a patient who has suffered an adverse medication event. The basic rule is to confine this to factual matters rather than opinion, but it is sensible to record the key points of any conversations with families and patients, including the fact that an apology has been given if one has. This type of writing, devoid of emotional content, may not be directly therapeutic but, as with other examples, simply participating in good practices may be of some therapeutic value, and the converse is also likely. Failing to manage the clinical processes that should follow an adverse event is unlikely to be good for a practitioner's self-esteem.

In Chapter 12, in our detailed discussion of the case of Dr. Bawa-Garba, we touch on the practice of written reflection after adverse events as part of the requirements for continuous professional development within the United Kingdom. If this is done in a truly confidential and protected manner, there may be considerable potential not only for learning but perhaps also for emotional benefit. Conversely, undue rumination on failure may be unhealthy. Unfortunately, documenting speculative opinions on the standard of care associated with an adverse event can create avoidable practical difficulties during later legal processes and thereby also add to the psychological challenges faced by a practitioner. One can only imagine the direct emotional effects on Dr. Bawa-Garba of first having this process influenced by her senior colleague and then having her reflective notes used to inform the prosecution's case against her during subsequent criminal proceedings (see Chapter 12). The extent to which these notes made a practical contribution to her subsequent conviction is a matter for speculation, but the point is clear: Great care is needed in any documentation related to an adverse event in healthcare.

5.5.4 Legal and Regulatory Consequences

We discuss legal and regulatory responses to avoidable adverse medication events in Chapters 11 and 12. Suffice to say at this point that they may be substantial. Again, the story of Dr. Bawa-Garba is a chilling example. We note, once more, that the impact on this doctor even of criminal conviction and suspension from practice do not rival that experienced by the patient (who died) and the patient's mother and other loved ones. Nevertheless, that fact does not in itself justify such an excessive response – justice should not be about vengeance.

5.5.5 Impact on Clinical Competence

In 2014, Stiegler interviewed Captain Chesley (Sully) B. Sullenberger III, whose aircraft was hit by Canadian geese and who then led a near-perfect response to this crisis and landed successfully on the Hudson River (41). This event did not involve any errors, and no one died. Nevertheless, Captain Sullenberger told her that all the crew suffered from post-traumatic stress disorder for several months.[3] Apparently, he himself could not sleep or concentrate for 3 months after the event and needed medication to control tachycardia. She cites Gazoni et al. who surveyed 1200 randomly selected members of the American Society of Anesthesiologists and found that 67% of respondents believed that their ability to provide patient care was compromised in the first 4 hours after their most memorable catastrophic event (interestingly, only 7% were given time off work). We already mentioned the survey Stiegler carried out with Dhillon and Russell, in which 5000 randomly selected members of the American Society of Anesthesiologists were surveyed. It

was found that almost half (49%) reported an effect on their confidence, performance, or both after experiencing an adverse event. Most (42%) reported recovering in a few days, but almost a quarter required 1 or more years to recover (27).

Clearly the actual effect of an adverse event on an individual will vary according to the nature and severity of the event and the capacity of the individual to cope with stress. There are in fact several good reasons for ensuring that an anesthesia provider who experiences a serious adverse medication event does not simply continue with the routine care of the next patient on the operating list, and we discuss these in Chapter 11. Foremost among them, though, is the very real possibility of impaired ability to practice. Stiegler makes the point that Captain Sullenberger and his crew were not expected to staff the next flight out of La Guardia or to continue working after pulling off "the miracle on the Hudson" (as this extraordinary event has become known). Apparently even the air traffic controller was excused from working for some weeks. In the same way, we suggest that it should simply be assumed that competence to practice might be impaired for some time in the immediate aftermath of any serious medication event, whether avoidable or not.

In the longer term, one might hope that most clinicians and institutions would learn from adverse events and thereby improve their practice(s). This is the concept that underlies incident reporting, mortality and morbidity meetings, root-cause analyses, and other approaches to audit, review, and quality improvement. Conversely, a complaint or legal action could lead to a loss of confidence and to changes in practice that amount to defensive medicine rather than better medicine (23,42). The range of possibilities can be seen in a study by Scott et al., who interviewed 31 health professionals involved with investigations of patient safety events in the United States. They identified three possible pathways for such professionals: "dropping out," "surviving," or "thriving" (43). Those described as thriving actually felt they had learned from the event and thereby became better clinicians, much as Hilfiker did in his essay. This is obviously an ideal outcome, but others did less well, surviving at much the same level of competence as before or perhaps even at a slightly lesser level of competence, while still others opted for dropping out and giving up practice altogether.

---

[3] Captain Sullenberger also found himself having to answer in a court of inquiry as to his decisions. As discussed earlier, this is understandable, but it would certainly have added to the stress he and others experienced.

5.5.5.1 Should Error-Prone Practitioners Stop Practicing?

It is worth considering in more detail whether *dropping out* is a good outcome for a practitioner who has made a serious medication error. It might be thought that this would reduce the number of incompetent practitioners, and ultimately reduce the number of future errors. One problem with this view is the sheer number of practitioners who make medication errors. Clearly it is not sustainable to invest substantial resources into training all the practitioners needed for the health workforce and then progressively remove them from practice as each in turn makes an inevitable error. On the other hand, the trauma and potential loss of confidence associated with a serious avoidable adverse medication event and the aftermath thereof are substantial and might well impact on a practitioners' self-confidence and future ability to practice safely.

The data on recidivist serious errors are interesting in this context. A recent survey of United Kingdom anesthesiologists by Hopping et al. explored attitudes to a safety initiative to reduce the incidence of wrong-sided regional blocks (44). One in four respondents had performed a wrong-sided block at some stage of their career. This high proportion supports our view that it would not be sustainable to remove all of these people from practice. On the other hand, it is a seriously troubling statistic. Although there are cases of wrong-side blocks having been done with what all believed to be an appropriate time-out to verify the side of the block, in many cases the practitioners had failed to conduct such a time-out. These time-outs are intended to identify the correct side for a block and are relatively straightforward, unlike making a diagnosis, which may involve considerable complexity. Choosing to not perform a time-out suggests a failure to adequately engage in sound approaches to avoiding a known and important problem. It is even more disconcerting that five respondents who had previously performed a wrong block indicated that they still do not perform the recommended check, called "stop before you block." It is also disconcerting that several respondents had performed more than one wrong-sided block during their career, and at least one had made this mistake four times (44). In Australia, Bismark et al. investigated a national sample of formal complaints against doctors to the health

ombudsman over an 11-year period. The distribution of these complaints was highly skewed: 3% of Australia's medical workforce accounted for 49% of complaints, and 1% accounted for a quarter of complaints. There was a strong relationship between the number of previous complaints and the likelihood of a further one. The interpretation of these findings is not straightforward, but clearly the majority of doctors who are the subject of a single complaint manage to continue practicing without generating further complaints, while a small proportion of them appear to practice medicine in a way that makes them prone to further complaints.

Taking all of this together, it seems as always that there is no simple answer to the question of what a single, avoidable adverse medication event might indicate about a practitioner's competence in the future, either because of underlying attitudinal or other problems or because of the practitioner's ability (or lack thereof) to learn from the experience. The answer presumably depends on the practitioner, the nature of the event, its consequences for the patient, and the subsequent responses to it. On one hand, it is hard to see how a conviction for manslaughter and a year of suspension from practice (as occurred with Dr. Bawa-Garba, see Chapter 12) can be expected to have a positive effect on a practitioner's self-confidence or competence. On the other hand, participating in a constructive process to learn from an event, particularly a less catastrophic event, might well improve a practitioner's ability to practice safely. It may also be therapeutic, through the sense of engagement in a meaningful effort to improve one's competence and hence the safety of one's future patients. We return to some of these themes in Chapters 11 and 12.

5.5.6 Impact on Career and Reputation

We discuss open disclosure in Chapters 4, 11, and 12 and emphasize that early and frank disclosure of the details of an adverse event is not only a legal requirement in many countries, but it is the right thing to do ethically. However, we also conclude that although it may be beneficial, it is difficult to predict the impact of open disclosure on the likelihood of subsequent complaints or litigation in any individual case. At an institutional level, the reaction of senior staff and managers to a medical error may also be inconsistent, and sometimes disapproving and blaming (45). Beyond the institution, litigation, prosecution, and adverse media publicity may all follow the disclosure or discovery of an error. There may be suspension from a salaried position and difficulty finding new employment, as happened with Kimberly Hiatt (the nurse mentioned earlier who went on to commit suicide) (33). One way or another, there is clearly potential for a serious adverse medication event to impact adversely on the reputation and future employment of a practitioner.

5.6 Caring for Practitioners

We end this chapter with a brief discussion of what should be done within institutions to mitigate the impact of adverse medication events on the practitioners who are involved in causing them.

The starting point of this discussion is surely that medication safety should be on the governance agenda of the boards of directors of healthcare institutions. It seems to us that those responsible for the governance of healthcare institutions, and those responsible for clinical leadership, should be engaged in the active management of all aspects of medication safety, including adverse medication events.

Repeated involvement of the same person in avoidable adverse medication events should raise a red flag and lead to a more detailed evaluation of the reasons for this. This should include consideration of the particular individual's willingness to engage in practices designed to ensure medication safety and perhaps also of basic competence to manage medications during anesthesia and the perioperative period. We do not rule out the possibility that, for a very small number of practitioners, a structured program of retraining may be required, and for some, it may even be that finding an alternative field of employment is in everybody's interests. Practitioners who persist in unsafe behaviors clearly fall within the willful violations category and should be managed as detailed in Chapters 11 and 12. For the majority of clinicians however, the aim should be the rehabilitation of the practitioners who have been involved in these events. Ideally, they should emerge stronger and more competent than before, having learned from whatever mistakes or systems failures have been identified through an appropriate review of the event and the implementation of actions arising from that review.

5.6.1 What Is Done Today

Procedural and legal support for practitioners involved in adverse events is often available through institutions' risk management departments. These departments tend to be broadly based in their expertise and processes, rather than focused on medication events. This is probably the only pragmatic way for most institutions to function in this context.

However, few institutions seem to have formal systems for looking after the emotional wellbeing of practitioners who are involved in adverse medication events. It seems that it is often left to each individual practitioner to seek help and support as needed and that the response of colleagues to such requests may be variable. There are some exceptions. Pratt et al. describe the development of a toolkit at the Beth Israel Deaconess Medical Center, Boston, Massachusetts, to help institutions develop programs of this type (46). The Brigham and Women's Hospital, Boston, Massachusetts, and the University of Missouri Health Care, Columbia, both have peer support programs for practitioners involved in events that harm patients (12). Krzan et al. describe a support program at the Nationwide Children's Hospital, Columbus, Ohio, for pharmacy employees involved in adverse medication events, patient-related injuries, and other traumatic work experiences (47). At the Johns Hopkins Hospital, Baltimore, Maryland, an initiative started in 2010 has led to the establishment of the RISE peer support program (48) to complement the existing staff support program. This program is worth discussing in more detail.

5.6.1.1 The Resilience in Stressful Events Program

The long-term goal of the RISE program is to develop a culture of mutual support and resilience among employees. This is consistent with the emerging ideas of resilience within the context of understanding healthcare as a complex system. It is interprofessional in nature, which is also consistent with current thinking on teamwork in healthcare (49).

Edrees et al. explain that the RISE program arose because a gap was recognized in the institution's capability to provide support to practitioners traumatized by adverse events to patients (48). Interestingly, this gap seems to have been recognized by "patient safety leaders" rather than clinical staff, which may be consistent with the observations outlined in Box 5.2, particularly in respect to physicians. It is interesting that the respondents to the assessment survey undertaken for the RISE program were predominantly registered nurses, and only one physician seems to have taken part. During the pilot phase of the program, 56% of 119 callers were nurses and 16.2% were physicians. In the absence of denominator data, these proportions are difficult to interpret, but it seems quite likely that the cultural shift needed for at least some physicians to feel comfortable about participating in a program of this sort is greater than that needed by other groups of practitioners.

An important point with the RISE program was the perception that "peers" should be the providers of support because they would understand the clinical context of adverse events. The term "peer" did not imply that responders need to share the same discipline as the person needing support, but it did imply that they would at least be fellow healthcare workers. It is interesting to speculate on whether it would make a difference if the responder was from the same primary discipline. For example, would a physician feel more comfortable talking to a fellow physician than to a nurse or pharmacist (and conversely)? In the context of perioperative medication management, there may well be a sense that the unique challenges faced by anesthesiologists in this regard would not be adequately appreciated by other groups of practitioners.

In the RISE program, responders are trained to listen to the person affected by the event and to focus on emotions rather than the details of the incident. The terms "psychological first aid" and "emotional support" are used to describe the immediate objectives. The responders also provide information on other resources available in the institution that might be of assistance. The interaction is confidential and presumed to be covered by patient safety privilege under Maryland State law. If the responder believes there is potential for self-harm or harm to others, an exception to these provisions allows communication for the purpose of managing this risk. At the end of the encounter, the responder also receives support from other members of the RISE team in a debriefing session, which simultaneously provides an opportunity for learning.

A mixed methods evaluation of the RISE program has been undertaken by Dukhanin et al. (50).

This provided some evidence for effectiveness (93% of respondents were likely to recommend the program to others) but also identified several barriers to such programs, including the need for more staff time to handle adverse events. There was considerable variation in respondents' opinions on desirable features of such a program, although there was general agreement with the principle that the respondents should be active listeners with expertise in clinical practice (50).

5.7 Conclusions

Some adverse medication events will occur despite the best efforts of all concerned, including some that should have been avoided. The evidence reviewed in this chapter suggests that these events may well have various and sometimes serious consequences for the practitioners responsible for caring for the patients who experience these events. It seems sensible to provide support for these clinicians. This should include practical support to facilitate excellent care for the harmed patient and to assist with the procedural aspects of the aftermath of any adverse event. On first principles, it seems that making emotional support available would also be appropriate. We have outlined one program and mentioned some others, but very few institutions currently provide this type of support in a systematic way. One of the problems is that the evidence to guide such support is limited. It is likely that to be effective, a support program would require considerable expert resources. The most important provision may be education, to create a better understanding of how things go wrong, and to develop an environment that is supportive in a general sense. Senior anesthesiologists can "set the tone" by speaking frankly with junior staff or trainees about the errors they may have made, thus opening a discussion about appropriate steps to be taken, and the very natural emotional responses to be expected. Such disclosures to junior peers begin to normalize both the inevitability of human error and the fact that there is a way through the aftermath. Monitoring staff involved in a preventable harmful event for signs of PTSD is obviously important, as is an institutional willingness to relieve staff from clinical duties during periods where the stress and distractions that may follow an adverse event might create an ongoing risk to patients.

In our view, initiatives to support practitioners should be instituted within a culture of efficacy using language to reflect the ultimate goal of improving patient safety and an expectation that practitioners will engage actively with efforts to achieve this. There should be no suggestion of a fatalistic acceptance that all that needs to be done for those practitioners who have somehow fallen foul of bad luck is to provide comfort to them. We concur with those who would prefer to avoid the term "second victim," but we would go further and emphasize the potential restorative and therapeutic value of learning from adverse events and continuously improving the processes by which medications are managed during anesthesia and the perioperative period. It may be that practitioners do need some resilience to the "heat of the kitchen," but it is also important to keep that heat as low as possible. A genuine commitment by all who oversee or deliver care within an institution to improving medication safety is surely the best way to achieve this. Reducing the likelihood of harm to patients is the best support that can be provided to both patients and practitioners.

References

1. Ameratunga R, Klonin H, Vaughan J, Merry A, Cusack J. Criminalisation of unintentional error in healthcare in the UK: a perspective from New Zealand. *BMJ*. 2019;364:l706.

2. Leape LL, Berwick DM. Safe health care: are we up to it? *BMJ*. 2000;320(7237):725–6.

3. Wu AW. Medical error: the second victim. *Br Med J*. 2000;320:726–7.

4. Gawande A. When doctors make mistakes. *The New Yorker*. 1999:41–55.

5. Gawande A. *Complications: A Surgeon's Notes on an Imperfect Science*. New York, NY: Metropolitan Books/Henry Holt; 2002.

6. Gomez-Duran EL, Tolchinsky G, Martin-Fumado C, Arimany-Manso J. Neglecting the "second victim" will not help harmed patients or improve patient safety. *BMJ*. 2019;365:l2167.

7. Russ MJ. Correlates of the third victim phenomenon. *Psychiatr Q*. 2017;88(4):917–20.

8. Denham CR. TRUST: the 5 rights of the second victim. *J Patient Saf*. 2007;3(2):107–19.

9. Martin TW, Roy RC. Cause for pause after a perioperative catastrophe: one, two, or three victims? *Anesth Analg*. 2012;1(3):485–7.

10. Clarkson MD, Haskell H, Hemmelgarn C, Skolnik PJ. Abandon the term "second victim." *BMJ*. 2019;364:l1233.

11. Tumelty ME. The second victim: a contested term? *J Patient Saf*. 2018;18:18.

12. Wu AW, Shapiro J, Harrison R, et al. The impact of adverse events on clinicians: what's in a name? *J Patient Saf*. 2020;16(1):65–72.

13. Hilfiker D. Facing our mistakes. *N Engl J Med*. 1984;310(2):118–22.

14. Shaban H. *Facebook to reexamine how livestream videos are flagged after Christchurch shooting. The Washington Post*. 2019. Accessed January 20, 2020. https://www.washingtonpost.com/technology/2019/03/21/facebook-reexamine-how-recently-live-videos-are-flagged-after-christchurch-shooting/?noredirect=on&utm_term=.6b9903d7c3b0

15. Benjet C, Bromet E, Karam EG, et al. The epidemiology of traumatic event exposure worldwide: results from the World Mental Health Survey Consortium. *Psychol Med*. 2016;46(2):327–43.

16. Mieder W. *The Politics of Proverbs: From Traditional Wisdom to Proverbial Stereotypes*. Madison, WI: University of Wisconsin Press; 1997.

17. American Psychiatric Association. *Diagnostic and Statistical Manual of Mental Disorders*. 5th ed. Arlington, VA: American Psychiatric Publishing; 2013.

18. Dieltjens T, Moonens I, Van Praet K, De Buck E, Vandekerckhove P. A systematic literature search on psychological first aid: lack of evidence to develop guidelines. *PLoS One*. 2014;9(12):e114714.

19. Spoont MR, Williams JW Jr, Kehle-Forbes S, et al. Does this patient have posttraumatic stress disorder?: rational clinical examination systematic review. *JAMA*. 2015;314(5):501–10.

20. Shalev A, Liberzon I, Marmar C. Post-traumatic stress disorder [Review]. *N Engl J Med*. 2017;1(25):2459–69.

21. Rose S, Bisson J, Churchill R, Wessely S. Psychological debriefing for preventing post traumatic stress disorder (PTSD). *Cochrane Database Syst Rev*. 2002(2):CD000560.

22. Hamilton L. *Independent Review of Gross Negligence Manslaughter and Culpable Homicide*. London: General Medical Council; 2019. Accessed January 3, 2020. https://www.gmc-uk.org/about/how-we-work/corporate-strategy-plans-and-impact/supporting-a-profession-under-pressure/independent-review-of-medical-manslaughter-and-culpable-homicide

23. Cunningham W, Wilson H. Shame, guilt and the medical practitioner. *N Z Med J*. 2003;116(1183):U629.

24. Busch IM, Moretti F, Purgato M, et al. Psychological and psychosomatic symptoms of second victims of adverse events: a systematic review and meta-analysis. *J Patient Saf*. 2019;3:26.

25. Localio AR, Lawthers AG, Brennan TA, et al. Relation between malpractice claims and adverse events due to negligence. Results of the Harvard Medical Practice Study III. *N Engl J Med*. 1991;325(4):245–51.

26. Skegg PDG. Criminal prosecutions of negligent health professionals: the New Zealand experience. *Med Law Rev*. 1998;6:220–46.

27. Dhillon AK, Russell DL, Stiegler MP. Catastrophic events in the perioperative setting: a survey of U.S. anesthesiologists. *Int J Emerg Ment Health*. 2015;17(3):661–3.

28. Hobgood C, Hevia A, Tamayo-Sarver JH, Weiner B, Riviello R. The influence of the causes and contexts of medical errors on emergency medicine residents' responses to their errors: an exploration. *Acad Med*. 2005;80(8):758–64.

29. Wu AW, Folkman S, McPhee SJ, Lo B. Do house officers learn from their mistakes? *JAMA*. 1991;265(16):2089–94.

30. O'Beirne M, Sterling P, Palacios-Derflingher L, Hohman S, Zwicker K. Emotional impact of patient safety incidents on family physicians and their office staff. *J Am Board Fam Med*. 2012;25(2):177–83.

31. Karga M, Kiekkas P, Aretha D, Lemonidou C. Changes in nursing practice: associations with responses to and coping with errors. *J Clin Nurs*. 2011;20(21–22):3246–55.

32. Cebeci F, Karazeybek E, Sucu G, Kahveci R. Nursing students' medication errors and their opinions on the reasons of errors: a cross-sectional survey. *J Pak Med Assoc*. 2015;65(5):457–62.

33. Grissinger M. Too many abandon the "second victims" of medical errors. *P T*. 2014;39(9):591–2.

34. Shanafelt TD, Balch CM, Dyrbye L, et al. Special report: suicidal ideation among American surgeons. *Arch Surg*. 2011;146(1):54–62.

35. Swanson SP, Roberts LJ, Chapman MD. Are anaesthetists prone to suicide? A review of rates and risk factors. *Anaesth Intensive Care*. 2003;31(4):434–45.

36. Coughlan B, Powell D, Higgins MF. The second victim: a review. *Eur J Obstet Gynecol Reprod Biol*. 2017;213:11–16.

37. May N, Plews-Ogan M. The role of talking (and keeping silent) in physician coping with medical error: a qualitative study. *Patient Educ Couns*. 2012;88(3):449–54.

38. Frisina PG, Borod JC, Lepore SJ. A meta-analysis of the effects of written emotional disclosure on the health outcomes of clinical populations. *J Nerv Ment Dis*. 2004;192(9):629–34.

39. Petrie KJ, Fontanilla I, Thomas MG, Booth RJ, Pennebaker JW. Effect of written emotional expression on immune function in patients with human immunodeficiency virus infection: a randomized trial. *Psychosom Med*. 2004;66(2):272–5.

40. Pennebaker JW, Beall SK. Confronting a traumatic event: toward an understanding of inhibition and disease. *J Abnorm Psychol*. 1986;95(3):274–81.

41. Stiegler MP. A piece of my mind. What I learned about adverse events from Captain Sully: it's not what you think. *JAMA*. 2015;313(4):361–2.

42. Cunningham W, Wilson H. Complaints, shame and defensive medicine. *BMJ Qual Saf*. 2011;20(5):449–52.

43. Scott SD, Hirschinger LE, Cox KR, et al. The natural history of recovery for the healthcare provider "second victim" after adverse patient events. *Qual Saf Health Care*. 2009;18(5):325–30.

44. Hopping M, Merry AF, Pandit JJ. Exploring performance of, and attitudes to, Stop- and Mock-Before-You-Block in preventing wrong-side blocks. *Anaesthesia*. 2018;73(4):421–7.

45. Sirriyeh R, Lawton R, Gardner P, Armitage G. Coping with medical error: a systematic review of papers to assess the effects of involvement in medical errors on healthcare professionals' psychological well-being. *Qual Saf Health Care*. 2010;19(6):e43.

46. Pratt S, Kenney L, Scott SD, Wu AW. How to develop a second victim support program: a toolkit for health care organizations. *Jt Comm J Qual Patient Saf*. 2012;38(5):P235–40.

47. Krzan KD, Merandi J, Morvay S, Mirtallo J. Implementation of a "second victim" program in a pediatric hospital. *Am J Health Syst Pharm*. 2015;72(7):563–7.

48. Edrees HH, Wu AW. Does one size fit all? Assessing the need for organizational second victim support programs. *J Patient Saf.* 2017;30:30.

49. Braithwaite J, Wears RL, Hollnagel E. Resilient health care: turning patient safety on its head. *Int J Qual Health Care.* 2015;27(5):418–20.

50. Dukhanin V, Edrees HH, Connors CA, et al. Case: a second victim support program in pediatrics: successes and challenges to implementation. *J Pediatr Nurs.* 2018;41:P54–9.

Why Failures Occur in the Safe Management of Medications

6.1 Introduction

Over the last 50 years or so, much progress has been made in the availability of the medications and technology used in anesthesia and the perioperative period. The training and expertise of anesthesiologists has also improved substantially. The risks of anesthesia are a fraction of what they once were, at least in high-income countries. Certain medication errors, notably those associated with the administration of oxygen, have been largely eliminated through improved engineering (e.g., the introduction of pin-indexing and antihypoxic delivery devices) and the advent of pulse oximetry, capnography, and the monitoring of gas mixtures delivered to patients. It is surprising, therefore, that almost all other types of medication errors continue to occur at unacceptably high rates during anesthesia despite repeated calls for action (1–5). Similarly, the focus on the preoperative assessment and postoperative management of patients undergoing surgery has vastly improved. Yet, as we have seen in Chapter 2, medication errors continue to plague their care.

We discussed some of the complexities involved in the perioperative management of patients' medications in the preceding chapters of this book. It may be thought that a substantial part of the problem of medication errors and adverse events lies in the ongoing, progressive increase in the number and potency of available medications. There is a counterpoise between the risks inherent in the increased number of medications in common use and the improvements in the manufacturing standards and the pharmacological characteristics of these medications, and in the technology to enhance the safety of their use. To illustrate these points, we begin this chapter with a synopsis of an adverse medication event that occurred during an anesthetic administered just over 50 years ago.

6.1.1 Two Cases of Poisoned Gas

On September 5, 1966, at the General Hospital, Bristol, a 39-year-old otherwise healthy women presented for a Wertheim hysterectomy (6). She had been premedicated with pethidine, promethazine, and atropine. At 9:05 a.m., Professor John Clutton-Brock (7) induced anesthesia with thiopentone, followed by nitrous oxide in oxygen, and then tubocurarine. The patient's lungs were ventilated by manual compression of a rebreathing bag using a face mask connected to a circle absorber circuit. Cyanosis developed and was attributed to inadequate ventilation, but efforts to improve this did not ameliorate the cyanosis. Her trachea was intubated and the concentration of oxygen in her inspired gas mixture increased to 50% and then 100%. Six minutes after the initial thiopentone, her pulse rate was 90 beats per minute and her blood pressure 75/60 mm Hg. The cyanosis had deepened, and she was described as starting to "look extremely ill." A differential diagnosis was made of coronary thrombosis or pulmonary embolus. An ECG and portable radiograph were obtained and a cardiologist consulted. The femoral artery was punctured to differentiate between central and peripheral cyanosis and produced blood that was "obviously cyanosed but also showed a distinct brownish color." The patient had undergone lymphangiography 5 days earlier with a solution containing chlorophyll, and the surgeon raised the possibility that this might be the cause of the discoloration. The blood was sent for analysis. The cardiologist arrived and decided that the most likely diagnosis was a pulmonary embolus, so the patient was transferred to the radiology department for pulmonary angiography. At this stage, x-ray showed several ill-defined opacities in the lung fields, and it was noted that the lungs were becoming more difficult to inflate. Angiography showed normal pressures in the right side of the heart, so the diagnosis of pulmonary embolism was excluded.

While these proceedings were continuing, the next case was called for. This turned out to be a young woman to be operated on for infertility who had experienced a cardiac arrest during induction of anesthesia some weeks earlier. Professor Clutton-Brock was asked to give this anesthetic as well because of his "considerable experience of anesthesia for cardiac surgery." A similar anesthetic to that described earlier was begun at about 10:40 a.m. This patient, like the previous one, became cyanosed soon after the start of manual ventilation of her lungs with nitrous oxide in oxygen. A diagnosis of poisoning was now considered obvious, but the source of the poison was still obscure. Her trachea was intubated, the anesthetic machine changed for a different one, the nitrous oxide turned off, and ventilation continued with 100% oxygen. The laboratory staff were asked to look urgently for abnormal pigments in the arterial blood taken from the first patient and quickly identified the presence of methemoglobin. Both patients were given injections of 10 mL of 1% methylene blue, and the color of each promptly turned to bright pink. A systematic evaluation of the candidate medications (in particular, the thiopentone, the curare, and the nitrous oxide) for the source of the poison followed. As part of this investigation, the cylinder of nitrous oxide was returned to the British Oxygen Company who found that it was contaminated with higher oxides of nitrogen. The contaminant was later confirmed to be nitric oxide (8).

Professor Clutton-Brock took steps to ensure that every cylinder of nitrous oxide in the country was recalled and that the use of nitrous oxide was stopped altogether until purity of supply could be assured.

The second patient, perhaps because of the very prompt response to the development of her symptoms, went on to recover. Tragically, the first patient continued to deteriorate. She had a cardiac arrest and died later that day. It was subsequently discovered that a third case of nitric oxide poisoning had occurred 2 days earlier, but the correct diagnosis had not been made because of a plausible coexisting cause for cyanosis. This patient had also died. Poisoning by higher oxides of nitrogen had not been reported for some 40 years prior to these events.

6.1.2 The Role of the System in the Safe Administration of Medications

The cases of poison gas illustrate graphically the vast number of interconnected elements within the complex system that subserves the delivery of healthcare in general and the use of medications during anesthesia and the perioperative period more particularly. Anesthesiologists should be able to expect that the commercially supplied medications they administer are of an acceptable purity and quality. The fact that this particular batch of nitrous oxide was contaminated presumably reflected a failure in the process of manufacturing (i.e., a "systems error"), which likely allowed an error by someone involved in that process to go undetected. This manufacturing failure, occurring temporally and physically at a distance from the tragedy, demonstrates the important point that many (and perhaps all) of the elements in a complex system are interrelated. This was famously characterized by the notion that the flapping of a butterfly's wing in Brazil could set off a tornado in Texas (9).

6.2 Medication Management and Types of Work

For many practitioners, the management of medications in the perioperative period often occurs under conditions that are far from ideal. Cognitive aids (e.g., barcodes, computerized decision support) are mostly absent. Look-alike ampules are presented containing sound-alike medications and then colocated in medication drawers to make mistakes in identification more likely. Instead of labels color coded according to a single international standard, some practitioners are still expected to use idiosyncratic labeling systems or are perhaps not even provided preprinted labels. Instead of sound being used to *assist* the process, operating rooms are often subject to extraneous and distracting sounds. There is often pressure of time, and often practitioners of all types are expected to work while fatigued.

Moppett and Shorrock have provided an interesting perspective on work (10). In their terminology, medication management according to guidelines and textbooks would be "work-as-prescribed" (Figure 6.1). "Work-as-imagined" might include a perception of an orderly operating room,

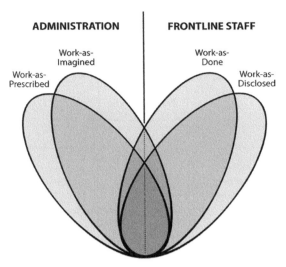

Figure 6.1 The four varieties of work. Reproduced with permission from Moppett and Shorrock 2017 (10).

in which silence is only broken by helpful and supportive comments and in which all factors are aligned to promote medication safety. However, "work-as-done" is very different from these ideals, as demonstrated by the empirical data reviewed in earlier chapters of this book. Finally, "work-as-reported" depends on who is doing the reporting and for what purpose, but it can be assumed that most failures to achieve work-as-prescribed go completely unreported in the context of medication safety.

It is appropriate to prescribe the way in which work should be done, but such prescriptions should be grounded in a sound understanding of the realities of the workplace and supported by all the required resources. Sadly, these two conditions are often not met. A major challenge in designing processes and procedures to enhance medication safety lies in aligning work-as-prescribed with what is reasonably possible and then working to ensure that work-as-done actually aligns with work-as-prescribed.

6.3 Complexity

A process or system can be simple, complicated, or complex (11–13). Counting a modest number of items is a simple task. Calculating the trajectory of a missile from its launching pad to the point at which it places a satellite into orbit is complicated. Nevertheless, both processes can

be replicated reliably, once understood. They are essentially deterministic and linear. Predicting the weather is complex and is quite different from the first two examples. It is beyond contemporary human capability to predict the weather more than a short period into the future – the longer the period, the greater the uncertainty. This is because of the number of elements at play, the number of interrelationships between these elements, and the nonlinear nature of some of the influences on the weather. These influences are still deterministic, not random, so short-term predictions can be reasonably accurate. The critical point is that for predictions to remain accurate, the calculations on which the predictions are based need to be repeated regularly at short intervals, resetting the baseline variables each time.

Complex systems are also difficult to influence. Attempts to do so need to be iterative, with frequent reassessments of the situation as it continues to develop, and consequent adjustments of whatever influences (or "levers") can be applied to the system. Our ability to manage complexity depends in part on the state of our knowledge and on our ability to understand the complicated interactions. Thus, we have become more successful at predicting the weather over time, but our ability to influence the weather is still very limited.

Bringing up a child is particularly illustrative of the nature of a complex process. A parent is not assured of success simply because of previous success. Indeed, it may even be difficult to define success. Nevertheless, there are effective ways to improve the chances of a child growing into a contributory and trustworthy adult with effective life skills. One can improve in one's ability to manage any process, complex or not, but simplistic linear approaches, no matter how logical they appear to be, cannot be relied on within complex systems.

Our cases of poisoned gas hinged on a failure in a process of manufacture. Many manufacturing processes lend themselves to linear solutions, and failures in the manufacture of anesthetic gases and vapors are now exceedingly rare, at least in high-income countries (but see our discussion of substandard medications in Chapter 10). By contrast, the clinical manifestation of the problem was complex in nature. It was essentially unpredictable, and its management had to be worked out from first principles in real time.

6.3.1 The Inevitability of Accidents in Complex Systems

In his book, *Normal Accidents* (14), Charles Perrow classified activities on two axes: complexity and coupling. In the cases of poisoned gas, the contamination of the nitrous oxide was tightly coupled to the consequences for the patients concerned. Intravenous medication errors are more variably coupled with consequences to patients – the consequences depend on the medication and the context. Fatigue is an example of an influence that is rather loosely coupled to the successful administration of medications and even more loosely to patient outcomes. (We discuss fatigue in detail in Chapter 8.) Fatigue may at times be a factor in the generation of an error, but many medications are administered accurately by fatigued practitioners (15), and many errors are made in the absence of fatigue. Furthermore, if a medication error does occur, it may or may not cause harm.

Perrow suggested all the components of a system should be considered in efforts to improve reliability. He identified these elements as design, equipment, procedures, operator, supplies, and environment, captured in the acronym DEPOSE. He emphasized that simply focusing on an individual who happens to be involved in the final stage of a series of events that culminate in a disaster is not likely to be effective in identifying ways to avoid recurrences of the same problem. At the same time, it is equally important to recognize that humans are part of the system – the operators in this list of elements. A distinction is sometimes made between a person-based approach to analyzing accidents and a systems-based approach. These may be thought of as distinct entities, with a systems-based approach automatically exonerating individuals from responsibility. On the contrary, a systems-based approach should be seen as more comprehensive in its scope, and all the elements of the system, including humans, should be considered (Figure 6.2).

Perrow argued that accidents are inevitable in systems that are both complex and tightly coupled, although the duration between accidents can be increased or decreased, depending on factors such as the resilience and inherent safety culture of the system. He was interested in the acceptability or otherwise of the risk of the nuclear industry. In considering this, he drew attention to the balance

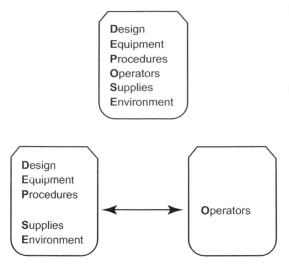

Figure 6.2 The elements of any system, making the point that operators (who are human) are a key part of the system and that any initiative to improve the system should include specific consideration of their role. After Perrow 1999 (14).

between the need for any particular activity and the severity of the consequences when an accident does finally occur. Perrow argued that potential consequences of an accident in a nuclear power plant are so severe that this industry cannot really be justified. This view is clearly controversial, but it makes an important point about the challenges of achieving safety in a complex system. Like the nuclear industry, anesthesia is complex and tightly coupled, with severe consequences for individuals when things go wrong. On the other hand, the net balance of benefits against harm is clear, and we think most patients today would refuse to undergo surgery without anesthesia if at all possible.

6.3.2 The Management of Perioperative Medications as a Complex Process

From the discussion so far, it can be deduced that we believe the overall management of perioperative medications to be complex, if only because it involves humans at multiple points in the process. However, this complexity may not be apparent on first inspection. In part, this is because individual parts of the process may not be complex. For example, a task analysis identified 41 steps in the administration of an intravenous medication in anesthesia (16). This number is not trivial but is not excessively large either. Furthermore, the individual steps all seem simple enough, and they interact in a way that seems to be linear. Thus, at the very least, it may seem that once a correct diagnosis has been made, it should be relatively straightforward to give the right medication to the right patient at the right time in the right dose by the right route and to record and monitor all of this correctly (see Box 2.2).

On superficial analysis, even the entire process by which a particular medication is taken from production through distribution to administration (Table 6.1 [17]) does have many hallmarks of linearity and may seem to be complicated rather than complex. We have already noted that modern medication production processes are highly automated with multiple quality checks and are very reliable. Unfortunately, there has been a failure to adopt this type of process engineering into the management of medications at the sharp end of clinical practice. In many hospitals, this is still done by humans who are subject to distraction, fatigue, and production pressure, often without double checks or cognitive aids or any other systematic approaches to ensuring high reliability. Furthermore, even when pro-

Table 6.1 The stages of medication management and some of the loosely connected processes by which medications are made, delivered to hospitals, selected by practitioners, and administered to patients, with examples of opportunities for the process to fail

Development	A pharmaceutical company develops a medication, undertakes clinical trials in human patients, and brings it to market. At this stage, relatively small numbers of patients have been exposed to it, so unusual side effects may not have been identified.
Manufacturing	This pharmaceutical company manufactures, packages, and labels medication in compliance with national regulations. This part of the process is usually highly reliable but can fail (e.g., through contamination of batches of medication). In some low- or middle-income countries, substandard or falsified medications put patients at considerable risk (see Chapter 10).
Distribution	The medication is distributed to retail organizations, perhaps crossing borders and requiring compliance with further regulations. This stage may involve repackaging and relabeling. In high-income settings, these processes are generally reliable, but errors can occur. Under pressures of medication shortage, in which a wider range of sources may be accessed for medications, a greater number of errors are likely. Look-alike labeling and illegible labeling are latent factors commonly introduced into the system at this stage.
Purchasing, stocking, and displaying	An institution purchases the medication, stores it, further distributes it to wards and operating rooms, and displays it in various forms and ways. Occasionally this part of the process involves repackaging (e.g., into prefilled syringes) or the use of technology to manage storage and dispensing. A common error is placing ampules in the wrong compartment of a medication drawer. Medication shortages often require rapid changes in medication supply, which may bring in vials or ampules that now look alike, when previously they did not.
Diagnosing	A clinician assesses a patient and determines the condition or state that requires pharmacologic intervention; if the diagnosis is in error, all subsequent stages will be wrong as well. Errors can reflect wrong information (e.g., wrong test results, omitted tests, unavailable results) and wrong conclusions.
Prescribing or selecting	This clinician chooses a specific medication to address the patient's condition or physiologic state; errors at this stage include wrong medication, wrong dose, wrong formulation, and prescribing a medication to which there are contraindications, including known allergies and interactions between medications and/or other medications.
Dispensing (preparing, compounding)	A clinician (either the same one or a different one) chooses a vial, ampule, or syringe and prepares the dose to be given. Errors include vial, ampule, or syringe swap; wrong concentration (wrong dilution); wrong compounding (e.g., use of water when saline is required); wrong labeling; and wrong patient (e.g., pharmacy-prepared medication delivered to wrong operating room).
Administering	This clinician now administers the medication to the patient. Errors include wrong medication (e.g., a syringe swap), wrong dose, wrong route, wrong time, wrong technique (e.g., bolus versus infusion), and omission.
Monitoring	The clinician may or may not recognize an adverse medication event or an inadequate or inappropriate response to the medication.
Recording	The administration is recorded; this may be done incorrectly or not at all.
Postmarketing surveillance	The pharmaceutical company, researchers, and various governmental and nongovernmental agencies monitor adverse events through numerous processes (including incident reporting), across the entire range of medication usage, and respond to evidence on adverse events.

Source: Modified and expanded from Wahr and Merry 2017 (17).

cess improvement measures are implemented, they are often not wholeheartedly adopted (we return to this problematic point in later chapters) (18).

6.3.3 Design and Administration of Medications

Objects have *affordances* (19) – they lend themselves to certain applications, and the way they are designed influences the way in which they will be used for these applications. For example, the natural response to a doorplate is to push it, whereas an intuitive response to a door handle is to pull it. The size of the knobs on the flowmeters of older anesthetic machines and their order from left to right influenced the likelihood of choosing the right one when wishing to give oxygen, for example. A stand-alone pulse oximeter is relatively easy to identify as such, but when incorporated into an integrated monitor display, the oximetry data may easily merge into a mass of other information. More generally, large text is easier to read than small text, yet the text on the labels of many medication ampules is small, and critical information is often lost among many facts that are of little use to the clinician.

Several engineering solutions designed to facilitate the safe administration of certain medications have been very successful, notably indexing systems for connectors to avoid incorrect connections between gas and vapor supplies and the anesthetic circuit (20). However, many other aspects of medication administration do not lend themselves to "fail-safe" solutions of this sort. In the overall perioperative environment, there seem to be more things designed to make medication administration errors more likely than those designed to avoid them.

One possible reason for this failure lies in an appreciation of the difference between hard and soft engineering. Norman (19) explains that humans are very good at certain activities, and machines are very good at other activities. A hard engineering solution is one that attempts to solve an entire problem through technology. A soft engineering solution is one that recognizes the different strengths of humans and machines and provides a solution in which those parts of a process that lend themselves to technology are supported by technology, in which the strengths of humans are facilitated and in which the weaknesses of humans are mitigated.

Reason provides further insight into this paradox when he describes the "catch-22 of human supervisory control" (21). Humans are not naturally good at spending long periods monitoring slowly evolving situations, such as the progressive development of hypovolemia during a long anesthetic. Machines, if well designed, are much better at this sort of activity than humans. However, machines are not distractible and remain rigidly focused on their assigned task. The fact that humans are distractible is actually an evolutionary advantage, in that it allows us to rapidly shift focus when the unexpected occurs. Thus, humans are better than machines at detecting unpredictable situations, such as a crisis during an anesthetic. They may also be better at managing such a situation once detected. This is because they have imagination, they can think from first principles and can draw from experience to interpret complex situations, and they can improvise on the fly. They can also bring judgement and empathy to decisions that may impact on the life or death of a patient. However, long hours spent on monitoring a patient (or on other routine forms of work) do little to develop or maintain the expertise of an anesthesiologist for managing the crises or difficult situations that actually call for human involvement. Furthermore, the designs of healthcare systems are often not as helpful in these difficult situations as they might be. At the very moment when the right medication is quickly needed in a clearly presented form, the anesthesiologist may be presented with a look-alike ampule placed precisely where he or she was expecting the desired medication to be.

6.3.4 Interrelationships, Society, the Human Factor, and Complexity

The processes shown in Table 6.1 do not occur in a sterile, robotic vacuum. Instead, they interact with each other within the real world, a world that involves humans in various ways and various contexts. National and organizational cultures and personal ethical and belief systems, competencies, health, and social experiences may all play a role at any stage. Commercial considerations are particularly important. These may manifest through pressures for hospitals to meet budgets, for companies or individuals to pursue profits, and through patients' varying ability to pay. It is expensive to provide highly trained practitioners to administer good-quality medications via modern technologically sophisticated systems. Thus, in some low-income countries, patients are required not only to pay for their medications but also to purchase them and bring them to hospital. Even in high-income countries, requests to invest in initiatives to improve safety (such as the use of prefilled syringes for intravenous medications or barcode scanning) are often rejected on economic grounds. We return to the topic of economic barriers to medication safety in Chapter 13.

The number of medications administered to or taken by patients is also relevant. For example, it has been estimated that anesthesiologists administer a mean of 10 medications to each patient (18), and in some patients the number is much higher. As outlined in Chapter 2, many other medications are also administered to patients before and after anesthesia, by routes ranging from intraspinal through rectal and transdermal to oral and intravenous. If one considers the number of patients operated on every day, the number of institutions in any particular country, and the large army of nurses and doctors involved in these activities, it becomes apparent that patients either take a medication themselves or have a medication administered to them an extraordinarily large number of times every day, let alone every month and year. It is one thing for one medication to be administered to a patient in accordance with the "rights" listed in Box 2.2. It is quite another to do this millions of times over, in different settings, under pressure of time, and in the presence of distractions.

In the end, whatever other aspects may or may not create complexity, the presence of humans within the system certainly does. The physiology and pharmacology of the patients themselves is both variable and complex and so are the cognitive processes of their clinicians. The story of the poisoned gas provides an interesting example of the role of human decisions in the generation of adverse events. With hindsight, one of the most interesting parts of this story was the decision to proceed with the second patient in the absence of a clear understanding of what had gone wrong with the first case. Furthermore, as we discussed in Chapter 5, an anesthesiologist who has just been confronted by a serious event is unlikely to be in the best emotional state to provide a safe anesthetic to the next patient. Times have changed, and the expectations placed on Professor Clutton-Brock were very different from those one might expect today. The introduction of human factors training

to anesthetic practice has made a decision to carry on with the next case on the list in circumstances of this sort less likely in a more modern context. However, even today, the perceived pressure to get on with the work of treating patients can be overwhelming, favoring productivity over patient safety.

If one considers the whole system by which medications are administered in anesthesia and the perioperative period, the number of interacting components within it, and the central roles of humans (both in prescribing and administering the medications and in receiving and responding to them), one must surely conclude that it is complex. In a sense, this is simply a reflection of the fact that healthcare as a whole is complex (13).

6.4 Mental Models and Hierarchies of Wisdom

The steps by which a clinician selects a medication and administers it to a patient (16) can be grouped into five essential components. First, someone has to *select* the medication to be administered and *plan* how this should be done (e.g., the dose, route, time of administration, etc.). Someone must then *implement the plan* by physically identifying the medication, preparing it, and administering it. The event should be *recorded*. Finally, the effect of the medication should be *monitored*, which may lead to a further iteration of this cycle. If the person administering the medication is not the same as the person prescribing it, then accurate and detailed *communication* of the prescription is also necessary. This transfer of responsibility creates its own opportunities for failure, but it also introduces the opportunity for certain checks to be made. The potential for each of these elements to fail depends as much on the inner workings of the human brain as on the physical features of the medications, the recipients, and the world in which they are administered.

6.4.1 How We Perceive the World: Schemata, Frames, and Mental Models

Humans make decisions and take actions on the basis of their mental representations of the situations in which they find themselves, rather than on the situations themselves as they exist in a physical sense in the so-called "real world." These mental representations may or may not be accurate, and they are seldom, if ever, comprehensive.

James Reason, in his classic book *Human Error* (21), emphasized that humans are first and foremost pattern matchers. They use *schemata* to store the key elements of a situation in memory in a way that facilitates pattern matching in the future. In a particular situation, one might synthesize several schemata into a more comprehensive overall picture, creating what is sometimes known as an individual's *mental model* of that situation (22,23). The term "frame" conveys the slightly different idea that people see the same situation from different perspectives, with each tending to believe that their frame is correct even though several individuals may apply very different frames to the same encounter (24). A decision can only be properly understood in the context of the perspective of the individual who made it and of that individual's mental model at the time.

6.4.2 Personal Knowledge: Data, Information, Evidence, Knowledge, Wisdom, and Enlightenment

In any patient care setting, clinicians bring with them the information and knowledge that is stored in their memory and a set of clinical skills which has been learned over time from reading, from educators, or from experience: Collectively, these elements can be thought of as *expertise* (we expand on the concept of expertise later in this chapter).

Some information is more reliable than other information. *Evidence-based medicine* encourages clinicians to use *evidence* – that is, scientifically sound and validated data from research that has been appropriately analyzed and interpreted (Box 6.1). Technically, one could argue that the evidence from a research study is the set of data itself, but raw data are of little direct value when making clinical decisions, so for practical purposes, it is easier to think of evidence as a particular type of information. Much of the information clinicians hold stored in their memories is not evidence in this sense.

The factual knowledge held in any individual's brain is immersed in a milieu of values, attitudes, or prejudices of various types that have also been implanted and modified over the years and which may be conscious or unconscious. Even factual knowledge is variably accessible to the conscious

---

Box 6.1 Evidence-based medicine

In recent decades, there has been a strong emphasis on "evidence-based medicine." Hierarchies have been described, with evidence from randomized controlled trials (RCTs), or meta-analyses of RCTs, at their pinnacle. In fact, Sackett et al. (25) defined evidence-based medicine as involving "tracking down the best external evidence with which to answer our clinical questions." These authors made the point that different research designs lend themselves to different questions. Such hierarchies of evidence were also challenged by Merry et al. (26) in the context of anesthesia, in an editorial in the same year. This editorial explicitly included qualitative research as an important source of evidence and emphasized the quality of the research as a key factor in determining the strength of evidence. Thus, evidence can be relied upon to the extent that studies are well designed, conducted, and reported whether these be RCTs, qualitative studies, or any other form of research. The converse is also true, and the world has seen many poor-quality RCTs.

Many but not all of the questions related to medication management in the perioperative period lend themselves to RCTs. For example, an RCT can provide information on the efficacy and side effects of a particular nonsteroidal anti-inflammatory medication (27). However, evidence about patients' likely perception of the relative importance of these risks and benefits would also be relevant to a decision on including such a medication in a hospital's routine postoperative multimodal analgesic regime. Evidence of the latter type would be qualitative in nature and, in the context of pharmacology, is often scantily available, if at all.

---

mind at any point in time. Several writers (28–30) have discussed an interrelated set of concepts including data, information, evidence, knowledge, and wisdom, and attempted to integrate these into various forms of hierarchy (e.g., the data, information, evidence, knowledge or DIEK hierarchy [30]). There is ongoing debate over detail, but a reasonable degree of high-level agreement can be discerned within this literature (Box 6.2). Thus, an individual's knowledge is broader, deeper, and richer than information or evidence. It is multifaceted, dynamic in nature, context-specific, subject to unconscious influences, and often imperfect. Yet clinicians, every day, bring all of their knowledge to bear in

---

Box 6.2 The "wisdom hierarchy": illustrative analogies

In 1987, Zeleney used beer and bread as analogies to illustrate the different elements of any decision (28). Here we have rephrased and expanded these analogies to reflect the context of medication management.

Data are like atoms or molecules of wheat or water, or the yeast bacteria – in their unprocessed state, they have no unified form or identity, but they could be used with other ingredients for making various things, including beer and bread. Similarly, molecules are at the heart of medication management and so are the individual data points in a research study in rats on the effects of a medication. Individual data points, unprocessed in a table, are of no direct use in making a clinical decision about a patient.

Information brings data together into substances with identities – flour, water, yeast; at this point, the possibilities are still multiple, but they are more limited: they are now less suitable for making beer, but can still be used to make bread, of many varieties. Similarly, appropriate statistical analysis of the data collected in the previous study and interpretation of these "results" in the context of other information (including information of the sort contained in textbooks of pharmacology, anesthesia, and internal medicine) turns the data into new information that can be used to inform a decision. Information derived from research data can be thought of as *evidence*, but we should recognize that, even as different individuals will make quite different breads from the same ingredients, individuals may and often do interpret the same statistical results in quite different ways.

Knowledge is the "know-how" to actually make the bread from the ingredients, perhaps using other things, such as an oven, to do so. Similarly, the expertise required to collect appropriate data, analyze them, and interpret them is knowledge. Information is one element of knowledge, but the interconnections and rearrangements that turn information into knowledge are dynamic, often "fuzzy" or ambiguous, and typically reflect experience and learning over time. Knowledge includes such things as knowing which medications are indicated for common medical conditions.

Wisdom concerns comparisons, choices, and judgments about what to do and indeed whether to do anything at all (e.g., should one make white bread or brown bread, or should one simply drive to the baker and buy a ready-made loaf?). Similarly, wisdom deals with questions such as "should we commercialize this molecule and make a patented pharmaceutical?" or "should I give this particular patient an extra dose of fentanyl?"

Enlightenment goes one step further than wisdom – it is value based and reflects ethics and integrity. Values matter in every walk of life. The discussion of research fraud (Box 6.3) provides just one illustration of the importance of values in underpinning decisions related to the management of medications. The clinical management of medications is predicated on trust in which patients rely heavily upon the integrity of their practitioners. Despite this, *enlightenment* is often dropped from so-called "DIKW" hierarchies.

---

developing mental models of successively evolving situations and make plans to manage these.

6.5 Assembling the Facts to Form a "Knowledge Base"

To develop a mental model of a particular situation, clinicians draw on information accessible "in the world" from various sources, starting with their eyes, ears, and other sensory organs. To this, they may add information that has been recorded in various ways and places, such as in patients' notes, in textbooks, in medical journals, on the World Wide Web, or on signs posted on the wall. They may also access information stored in other people's minds, including, for example, the minds of patients, family members, other clinicians, and anyone else who is on hand. They round off all of this information with excerpts from their personal knowledge.

The totality of the information an individual accesses and brings into the making of any particular decision is sometimes called the "knowledge base" of that decision (21). From this knowledge base, the individual must construct a "mental model" of the situation. As explained, decisions are made on the basis of mental models rather than reality. Given that individuals bring different knowledge to exactly the same situation and perceive situations from different frames, there may be several mental models on which individuals act even when they are side by side in the same operating room.

6.5.1 Accessing, Interpreting, and Storing the Facts

There are many challenges to forming a sound mental model on which to make a decision. There is typically just too much information to handle, clinical situations change continuously, important facts are often missing or incorrect, correct information may be misinterpreted, memory may be imperfect, and unconscious emotional reactions may lead an individual to frame a situation in a manner that might be partially or completely unfounded.

6.5.1.1 Information Overload: The Need to Filter, Find, and Verify

Each of us is perpetually bombarded with an excess of sensory input. Only a small portion of the information that is available in the world from various sources is typically necessary for our immediate purposes. Similarly, although we always seem to wish we knew more (particularly about difficult and rapidly advancing subjects such as pharmacology), the real challenge lies in being able to recall the right information at the right time. In order to function effectively, we have to access and select the information that is really needed to form a mental model that is sufficiently complete and accurate for us to be able to make a sensible and timely decision.

A person fishing off a rock near the mouth of an estuary in Africa might have to balance the objective of catching fish with certain risks. Advantages of a prime position on the bank of the estuary might warrant accepting a degree of risk – in relation to crocodiles, for example. It would then be necessary to pay considerable attention to relevant potential hazards, such as half-submerged "logs," any one of which might turn out to be a crocodile. A high state of vigilance would be appropriate. The difficulty would lie in deciding which of a large number of logs really needed attention. Logs more than a certain distance away could be ignored so that all mental resources could be directed to those logs that might really matter. But, although crocodiles may be front of mind, there may also be other risks that might easily be overlooked, such as that posed by a venomous snake dozing on a nearby rock, for example.

Similar comments can be made about medications. In a parallel way, one has to balance the potential benefits of any medication with potential risks, which may be direct risks of known side effects or indirect risks associated with errors in medication management. As discussed in Chapter 2, despite a veritable torrent of peer-reviewed papers in the relevant literature (Box 6.3), the strength of evidence for most of the issues about which decisions need to be made in the management of patients and their medications is quite variable (31–33). Also, context matters, and there may be doubt about whether the results of any one research study apply to a particular patient in a particular situation. It would not be difficult to focus on one aspect of safe medication management while ignoring another equally important aspect.

6.5.1.2 Changing Situations

Medication management in the perioperative period is often undertaken in patients whose physiologic and clinical state is continuously changing, particularly during anesthesia. It turns out that humans have difficulty in identifying slow and progressive changes in their surroundings, particularly changes they are not explicitly focusing on. There are various demonstrations of animated pictures that slowly change in some important way: most people find it difficult to identify the change until it is explicitly pointed out to them. Thus, in our example of an angler in Africa whose attention was focused on distinguishing logs from crocodiles and perhaps keeping an eye out for snakes, it would not be difficult to miss the threat posed by a gradually rising tide that might potentially block the only route of exit. Similarly, important changes in the physiology of anesthetized patients (such as an increasing temperature and other signs associated with malignant hyperthermia) may develop gradually and be missed.

6.5.1.3 Incorrect or Missing Information

The mental models on which decisions are made are frequently both *imperfect* and *bounded* (21), in that key knowledge and information is often incorrect or incomplete.

Even expert physicians have gaps and misconceptions in their personal knowledge. In addition, information obtained from external sources is often deficient. Even when it is correct, it may be

---

Box 6.3   Some of the challenges associated with keeping up with the literature

- Far too many journal articles are published, even in specialty journals, for any individual to read them all (32).
- Information on the Internet is also excessive, and sources such as Wikipedia, although often very helpful, may, at times, be unreliable.
- Too many textbooks are published for any individual to read them all, and the publication process is slow enough for at least some of the information to be out of date by the time a textbook is published.
- There are flaws in the design or execution of many published studies or in the statistical analysis of their data.
- Much research is subject to commercial or other influences, notably of pharmaceutical companies and medical device companies. Individual researchers are also subject to the desire for recognition, or the need to publish to advance one's career: Authors may be unconsciously biased to present their work in the most striking fashion possible, whether or not that accurately represents all of their results (33–35).

- Outright research fraud by apparently reputable individuals has increasingly been identified. Fraud undermines the integrity of the fraudulent articles themselves and of reviews or book chapters that cite them, or meta-analyses that include their data. Much of this fraudulent research has concerned medications commonly used during anesthesia and the perioperative period, including beta-adrenergic blockers, colloids for volume replacement, and anti-inflammatory medications (35–41).
- Secondary sources (e.g., reviews and book chapters) often provide summaries of the literature that reflect the opinions of the secondary source authors. These sources are also sometimes simply erroneous. It is common for secondary sources to be re-cited, so erroneous views may be perpetuated iteratively through multiple publications. In this way, textbooks often repeat dogma, without qualification, for which evidence is lacking.
- Media reports often slant the messages from research and may frequently be misleading.

---

inaccurately assimilated. One reason for this is the interpretative way in which mental models are constructed. People tend to see what they expect to see, notably when reading the labels on syringes and ampules (see next section).

The information used to make a clinical decision is seldom complete. A commonly used analogy to illustrate the concept of the bounded nature of the information used in many decisions is that of the beam of a torch. At any moment, the beam can illuminate only a small part of a dark room, a passage of text on a blackboard, or an object at night. The revealed information may be accurate, but it is incomplete. It may, therefore, be very difficult to interpret. In a similar way, there may be gaps in the scientific evidence needed to guide a clinical decision about a patient's medications or in a clinician's personal knowledge of that evidence, or there may be missing facts in the information obtained during reconciliation of the patient's medications. Biopsies or tests typically provide some but not all the information needed for a diagnosis. As another example, images obtained by perioperative transesophageal echocardiography provide only part of the overall clinical picture, and it is wise to integrate this information with other sources of information to form a more comprehensive assessment of the patient's condition before deciding on therapy (42). As a further example, not all patients presenting with anaphylaxis have a rash. This sign may be missing, or it may be present but missed (e.g., it may be hidden under drapes and clothes, and clinicians may fail to look for a rash). Similarly, there might be no prior history of penicillin allergy, or a prior history might have been missed in a very large and complicated set of notes, or a patient may fail to accurately list all known allergies. Alternatively, a correct history might have been accessed by one clinician but not conveyed to another.

6.5.1.4 Labels and Cognition: Size, Shape, Color, and Sound

Some anesthesiologists have used the size and shape of syringes or ampules as an aide to identifying their contents. There is little evidence either way on this approach. There would seem to be no harm in using it to supplement labeling, but the consensus on labeling is clear: All medications and syringes should be clearly labeled (31).

97

Unfortunately, even when labels are used, failures to read them correctly, or at all, provide a classic example of bounded and imperfect mental models. It has been suggested that such failures amount to negligence, when in truth, they often arise, despite the best efforts of practitioners, from the cognitive processes by which we access information. Because humans are natural pattern recognizers, we tend to read text by recognizing the general shape and form of words and phrases rather than by evaluating each letter in turn. We may also be influenced by suggestion, and we tend to interpret text in the light of what we expect to see. If we have reached for what we believe is an ampule of doxapram and we see a word like "dopamine," we may well read it as "doxapram" (see the story at the beginning of Chapter 7), particularly if the label background color is the same (usually white) or vial caps are the same color.

Some insight into this can be obtained from an interesting online discussion by Matt Davis of Cambridge University (www.mrc-cbu.cam.ac.uk/people/matt.davis/cmabridge/, accessed July 17, 2020). "Raeding wrods with jubmled lettres" (43) can be done, sometimes surprisingly easily, particularly if the first and last letters of each word are retained so that the general shape of the word is preserved. However, the extent to which this is possible varies with the specifics of each example, and it takes longer to read the jumbled words than to read correctly ordered text.

Some commentators, notably some pharmacists, have suggested that color-coding of labels make certain types of error more likely and have the overall effect of promoting error, particularly certain categories of error (44,45). There is a possibility that color-coding might be used as a substitute for reading the label, and it is important that this does not happen. In Chapter 9, we discuss the evidence on color-coding of labels in detail and conclude that color-coding according to an agreed international standard is, on balance, useful within a multifaceted approach to improving medication safety. Nevertheless, there are ways in which color-coding can contribute to medication errors.

In 2002, Christie and Hill published the results of a postal survey of College Tutors of the Royal College of Anaesthetists. At this time, different hospitals used different color-coding systems, although one was used considerably more commonly than various others (46). This variation was difficult for those who moved between hospitals or between countries (e.g., to undertake training fellowships) and would almost certainly have contributed to errors. It seemed clear that a change was needed and the Councils of the Royal College of Anaesthetists, the Association of Anaesthetists of Great Britain and Ireland, the Faculty of Accident and Emergency Medicine, and the Intensive Care Society agreed to implement a single international standard for syringe labeling (47). This change created its own challenges, with an increase in latent errors (or near misses) reported during the period of transition (48). Interestingly, the only factor that appeared to reduce the risk of these latent errors was prior experience with the international coding system. In 2012, a survey of members of the European Society of Anaesthesiology showed that there was still considerable variation in the use of colored labels between countries in Europe, with about a third of countries using the international standard (49). Once again, it would seem likely that anesthesiologists moving from one country to another might well be lured into error by thinking that a color implied one class of medication, when in the particular country or institution it was being used to indicate a different one.

With medication shortages, local pharmacies often take a multidose vial and divide it into multiple syringes to conserve supply. These syringes, although they contain familiar medications (e.g., neostigmine, hydromorphone), may not have the expected colored label. This increases the possibility of confusion, especially since the medications involved in shortages change with regularity. Thus, a white label one week might be for neostigmine and for hydromorphone the next.

Of course, the use of prefilled syringes actually provides an opportunity to manage this problem by adopting a standard presentation with appropriately color-coded labels regardless of which supplier has provided the particular medication. This raises a rather different contributing factor to medication error – the failure of different departments within an institution to align their approaches to managing particular systemic aspects of the medication process. We accept that the evidence on color-coding is not unequivocally clear – but that caveat applies as much to the suggestion that it promotes error as to the view that it reduces error. Therefore, given that anesthesiologists actually administer these medications, and that it is, therefore, anesthesiologists who will be held accountable for errors in doing so, we take the view that, within institutions, anesthesiology departments should make the final decision on this issue and be supported by their pharmacy departments on whichever decision they make.

Given that labels may be difficult to read, and that color-coding is clearly not enough on its own to ensure accurate identification of medications within syringes, it seems logical to suggest that double-checking should be part of the standard practice of selecting and administering intravenous medications. Double-checking with another human is not entirely reliable, because the second human may also be influenced by expectations of the medication to be given and tend to read what is expected to be on the label rather than what is actually on it. Nevertheless, the fact that such double checks occasionally fail does not imply that they are not worthwhile overall. A study in England in 2010 concluded that the introduction of a two-person confirmation for every medication administration would contribute to reducing medication errors but that this would be difficult to achieve (50). They suggested that the use of barcoding technology for double-checking the identity of each intravenous medication, supported by audible as well as visual prompts (see Chapter 9) would be more feasible. Furthermore, a computer is not suggestible and will enunciate the name of the medication that is actually swiped past a barcode reader (17,51,52). The fact that *neither* suggestion has been widely adopted illustrates a major reason that failures continue to occur in medication management. This reason is that practitioners tend to continue to practice as they have always done, and that there seems to be substantial cultural inertia that inhibits efforts to adopt practices or innovations that have the potential to improve medication safety.

6.5.1.5 Storing the Facts: Memory

Having acquired information from the world, a clinician has to retain it in working memory for long enough to use it, integrate it with information and knowledge stored in long-term memory, and then draw on previously learned skills to undertake whatever actions are decided on. It is also desirable for clinicians to progressively increase and enhance the knowledge held in their long-term memories.

Memory may be *declarative* or *nondeclarative*. Declarative memories can be accessed consciously

and expressed in words. One example would be a memory of an event, such as an anaphylactic reaction by a specific patient to whom one had administered a particular medication. This is called *episodic* memory. Some declarative memories are more conceptual. Knowledge of pharmacology is largely of this type and varies from simple facts (e.g., that rapid administration of propofol may lead to a fall in the patient's blood pressure) to complex concepts about pharmacodynamics and pharmacokinetics, made worse by the variability of the data (e.g., the half-life for methadone varied between 13 and 47 hours in one study [53]). This type of memory is called *semantic*. Nondeclarative memory relates to procedural skills, such as inserting an intravenous cannula or intubating the trachea of a patient. These skills may be difficult to acquire, but once acquired they are usually retained.

Working memory (which is declarative in nature) is retained in the conscious mind for short periods, perhaps up to a minute or two. The quantity of information that can be held in working memory varies between individuals, but many people can keep six or seven digits in mind by repeating a number over and again. In a similar way, immediately relevant information about a medication or a patient must be kept actively in working memory while decisions are made about how to respond to an evolving situation. On the other hand, it may be very difficult to recall many details about a long and somewhat routine anesthetic after it is over and even more so after a lapse of days or weeks. Similarly, facts learned through reading a patient's notes, taking a history, or talking with a colleague might fail to embed in even medium-term memory and may be forgotten by the time they are needed.

The process of forming and then retaining *long-term memory* is complicated (to say the least). It involves iterative cycles of recalling the memory, retelling the "story" to oneself, and then resaving the memory. This process may be influenced by the emotional significance of the memory and through suggestion from other external sources of information, such as media stories on similar topics. In this way, it is possible for *false memories* to be created, which the individual is convinced are true (54,55). It is becoming more widely recognized that the accounts of different eyewitnesses of an accident or crime may vary, partly because of the way memories are created and modified and partly because of the way in which we assimilate information from the world around us (56). This phenomenon is of obvious importance to evidence given in courts of law, but it can also be relevant to anesthesia and perioperative medicine. For example, it is quite possible for the key features of a complex patient assessed a few days prior to have undergone some reformulation in the interim period. The features of one patient may even become merged with those of another seen at the same clinic or on the same visit to a ward.

A large store of long-term knowledge is essential for any clinician. Active techniques can be used to facilitate learning. Interestingly, it seems that information may sometimes be stored unconsciously as well as consciously, perhaps even while under anesthesia (57).

As explained, the knowledge base for a decision typically involves adding knowledge from memory to knowledge acquired from the word at the time the decision is made. This requires not only that the pertinent information has been stored in memory but also that it can be recalled at the precise time it is needed. The fact that something has been stored in long-term memory does not necessarily mean that it can be recalled when needed, and the converse is also true. For example, it may sometimes be difficult to recall the name of a well-known person or the name or dose of a medication that one has learned and used in the past. This *blocking* may be spontaneous or may be triggered by a competing thought that seems to get in the way of recalling the desired fact. Blocking does not imply that the memory has been lost. Often it will return later, after one has moved on to think about other things. This phenomenon appears to increase with age.

6.5.2 The Sixth Sense and Situational Awareness

Experienced anesthesiologists sometimes seem to have a sixth sense that allows them to distinguish situations that are safe from those in which something is going wrong, even when they may have difficulty articulating the precise source of their anxiety. Gary Klein and others have studied decision-making by experts under pressure in contexts such as firefighting and armed combat (58). *Naturalistic* decision-making reflects the way people function in the field (rather than in a laboratory), under pressure of time, with limited and imperfect information.

The importance of *situational awareness* becomes obvious in this context. Situational awareness implies the keeping of a bird's-eye (or helicopter) view of the big picture, often while simultaneously resolving matters of detail. It also becomes clear that a considerable degree of pragmatism is essential for success in a crisis. *Satisficing* is the process of finding a workable solution quickly. Instead of comparing all alternatives in pursuit of an optimal solution, a pragmatic approach is taken to reach a *recognition-primed decision* (58–60). When making rapid decisions under pressure, it sometimes seems that experienced operators have a sense of *déjà vu* – of having lived through the same situation before. They often seem to make great decisions that less experienced members of the team find difficult to understand but which (usually) prove to be correct. In retrospect, it seems that these decisions reflect a greater than average store of learned patterns from which these experts can recognize subtle nuances in complex situations and know from experience what needs to be done. Subjectively, these decisions often seem to arise from a sense of unease or anxiety that "something was not quite right."

In a more general way, Malcolm Gladwell has explored this ability to respond to situations or things on the basis of subconscious pattern recognition in his book *Blink* (61). He argues that first impressions are often trustworthy but not always. Examples can be found in stories of an art expert's sense that something about an apparently authentic painting is suspect (and so does not buy what turns out to be a fake) or a fire-chief's sense that a burning house just feels wrong (and so orders its evacuation minutes before it collapses). In the same way, an anesthesiologist may sometimes develop an inexplicable sense that a patient is bleeding covertly more than the evidence from the blood in the drains would suggest and order units of blood before the need for this becomes overt.

A critical implication of naturalistic decision-making is that its success depends on experience. In this regard, there is a distinction between real-life experience and simulation-based experience. Simulation has many advantages for training, but it is difficult to accurately capture the variations in individual patient's responses to different clinical situations. One might say that real patients do not read the textbooks. One can develop a substantial store of useful schema and rules from simulation training, but expertise developed in real life is more valuable. Thus, a key element to becoming and staying an excellent clinician (in any discipline) is extensive clinical experience.

6.5.2.1 Déjà vu: Friend or Foe?

Unfortunately, it is difficult to gain experience of rare situations through clinical practice and even more difficult to learn appropriate lessons from events in real life. The rules one lays down from experience are typically weighted by the emotional associations they evoke more than by any logical evaluation of what happened and why. On one hand, a poor decision may turn out well; on the other hand, a patient may die despite perfectly reasonable care. There is a risk of storing poor rules into memory. Thus, the sense of *déjà vu*, of having seen the situation before and recalling how one handled it on the previous occasion and whether that worked or not, may, at times, lead one astray.

For example, soon after receiving induction agents, a patient might become hypotensive and difficult to ventilate, with air trapping and reduced or absent peaks of carbon dioxide on the capnography trace. There may be no obvious urticarial rash, but these signs could, nevertheless, indicate developing anaphylaxis. Anaphylaxis is not frequently encountered. Faced with an urgent need to respond, one might decide to administer epinephrine and take other steps that would be appropriate for treating anaphylaxis, but without taking the time to rule out alternatives. One such alternative would be an obstruction to the expiratory limb of the anesthetic circuit, a very rare but potentially lethal problem that can present in a similar way.

An active decision to assume that one is dealing with the most likely of two or more alternative diagnoses is known as *frequency gambling*. Medical students are often told that "common things commonly occur" and that if one hears the sound of hoofbeats one should think of horses, not zebras. Unfortunately, zebras do turn up from time to time, as well as even more unusual "animals," and the unexpected does occur in clinical practice (62). If we return from metaphor to anesthesia, we can see that this point is very well illustrated in the cases of poison gas. For Professor Clutton-Brock, the contaminated nitrous oxide was without precedent in his practice, and it seems unlikely that he would have received any training directed at dealing with such an eventuality, particularly in his era. In circumstances such as these, there is a real danger

of failing to consider some of the less likely possibilities and *fixating* on the first thing that comes to mind, using what is sometimes called an *availability heuristic*. Furthermore, having once made a diagnosis, there is a tendency to interpret new information as supporting that diagnosis, whether it does or not, a phenomenon termed *confirmation bias*.

Thus, frequency gambling and pattern recognition are fast but not highly reliable. It is because humans are not naturally inclined to use logic, at least under pressure of time, that cognitive aids can be so useful. A real strength of simulation lies in the ability to create rare scenarios on demand and then repeatedly practice different responses, debrief, and learn without putting patients at risk.

6.5.2.2 Prejudice and Bias

Prejudice and bias are powerful and insidious elements of human cognition. They may generate responses to the race, accent, gender, age, weight, height, social class, and many other characteristics of a person, often unconsciously (61,63,64). Marketing experts understand that subtle clues may influence the behavior of their customers. The removal of cigarettes from display in the shops of some countries testifies to the temptation to buy that arises from simply seeing a product. The positioning of products on the shelves in a shop, the order in which information is presented, the weight that a senior team member's opinion carries, and the fear of embarrassment may all influence our decisions. Marketing by pharmaceutical companies can have a profound influence on physicians' decisions. Even factors such as how recently one has seen information about a medication and where one has seen that information can influence the likelihood that one will select or prescribe it: recency of experience is an important driver in the selection of rules (21). Many postmarketing medication trials are funded from the marketing budgets of the companies concerned, and their purpose may be as much to give the impression that reputable, even famous, institutions have undertaken research into these agents as to truly advance knowledge about their safety or pharmacology. Understandably, the funding for investigations of products under patent far exceeds that available for older, less expensive analogs, so the weight of published studies tends to favor the former. It is for these reasons that increasing importance is placed on the declaration of all potential conflicts of interest by speakers at conferences.

Numerous other biases influence our decisions (65,66). For example, it seems unlikely that 50% of anesthesiologists believe they are below average in their field and yet this must be true, statistically. This observation reflects *optimist bias*. *Outcome bias* is bias generated by knowledge of the outcome of an event. The opinion of reviewers on the standard of care differs between groups sent summaries that included a bad outcome and those sent the same summaries with a good outcome (67).

Kahneman's book, *Thinking, Fast and Slow* (63), provides an in-depth exploration of these subtle influences on our decisions. An understanding of these factors has profound implications for the courts, and this subject has also been discussed in detail elsewhere (68). The point here is that bias and prejudice may have powerful effects on our choice of medications (and hence on safe medication management), whether intentionally or unintentionally. On the positive side, there is considerable potential to utilize the principles of social engineering (21) to advance the cause of safe medication management.

6.5.3 Expertise

We argued that substantial clinical experience is of real value. However, experience on its own is not sufficient to ensure an optimal response to any particular situation. Some events are so infrequent that it is not practicable to gain experience with them – poisoned nitrous oxide, for example. Even for more common events, the practices we learn through experience may not be ideal, and our choice of a suitable rule may be influenced by various biases of which we may not even be aware.

It follows that experience should be supplemented with other, more systematic, forms of learning. Furthermore, when confronted with a difficult situation in the operating room or on the ward, instinctive, recognition-primed decisions should be supported by more structured and systematic approaches to management. This is where cognitive aids, such as checklists and algorithms, have much to offer, but these are just tools, and their value lies in the facilitation of expertise, not in substituting for it.

Expertise can be thought of as the skill and knowledge associated with being an expert. Neither skill nor knowledge on their own is enough. Even in highly conceptual fields, such as philosophy, there is more to expertise than simply knowing a large number of facts: the ability to make sense out of information, and to communicate that sense, are essential components of expertise.

The safe management of medications in the perioperative period certainly requires a substantial body of knowledge, various skills, *and* the ability to apply both effectively. Skills may be technical (e.g., the ability to intubate the trachea of a patient) and nontechnical (e.g., the ability to communicate effectively with an entire team in a crisis). The evaluation of a situation is also an important skill, one that includes the ability to acquire the requisite information and then interpret it, come to a decision, and, if appropriate, take action. For example, both technical and nontechnical skills are required to successfully manage a patient with a difficult airway, particularly if a "can't intubate, can't oxygenate" crisis develops unexpectedly.

The term "clinical skills" is in common usage to describe the process of obtaining a history and undertaking a clinical examination of a patient and then combining the information thus acquired with the results of investigations in order to make a diagnosis and devise a plan of management. Evaluating a clinical situation that has arisen during an anesthetic or on the wards and then formulating an appropriate response to it, is an extension of this type of skill. Undertaking the actions that may be needed to execute the response also requires skill. A high level of skill is obviously required for inserting a central venous line, or for the acquisition of useful ultrasound images of the beating heart. It may be less obvious that considerable skill is also required for the drawing up of multiple medications from ampules into syringes and then administering these medications to many successive patients over the extent of an anesthesiologist's career, always in accordance with the "rights" listed in Box 2.2. In fact, success in this takes considerable expertise, yet few anesthesiologists receive any formal training in this specific aspect of their work.

Clinicians of many other disciplines are also involved in the safe administration of medications in anesthesia and perioperative medicine. These include nurses, pharmacists, surgeons, and interns, all of whom bring their own expertise to the task of managing the medications of a particular patient. Each will have particular strengths and weaknesses in this expertise. It is to be hoped that where there is overlap in areas of expertise, this overlap will be congruent. The tendency in healthcare is for the training of different professional groups to occur separately, in educational silos as it were. Their background experience also differs in detail and in nature. There is a real possibility that at least some of these different individuals' stored schemata and rules in relation to any particular issue will differ. There are many other reasons why their medical models of a particular situation may not be aligned. Thus, the ability to communicate effectively with other members of a team should be a core part of the expertise of any healthcare professional.

6.6 Conclusions

In earlier chapters, we reviewed a large body of empirical evidence that adverse events occur in the perioperative period, only too commonly. Many of these are at least potentially avoidable. Medication safety depends on systemic factors, some of which involve processes far from the clinical interface (as illustrated by our opening story). The system in which medications are managed is complex, if only because humans are a key part of this system. The processes of human cognition are particularly complex. An understanding of complexity and human cognition may often provide an explanation for failure in healthcare, and these concepts will inform our analysis of human error in Chapter 7. More importantly, such an understanding provides a foundation for our overall pursuit of medication safety.

References

1. Merry AF, Anderson BJ. Medication errors: time for a national audit? *Paediatr Anaesth.* 2011;21(11):1169–70.

2. Llewellyn RL, Gordon PC, Reed AR. Drug administration errors – time for national action. *S Afr Med J.* 2011;101(5):319–20.

3. Merry AF, Webster CS. Medication error in New Zealand – time to act. *N Z Med J.* 2008;121(1272):6–9.

4. Orser BA. Medication safety in anesthetic practice: first do no harm. *Can J Anaesth.* 2000;47(11):1051–2.

5. Eichhorn J. APSF hosts medication safety conference: consensus group defines challenges and opportunities for improved practice. *APSF Newsletter.* 2010;25(1):1–7. Accessed January 3, 2020. https://www.apsf.org/article/apsf-hosts-medication-safety-conference/

6. Clutton-Brock J. Two cases of poisoning by contamination of nitrous oxide with higher oxides

of nitrogen during anaesthesia. *Br J Anaesth.* 1967;39(5):388–92.

7. Obituary. Professor John Clutton Brock, MA, MB, BChir, DA. *Bristol Med Chir J.* 1987;102(1):26–7.

8. Taylor MB, Christian KG, Patel N, Churchwell KB. Methemoglobinemia: toxicity of inhaled nitric oxide therapy. *Pediatr Crit Care Med.* 2001;2(1):99–101.

9. Lorenz E. Does the flap of a butterfly's wings in Brazil set off a Tornado in Texas? Paper presented at: American Association for the Advancement of Science, 139th Meeting; December 29, 1972; Cambridge, MA. Accessed January 16, 2020. http://eaps4.mit.edu/research/Lorenz/Butterfly_1972.pdf

10. Moppett IK, Shorrock ST. Working out wrong-side blocks. *Anaesthesia.* 2017;27:1–5.

11. Glouberman S, Zimmerman B. *Complicated and Complex Systems: What Would Successful Reform of Medicare Look Like?* Commission on the Future of Health Care in Canada; 2002. Discussion Paper No. 8. Accessed January 2, 2020. https://www.alnap.org/system/files/content/resource/files/main/complicatedandcomplexsystems-zimmermanreport-medicare-reform.pdf

12. Gawande A. *The Checklist Manifesto.* New York, NY: Metropolitan Books; 2009.

13. Braithwaite J, Churruca K, Ellis LA, et al. *Complexity Science in Healthcare – Aspirations, Approaches, Applications and Accomplishments: A White Paper.* Australian Institute of Health Innovation; 2017. Accessed July 17, 2020. https://www.mq.edu.au/__data/assets/pdf_file/0003/680754/Braithwaite-2017-Complexity-Science-in-Healthcare-A-White-Paper.pdf

14. Perrow C. *Normal Accidents: Living with High Risk Technologies.* 2nd ed. Princeton, NJ: Princeton University Press; 1999.

15. Webster CS, Merry AF, Larsson L, McGrath KA, Weller J. The frequency and nature of drug administration error during anaesthesia. *Anaesth Intensive Care.* 2001;29(5):494–500.

16. Fraind DB, Slagle JM, Tubbesing VA, Hughes SA, Weinger MB. Reengineering intravenous drug and fluid administration processes in the operating room: step one: task analysis of existing processes. *Anesthesiology.* 2002;97(1):139–47.

17. Wahr JA, Merry AF. Medication errors in the perioperative setting. *Curr Anesthesiol Rep.* 2017;7(3):320–29.

18. Merry AF, Webster CS, Hannam J, et al. Multimodal system designed to reduce errors in recording and administration of drugs in anaesthesia: prospective randomised clinical evaluation. *BMJ.* 2011;343:d5543.

19. Norman D. *Things That Make Us Smart: Defending Human Attributes in the Age of the Machine.* Reading, MA: Perseus; 1993.

20. Craig DB, Longmuir J. Implementation of Canadian Standards Association Z168.3-M 1980 Anaesthetic Gas Machine Standard: the Manitoba experience. *Can Anaesth Soc J.* 1980;27(5):504–9.

21. Reason J. *Human Error.* New York, NY: Cambridge University Press; 1990.

22. Lipshitz R, Ben Shaul O. *Schemata and Mental Models in Recognition-Primed Decision Making. Naturalistic Decision Making.* Mahwah, NJ: Lawrence Earlbaum Associates; 1997:293–303.

23. Nakarada-Kordic I, Weller JM, et al. Assessing the similarity of mental models of operating room team members and implications for patient safety: a prospective, replicated study. *BMC Med Educ.* 2016;16(1):229.

24. Rudolph JW, Simon R, Dufresne RL, Raemer DB. There's no such thing as "nonjudgmental" debriefing: a theory and method for debriefing with good judgment. *Simul Healthc.* 2006;1(1):49–55.

25. Sackett DL, Rosenberg WM, Gray JA, Haynes RB, Richardson WS. Evidence based medicine: what it is and what it isn't. *Br Med J.* 1996;312(7023):71–2.

26. Merry AF, Davies JM, Maltby JR. Qualitative research in health care. *Br J Anaesth.* 2000;84(5):552–5.

27. Merry AF, Webster CS, Holland RL, et al. Clinical tolerability of perioperative tenoxicam in 1001 patients – a prospective, controlled, double-blind, multi-centre study. *Pain.* 2004;111(3):313–22.

28. Zeleney M. Management support systems: towards integrated knowledge management. *HSM.* 1987;7(1):59–70.

29. Ackoff RL. From data to wisdom. *J Appl Syst Anal.* 1989;16:3–9.

30. Dammann O. Data, information, evidence, and knowledge: a proposal for health informatics and data science. *Online J Public Health Inform.* 2018;10(3):e224.

31. Wahr JA, Abernathy JH 3rd, Lazarra EH, et al. Medication safety in the operating room: literature and expert-based recommendations. *Br J Anaesth.* 2017;118(1):32–43.

32. Bawden D, Robinson L. The dark side of information: overload, anxiety and other paradoxes and pathologies. *J Inf Sci.* 2009;35(2):180–91.

33. Loadsman JA. Dilemmas in biomedical research publication: are we losing the plot? *Curr Opin Anaesthesiol.* 2012;25(6):730–5.

34. Moore RA, Derry S, McQuay HJ. Fraud or flawed: adverse impact of fabricated or poor quality research. *Anaesthesia.* 2010;65(4):327–30.

35. Merry AF. Ethics, industry, and outcomes. *Semin Cardiothorac Vasc Anesth.* 2008;12(1):7–11.

36. Shafer SL. Tattered threads. *Anesth Analg.* 2009;108(5):1361–3.

37. Loadsman JA, McCulloch TJ. Widening the search for suspect data – is the flood of retractions about to become a tsunami? *Anaesthesia.* 2017;72(8):931–5.

38. Carlisle JB. Data fabrication and other reasons for non-random sampling in 5087 randomised, controlled trials in anaesthetic and general medical journals. *Anaesthesia.* 2017;72(8):944–52.

39. Kharasch ED, Houle TT. Seeking and reporting apparent research misconduct: errors and integrity. *Anaesthesia.* 2018;73(1):125–6.

40. Carlisle JB. Seeking and reporting apparent research misconduct: errors and integrity – a reply. *Anaesthesia.* 2018;73(1):126–8.

41. Runciman B, Merry A, Walton M. *Safety and Ethics in Healthcare: A Guide to Getting It Right.* Aldershot, UK: Ashgate Publishing; 2007.

42. Sidebotham D, Merry AF, Legget M, eds. *Practical Perioperative Transoesophageal Echocardiography.* London, UK: Butterworth-Heinemann; 2003.

43. Rayner K, White SJ, Johnson RL, Liversedge SP. Raeding wrods with jubmled lettres: there is a cost. *Psychol Sci.* 2006;17(3):192–3.

44. Rupp SM. Color-coding of syringes may not enhance safety. *Reg Anesth Pain Med.* 2005;30(6):589–90.

45. Grissinger M. Color-coded syringes for anesthesia drugs – use with care. *P T.* 2012;37(4):199–201.

46. Christie W, Hill MR. Standardized colour coding for syringe drug labels: a national study. *Anaesthesia.* 2002;57:793–8.

47. International Organization for Standardization. *Anaesthetic and respiratory equipment – user-applied labels for syringes containing drugs used during anaesthesia – colours, design and performance. ISO 26825:2008.* Accessed January 20, 2020. https://www.iso.org/standard/43811.html

48. Haslam GM, Sims C, McIndoe AK, Saunders J, Lovell AT. High latent drug administration error rates associated with the introduction of the international colour coding syringe labelling system. *Eur J Anaesthesiol.* 2006;23(2):165–8.

49. Wickboldt N, Balzer F, Goncerut J, et al. A survey of standardised drug syringe label use in European anaesthesiology departments. *Eur J Anaesthesiol.* 2012;29(9):446–51.

50. Evley R, Russell J, Mathew D, et al. Confirming the drugs administered during anaesthesia: a feasibility study in the pilot National Health Service sites, UK. *Br J Anaesth*. 2010;105(3):289–96.

51. Jelacic S, Bowdle A, Nair BG, et al. A system for anesthesia drug administration using barcode technology: the Codonics Safe Label System and Smart Anesthesia Manager. *Anesth Analg*. 2015;121(2):410–21.

52. Merry AF, Webster CS, Mathew DJ. A new, safety-oriented, integrated drug administration and automated anesthesia record system. *Anesth Analg*. 2001;93(2):385–90.

53. Inturrisi CE, Verebely K. The levels of methadone in the plasma in methadone maintenance. *Clin Pharmacol Ther*. 1972;13(5):633–7.

54. Loftus EF. Memory distortion and false memory creation. *Bull Am Acad Psychiatry Law*. 1996;24(3):281–95.

55. Loftus EF. Planting misinformation in the human mind: a 30-year investigation of the malleability of memory. *Learn Mem*. 2005;12(4):361–6.

56. Loftus EF. 25 Years of eyewitness science … finally pays off. *Perspect Psychol Sci*. 2013;8(5):556–7.

57. Veselis RA. Memory formation during anaesthesia: plausibility of a neurophysiological basis. *Br J Anaesth*. 2015;115(suppl 1):i13–i19.

58. Klein G. *Sources of Power: How People Make Decisions*. Cambridge, MA: MIT Press; 1999.

59. Simon HA. Rational choice and the structure of the environment. *Psychol Rev*. 1956;63(2):129–38.

60. Endsley M. The role of situational awareness in naturalistic decision making. In: Zsambok CE, Klein G, eds. *Naturalistic Decision Making*. Mahwah, NJ: Lawrence Erlbaum Associates; 1997:269–83.

61. Gladwell M. *Blink. The Power of Thinking Without Thinking*. New York, NY: Little, Brown and Company; 2005.

62. Rotella JA, Yeoh M. Taming the zebra: unravelling the barriers to diagnosing aortic dissection. *Emerg Med Australas*. 2018;30(1):119–21.

63. Kahneman D. *Thinking, Fast and Slow*. London: Penguin Books; 2011.

64. Thaler R, Sunstein C. *Nudge: Improving Decisions about Health, Wealth and Happiness*. New Haven, CT: Yale University Press; 2008.

65. Stiegler MP, Neelankavil JP, Canales C, Dhillon A. Cognitive errors detected in anaesthesiology: a literature review and pilot study. *Br J Anaesth*. 2012;108(2):229–35.

66. Stiegler MP, Tung A. Cognitive processes in anesthesiology decision making. *Anesthesiology*. 2014;120(1):204–17.

67. Caplan RA, Posner KL, Cheney FW. Effect of outcome on physician judgments of appropriateness of care. *JAMA*. 1991;265(15):1957–60.

68. Merry AF, Brookbanks W. *Merry and McCall Smith's Errors, Medicine and the Law*. 2nd ed. Cambridge, UK: Cambridge University Press; 2017.

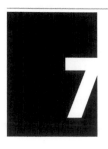

Errors in the Context of the Perioperative Administration of Medications

7.1 Introduction

In 1994, in an influential paper entitled "Error in Medicine," Lucian Leape made the following comment: "All humans err frequently. Systems that rely on error-free performance are doomed to fail" (1). One of the themes of this book is that many initiatives to reduce reliance on error-free performance require the active engagement of clinicians to be effective – and that it is sometimes surprisingly difficult to get that engagement. Thus, we begin this chapter with a story in which a system introduced to reduce reliance on error-free performance also failed. Conversely, the story also illustrates elements of resilience in a strong and well-resourced contemporary clinical setting.

7.1.1 Dopamine Strikes Again: A Failure to Learn from History

A few years ago, a well-regarded anesthetic resident of several years' experience was working under the supervision of a senior attending in a large urban hospital in New Zealand, caring for a patient undergoing a prolonged resection of a malignant tumor. An arterial line had been inserted to facilitate the management of the anesthetic.[1]

In New Zealand, most medications are procured by a central, government-owned purchasing agency called *Pharmac* (see www.pharmac.govt.nz/, accessed January 20, 2020). Many of these are generic and are purchased in bulk and repackaged. This has resulted, from time to time, in different intravenous medications being presented in ampules of similar appearance. For example, magnesium and dopamine have been provided in

similarly sized ampules, each with plain black lettering on transparent glass.

In this particular hospital, a multifaceted system for safer administration of anesthesia was in routine use. This system is mentioned in Chapter 9 and has been described in detail elsewhere (2). A randomized controlled trial (RCT) had shown it to be effective in reducing errors in the administration and recording of intravenous medications, particularly if used as intended (3). Among other things, the system provides purpose-designed user-applied syringe labels with barcodes. When these labels are swiped with a barcode reader, a computer announces the name of the medication and also displays it clearly on a screen. On both the screen and the labels, color-coding is used to distinguish between the main classes of medication commonly used in anesthesia. Thus, medications can be checked just before their administration.

At a point during the case when the attending anesthesiologist was out of the operating room, a transient increase in the patient's blood pressure occurred. The resident decided to administer a bolus of magnesium. He drew up what he thought was magnesium and administered it without applying a label to the syringe and, therefore, without swiping the barcode or carrying out any other check before doing so. The systolic blood pressure promptly increased to more than 300 mm Hg. On inspecting the ampule, the resident realized that he had, in fact, administered 200 mg of dopamine as a bolus injection.

The attending, returning to the operating room at that moment, was quickly appraised of the situation. He immediately administered aggressive and repeated doses of nitroglycerin and succeeded in bringing the blood pressure back under control very quickly. No permanent harm occurred to the patient. The resident was asked to participate in a substantive debriefing at a departmental meeting

---

[1] The details of this case are not in the public domain, but they are well known to one of the authors (AM). We have chosen to present only enough information to illustrate certain interesting points.

and to take part in a process of full disclosure to the patient. There were no legal or disciplinary consequences.

This case is particularly interesting because it closely resembles a seminal case that occurred two decades earlier, in a small rural hospital in New Zealand. On that occasion, dopamine was inadvertently given instead of the analeptic agent doxapram, to a patient who was becoming hypoxic in the process of emergence from anesthesia. No arterial line was in place, and the principal manifestation of the error was a cardiac arrest. The error was only discovered later, after the anesthesiologist returned to the operating room having transferred the patient to the intensive care unit of the closest major hospital. The patient went on to die. The anesthesiologist, who himself disclosed the error, was subsequently convicted of manslaughter. This event has been described in detail elsewhere (4). One of the major motivations for the development of the multifaceted system for safer administration of anesthesia (that the resident had chosen to bypass) was to prevent a recurrence of this particular type of error.

7.1.2 Making Medical Errors into Medical Treasures

Leape's paper, "Error in Medicine" (1), was accompanied by an editorial by David Blumenthal, entitled "Making Medical Errors into 'Medical Treasures'" (5). Blumenthal referred to the "extraordinary autonomy and power" traditionally granted to physicians by the public and went on to describe the corresponding expectation that "among other things, physicians would guarantee the quality of care patients receive." A guarantee of this sort could, of course, be pursued in different ways. Ideally, its pursuit would apply principles of systems engineering to the practice of medicine to compensate for human fallibility in the complex system of patient care. In stark contrast, however, Blumenthal explains that a more simplistic construct has been adopted: that of an expectation of perfect performance. He writes, "Implicit in this social contract was the belief on both sides that physicians have the capability to practice error-free or nearly error-free medicine themselves and to ensure that the rest of the system functions just as well" (5). It is certainly true that anesthesiologists, surgeons, and nursing staff working in

high-income countries today are highly trained in the theoretical aspects of their fields, notably pharmacology, particularly in the case of anesthesiologists. When medication errors occur, these do not typically arise from deficiencies in technical knowledge about medications. Instead, they usually arise through well-characterized failures in the processes by which decisions are made and implemented. It seems to us that, nearly 25 years later, the self-evidently incorrect construct that physicians and other clinicians have the capability to practice error-free medicine still underpins the predominant approach to the administration of medications. Instead of adopting the many recommendations that have been made for improving the design of the system and processes of medication administration, many practitioners and institutions have been resistant to change. There seems to be a widespread fixation on *having expert knowledge* and *being careful* and *reading the label* in the expectation that greater effort of this type will somehow suddenly become effective after years of empirical evidence to the contrary. Unfortunately, a prerequisite for obtaining different results from a system or process is change of that system or process. Therefore, it not surprising that the empirical evidence (outlined in Chapters 2 and 3) demonstrates that errors continue to be rife in the management of patients' medications during the perioperative period. What is perhaps more surprising is the ongoing widespread failure to appreciate the unassailable logic that links cause to effect in this context. Not all preventable adverse medication events are attributable to errors. As we discuss in Chapter 8, violations at the individual level (e.g., failure to apply and use a barcoded label) and at the institutional level (e.g., failure to invest in initiatives to promote medication safety) also play a very important part in undermining medication safety. Either way, if we continue to approach the administration of medications on the basis of reliance on flawless human performance, we will be doomed to continue experiencing unacceptably frequent failures in medication safety.

In Chapter 6, we described the ways in which clinicians working in a complex system acquire, interpret, and store information in memory. We outlined some of the vulnerabilities inherent in these processes. We now turn to the subject of decisions, actions, and human error. A fundamental conclusion of the discussion in this chapter and the previous one is that errors, as defined in this book, are intrinsic to human cognitive processes and not blameworthy. Like Blumenthal, we advocate a culture that emphasizes the open reporting of errors with a view to learning from these "medical treasures." At the same time, we recognize that there is a question that must be addressed with this approach. Blumenthal asks, "How can mistakes that may endanger the health of human beings ever be regarded as 'treasures'? For physicians to adopt such an attitude seems not only unethical but also professionally dangerous given the modern malpractice climate" (5). This is an important question. The problem of medication errors, described in Chapters 2 and 3, is a serious one and clearly demands a response. Calls for accountability are understandable. It is not surprising that the courts and disciplinary authorities often seem to take the view that such failures in the expected standard of medical practice are indefensible.

We accept that some medication errors will always occur despite all possible efforts to practice safely. However, we believe that the current rate of medication errors is unacceptably high and that much more could be done to improve medication safety. Care and conscientiousness certainly do have a place, but they need to be applied in ways that take into account the human and systems factors that predispose to error. This implies greater investment in well-designed initiatives to improve the safety of practice. Collectively, clinicians need to do more to insist on, embrace, and support such initiatives. Furthermore, violations (often thought of as "minor") play a role in the genesis of failures in medication safety, and their widespread acceptance in healthcare needs to be addressed.

In this chapter, our interest is in error. In Chapter 8, we discuss violations and expand on their role in predisposing to error and exacerbating the consequences when error occurs. In the latter part of the book, we turn to the changes in practice and attitude that will be required if we are to succeed in improving medication safety for patients during anesthesia and the perioperative period.

7.2 Definition of Error

In Chapter 1, we defined an error as follows: An error is unintentional; it involves either the use of a flawed decision or plan to achieve an aim, or the failure to carry out a planned action as intended.

More informally, one might say that an error is when one tries to do the right thing but actually does the wrong thing. The justification for preferring this definition to various alternatives has been discussed in considerable detail elsewhere (4), but some explanation of two key elements of this definition is warranted here.

7.2.1 Element 1: Errors Are Unintentional but Reflect an Intention

The first element is, on first appearances, paradoxical. With an error, there is a disconnect between a general intention to do one thing and the decision or action that, unintentionally, results in doing something different.

The concept of error can only really be understood in relation to an intention to achieve a particular result or outcome. A reflex action is a different thing altogether. Imagine that a surgeon receives a burn from a surgical cautery and, in the reflex action of withdrawing his hand, tears a blood vessel or causes some other damage to the patient. Reflexes of this type are subserved by neural paths at the spinal level – the hand would be withdrawn before the pain was felt, let alone before any central cognitive process could be employed, or any intention formulated, even subconsciously. It is worth noting that, in many countries at least, the law recognizes this type of "automatic" act as such, and typically treats such acts as blameless.

A criminal might have the intention of doing something that would be viewed as morally wrong (and this intention could go astray through the making of an error). By contrast, in the context of medication practice, the intention is generally to do the right thing. The informal version of our definition makes this point very clearly. For example, it is reasonable to presume that most anesthesiologists would embrace the intention to administer an antibiotic prophylactically to all patients in which this is indicated before the surgical incision. The underlying intention in doing this, one may presume, is to reduce the risk of postoperative infection. If, on a particular occasion, an anesthesiologist were simply to forget to administer the antibiotic at the right time, this failure would be unintentional.

The nature of the primary intention differentiates between an error and a violation. In a violation, a deliberate decision is taken by an individual to deviate from a practice widely accepted as optimal. This is not "doing the right thing," even if the individual hopes that no material harm will result, as is normally the case with violations. An explicit intention to cause harm is called "sabotage" by James Reason (6), but we believe this is very uncommon in the context of the perioperative management of medications (and indeed in healthcare more generally).

It can be difficult to distinguish between an error and a violation (Box 7.1). Even when it is clear that an action was deliberate and contravened optimal practice, and was, therefore, a violation and not an error, there may be gradations of reasonableness in the associated decision. At one extreme, there may be a flagrant and repeated lack of concern over the extra risk created for a patient. At the other extreme, there might be a well-articulated justification for the decision to break a rule or deviate from normal practice. To make matters more

complicated, it is also possible for errors to occur in the execution of an intended violation. We discuss violations in more detail in Chapter 8.

7.2.2 Element 2: A Decision or Act Should not Be Judged by Its Outcome

The second important element in our definition of error is that it is not predicated on outcome. Our definition, unlike many other definitions of error, makes no reference at all to outcome. This is because an error may have no outcome (at least in the sense of an outcome that a patient would relate to), or it may even have a positive outcome.

In the first example in Box 7.1, an anesthesiologist might forget to administer a prophylactic antibiotic to a patient (which would be an error). The patient may, nevertheless, experience no postoperative infection. Thus, this error would be of no consequence. This is true of many medication errors.

Box 7.1 Examples illustrating how the same action (e.g., failing to administer an indicated medication) may represent either an error or a violation; in evaluating a failure of this type, it is necessary to understand the mental model (or frame) from which the practitioner has been operating, but this may not always be easy to establish

In a case reported to the management of a hospital, an anesthesiologist failed to follow institutional policy and administer prophylactic antibiotics to a patient undergoing a total hip replacement. The following possibilities exist (among others):

1. He had intended to give the antibiotic but simply forgot, because he was distracted by some difficulty in managing the patient at the critical time. This action was uncharacteristic in that he was known by nursing staff and surgeons to be generally careful and conscientious in this particular aspect of his practice.
2. He had decided not to give the antibiotic on this one occasion, for one of two reasons:
   a. He thought the effort involved in doing so was excessive and did not believe it was worth the trouble – he knew that only about 1% of patients undergoing joint arthroplasty get infected anyway, he did not believe this patient had any particular risk factors, and he did not believe the antibiotic would make very much difference.
   b. This particular patient had a phobia of Stevens-Johnson syndrome and had expressed a preference for accepting the increased risk of infection to avoid the possibility that an antibi-

otic might precipitate this syndrome in her. He had discussed this with all concerned (including the surgeon) and formed the view that he should respect her wishes.
3. He often failed to give antibiotics to patients undergoing hip replacement because he was too lazy to ensure that he always did this, and he personally thought the risk of infection in these patients was more closely related to surgical and patient factors than to the use of prophylactic antibiotics.

Possibility 1 is an error. Possibilities 2a, 2b, and 3 are all violations, even though they differ considerably in their associated culpability. Example 2b actually occurred in one of the authors' institutions, although for a different operation. The difficulty here was balancing a strong belief by both the surgeon and the anesthesiologist that withholding antibiotics constituted a serious risk and that the chances of Stevens-Johnson syndrome occurring were remote, whereas the chance of infection was considerable. The decision to respect the patient's wishes could be viewed as sound (i.e., neither an error nor a violation) but is probably better characterized as a justifiable violation (see Chapter 8).

One can extend this idea further and contemplate the possibility of a "fortunate error" from which the outcome is, paradoxically, desirable. Thus, in our present example, it could happen that, unbeknownst to the anesthesiologist, the patient was allergic to the intended antibiotic. In this case, the error would avert the potential for serious harm in the form of anaphylaxis, albeit that this fact might not be apparent to anyone. Conversely, the successful administration of the antibiotic as intended might have precipitated a serious adverse medication event, despite perfectly correct practice. The outcome of a decision or action may be influenced by many factors beyond the control of the actor.

The central point is clear: Many errors, including many medication errors, are without material consequence, while some adverse medication events occur in the absence of error. Outcome does not distinguish the former from the latter. Decisions and actions should be judged on what should reasonably have been done on the basis of what could reasonably have been known about the situation at the time they were taken. This information would not include their outcome.

The concept of a "number needed to treat" (NNT) adds color to this discussion of the interpretation of the outcome of administering a medication. As an example, not every depressed patient who receives an antidepressant agent experiences a reduction in depressive symptoms. Thus, it might be necessary to treat several patients to achieve one positive outcome. Although our anesthetic agents are so reliable that a weight-based dose of propofol may confidently be expected to result in anesthesia (the NNT = 1), the effects of this dose on the patient's cardiac output, pulse rate, blood pressure, coronary circulation, and myocardium are more variable. These effects will be influenced by the patient's physiologic state at the time, and the factors at play may be both complex and dynamic. Furthermore, the continued occurrence of awareness under anesthesia in some patients (7) shows that even the primary outcome (anesthesia) may vary, notably in its duration. The results of treatment are seldom entirely binary, and the definition of the response to a medication needs to include consideration of its extent and duration as well as its nature.

If an adverse medication event, including a failure to respond to a medication (as with awareness), does occur, it would be reasonable to ask whether an error had been made. The answer to this question would hinge on several points. First, one might ask whether the anesthesiologist had successfully administered the intended dose. If not, one would likely be dealing with a slip or lapse, or possibly a technical error (see later). If so, one would likely be dealing with a mistake. A mistake might have occurred in calculating the dose or in choosing the dosing schedule. One would need to ask whether the intended dose or rate of infusion was in line with accepted guidelines, given the age, weight, height, and gender of the patient, and perhaps other information such as any previous history of medication and substance use. More generally, to determine whether a mistake had been made, the line of questioning should be as follows: Was the decision one that a reasonable anesthesiologist in the position of that particular anesthesiologist in that particular situation might have made? If not, and if the failure was unintentional, then that failure was a mistake, whatever the outcome. Importantly, the converse also applies: it would be quite possible for an adverse event to have occurred without any kind of error having been made.

7.2.3 Definitions of Medication Errors and Adverse Medication Events

Many writers have provided specific definitions of various types of medication error. It seems simpler to agree on a definition of error, such as the one given earlier, and then define a *medication error* as any error in any part of the medication process (per Table 6.1 and the definition in Chapter 1). *Medication administration* errors can then be thought of as a subset of medication errors, namely, those errors involving the administration of a medication. In a similar way, one can refer to errors in the *prescribing* and *recording* of medications and so forth.

An adverse medication event (AME) is defined in Chapter 1 as "a response to a medication that is undesired and causes harm," where we note that undesired or harmful effects of the failure to administer an indicated medication should be included in AMEs. In Chapter 1, we also note that AMEs may or may not be avoidable. AMEs associated with errors should be avoidable in theory. In practice, human error cannot be eliminated, but with redesign of the system it should be possible to reduce the frequency of AMEs associated with errors. Those associated with violations should certainly be avoidable, although even some of these may be best addressed through redesign of the system (we go into more detail on the different types of violations and the reasons for them in Chapter 8).

7.3 Decisions and Actions

In Chapter 6, we discussed the ways in which people access information from various external sources ("information in the world") and integrate this with information stored in their memory to form conceptualized mental models of particular situations. We turn now to the next steps – deciding what to do on the basis of this mental model and then doing it. We also consider some of the ways in which these steps can go wrong.

7.3.1 Fast and Slow Thinking

In his classic book, *Human Error* (6), drawing on work by Jens Rasmussen, James Reason presented a generic error modeling system (GEMS) in which he divided errors into subconscious failures of action (called "skill-based errors," also known as "slips" or "lapses") and failures in decisions ("mistakes"). He further divided mistakes into those that are "rule based" and those that are "knowledge based."

A fundamental assumption of the GEMS is that of reluctant rationality. In Reason's words, "human beings are furious pattern matchers." (6). And in Rouse's words, "humans, if given a choice, would prefer to act as context-specific pattern-recognizers rather than attempting to calculate or optimize" (8). In Chapter 6, we introduced the notion of mental models, and that of schemata that capture the key elements of any situation. Where possible, humans draw on their memory of situations they have seen previously (and stored as schemata) to find one that best matches their mental model of the current situation. This action is subconscious, and humans are typically unaware of how the chosen remembered schemata matches the current situation or the exact ways in which the two do not match. To decide what to do, they seek preferentially to apply rules learned from experience (or in other ways). Under ideal circumstances, this is done quickly, effortlessly, and almost unconsciously. A common cause of failure in this process lies in the application of a rule that is inappropriate or defective – hence the term "rule-based mistakes."

Sometimes a person meets difficulty in this matching of patterns or in finding an appropriate rule. Under these circumstances, it is necessary to think effortfully and logically, from first principles. This active cognitive process uses as its building blocks the knowledge base that has been assembled for the particular problem. A common cause of failure in such a decision is an incomplete or incorrect knowledge base (or mental model) – hence the term "knowledge-based mistakes."

In Chapter 6, we explained that all decisions are made on the basis of mental models of situations rather than on the hard reality of the situations themselves. Thus, an inaccurate or incomplete mental model (or knowledge base) is just as likely to result in the application of a wrong rule as it is to result in a failure in thinking from first principles. The key difference between rule-based and knowledge-based decisions actually lies in the cognitive processes by which they are made, and in the distinction between what Kahneman (9) (and others [10]) call "fast" and "slow" thinking. Stanovich and West used the terms "System I" and "System II" (11,12). System I thinking is fast, associative, unconscious, effortless, and rule based, while System II thinking is slow, deductive, conscious, effortful, and logical (Table 7.1). System II thinking is very powerful, underpins the scientific method, and is essential for making difficult

Table 7.1 The two systems that describe the ways in which we think, and their relationship to the terminology used by James Reason

System I: Fast and Automatic	System II: Slow and Reflective
Associative	Deductive
Unconscious	Conscious
Effortless	Effortful
Uses pattern recognition and rules	Uses logic and works from first principles
Feed-forward	Feed-back
Informed by the individual's mental model of the situation	Informed by the individual's mental model of the situation

Terminology used in Reason's Generic Error Modeling System		
Skill-based	Rule-based	Knowledge-based

Source: Synthesized from various sources: Reason 1990 (6), Kahneman 2011 (9), Thaler and Sunstein 2008 (10).

decisions about unusual situations. For example, it might well be needed in a preassessment clinic to decide on changes in a patient's medications preoperatively. However, in the dynamic context of managing the medications of an unstable patient during anesthesia (for example), the time required for System II thinking can be a major limitation.

In patients under anesthesia and often at other times in the perioperative period, many decisions and actions may be needed in quick succession about medications (and other things). These are not taken or executed in isolation but in the context of an evolving situation informed by what has gone before and what is expected in the near and more distant future. Further complexity arises from the teamwork inherent in hospital medicine – many decisions and actions involve interactions between individuals, so errors that appear to have been made by one individual may have several origins involving various people and various aspects of the systems and processes by which healthcare is delivered. It is sometimes helpful to think about an individual event in relation to a particular category of error (such as a slip or lapse or a rule-based error). However, it is often better to conceptualize the way practitioners think about and administer medications by reference to a continuum on which cognition shifts iteratively between being very fast, automatic, and subconscious at one extreme to being effortful and slow at the other than by trying to capture each decision and action into a circumscribed category. Thus, an anesthesiologist's brain must move dynamically from conscious thought to automatic actions and back again. All these actions (notably those involving medication administrations) must be monitored on the fly, even those that are automatic and unconscious. This involves *metacognition,* or thinking about thinking, during which practitioners must also maintain what is often called *situational awareness.* This dynamic process also involves communication with other members of the team.

7.3.2 Classifying Failures in the Management of Perioperative Medications

An understanding of the cognitive processes at play in the generation of an adverse medication event is critical for an understanding of the extent to which blame is justified and for distinguishing situations involving *behaviors* that could reasonably be expected to change from situations where prevention depends primarily on improving the *system.*

We return to these themes in later chapters. However, as outlined in Chapter 2, in larger studies involving many events, this type of classification is seldom used. In particular, it seems to be uncommon in such studies for any distinction to be made between errors and violations. A phenomenological approach is typically chosen over a cognition-based analysis (see Table 2.2). Toward the end of this chapter, we present a framework for categorizing medication errors that integrates the phenomenological categories of medication errors with the cognitive processes involved in their genesis.

Reports of medication errors may also include secondary analyses of *contributory* or *predisposing factors* (see Table 2.3). Identifying contributory factors can assist in understanding the mechanisms by which an error has occurred and for finding ways to make errors less likely. For example, distraction predisposes to skill-based errors (slips and lapses) and recommendations to reduce the risk of distraction during the drawing up and administration of medication are currently enjoying a vogue. Reason emphasizes the importance of *latent factors* in the system in the causation of accidents (13). He also argues that single failures seldom result in serious harm because they are usually captured by one or more of the multiple defenses present in any system. These ideas have been depicted in the image of slices of Swiss cheese, which represent layers of defense against accident trajectories (14). The holes in each slice represent the latent factors that threaten the integrity of these defenses. Harm occurs when a series of these holes line up and can, therefore, be traversed by an "accident trajectory." Unfortunately, in the operating room, for a given single anesthesiologist, many of the normal defenses for medication management are not present, and latent factors abound.

The intelligent use of multiple defenses is the key to improving safety in complex processes. Harm may be averted even after an accident by virtue of post-accident defenses. Thus, airbags may save a driver's life after a motor vehicle accident, and the presence of arterial line monitoring and the timely availability of a competent supervisor came to the rescue of the resident who inadvertently administered dopamine instead of magnesium.

The identification of contributory factors can certainly inform initiatives to improve medication safety. However, a considerable number of contributory or latent factors may be identified for any reported medication event. Furthermore, factors reported as contributory may or may not have been relevant to the particular event: An association between two things does not in itself mean that one has caused the other or even contributed to it. For example, many reports of medication errors suggest that the anesthesiologist was fatigued at the time an error was made. More sophisticated analysis is required to assess whether the fatigue contributed to the error or not (see the discussion of fatigue and of the Libby Zion case in Chapter 8).

In summary, errors range from simple skill-based slips and lapses in which an action, such as picking up a syringe and administering its contents to a patient, seems to go wrong without any conscious cognitive input to mistakes in laboriously considered decisions made collectively over time by teams of people. Although we have emphasized a continuum in the underlying cognitive processes that lead to errors, there are also important differences in errors at different parts of this continuum. We now explore these differences in greater depth, starting with mistakes.

7.4 Mistakes

Every action taken in the management of patients' medications during the perioperative period arises from a decision reflecting an immediate intention (e.g., to induce anesthesia) as a step toward an overall intention (e.g., to facilitate successful surgery for a patient in the safest, most pain-free manner possible). The achievement of even an immediately intended outcome may require several linked decisions that go beyond the choice of medications and doses to many secondary aspects of the processes by which these medications are to be administered and recorded and their effects monitored.

The processes of communication can also be considered as actions. Thus, decisions may also be needed about appropriate communication with relevant people (e.g., patients, their families, other members of staff). This applies to reviewing, rationalizing, and administering patients' medications preoperatively, to administering anesthesia

and to managing medications postoperatively in the postanesthetic care unit (PACU), in the intensive care unit (ICU), on the ward, and at time of discharge from hospital. Failures in communication are common and include failures to communicate with the patient. For example, as explained in Chapters 2 and 3, it is common for patients to leave hospital with inadequate information about the medications they are expected to continue taking.

Errors that occur during the perioperative management of patients' medications can be divided into mistakes in *prescribing* (i.e., choosing the most appropriate medications and dosages for the circumstances) and mistakes or other errors in translating prescriptions into effective and safe therapy (Table 7.2). One factor that differentiates anesthesia from most (but not all) other fields of healthcare is that anesthesiologists and anesthetists typically choose, draw up, and administer medications themselves, with no contribution to the process from any other health professional, such as a pharmacist or ward nurse, in the way that would occur in most other settings. Thus, their "prescriptions" are not usually written down before the medication is administered, and the safeguards that are often present in other settings (such as second person check, or electronic checking of dose and for medication interactions) are typically omitted in the setting of anesthesia.

7.4.1 System I Decisions and Mistakes

We have already noted that there may not be time to think through every decision about medications while managing a dynamically changing clinical situation, as is often the case under anesthesia. In fact, it is one of the characteristics of medicine in general that the pressure of clinical work is often too great for System II thinking. In practice, most decisions have to be made in a timely fashion, even in the context of the clinic or the ward. It is not practicable to refer to a textbook every time a medication needs to be prescribed, chosen, or given. Reasonable pharmacological expertise is expected of most physicians, and considerable expertise is expected of some, including anesthesiologists. In earlier chapters, we have seen just how complicated this pharmacology can be. Add to this the human inclination to prefer the quick and effortless System I thinking to the more laborious and effortful System II thinking (see Table 7.1), and it becomes apparent that

Table 7.2 Decisions and actions involved in the perioperative management of patients' medications. Errors occurring in decisions are mistakes. Those occurring in actions are often skill based but may also be technical, or may involve mistakes in deciding how actions are to be carried out

Decisions that need to be made	• How far one should pursue every possible piece of information about a patient and the medications to be used before prescribing a medication
	• The information that should be given to the patient about the proposed medication – including how much information, when it should be given, and in what manner
	• The choice of medication – considering the patient's wishes, including about whether any medication should be administered at all[a]
	• The dose, formulation, route, and frequency and timing of medication
	• Safeguards to ensure safe administration (e.g., labeling syringes, aseptic methods of drawing up medications, etc.)
	• How to monitor the effects of the medication
	• Potential interactions between medications
	• Patient factors that should be considered
Actions to be undertaken	• Communicating with the patient and other clinicians[b]
	• Writing the prescription (a step that is usually omitted during anesthesia)
	• Selecting the medication (from a stock of tablets, liquids, ampules, or other forms of medication); this may involve dispensing by a pharmacist
	• Preparing the medication for consumption or administration (e.g., taking a tablet out of its wrapping or drawing an intravenous medication into a syringe and labeling the syringe)
	• Administering the medication
	• Making an appropriate and accurate record
	• Monitoring the effect of the medication administered

[a] It is clearly not practical to ask an anesthetized patient about which muscle relaxant would be preferred; on the other hand, a patient may very well wish to be involved in many decisions about medications (especially postoperative opioids) and anesthesia more generally, and the point here is that the anesthesiologist needs to decide what to ask a patient.

[b] Communication is a complex and dynamic process that involves listening as well as talking and may be supported by written or illustrative materials.

many decisions about medications in the perioperative period will be rule based.

For example, a rule could be in the following form:

If a patient's blood pressure falls after induction of anesthesia, then administer 1 mg of metaraminol; or
If a patient is vomiting postoperatively, then prescribe 8 mg dexamethasone intravenously.

These rules would be associated with learned caveats. For example, the first rule might be subconsciously understood to be the first step in a sequence of possible responses. If the hypotension resolves, no further thought would be necessary. If the problem persists, System II thinking will probably be required, although there may well be subsequent rule-based steps that could be implemented first. Other automatic or semiautomatic steps might lie more in the System I part of our cognitive spectrum than in the System II part. In the example of managing nausea and vomiting, a particular anesthesiologist might administer ondansetron and metoclopramide as standard antiemetic agents during every anesthetic. Thus, if asked to see his own patient postoperatively, it would not be necessary for this anesthesiologist to work out what had already been given before prescribing dexamethasone. However, if he had been called to see a patient who had been anesthetized by someone else, the rule about dexamethasone would not be applicable. Instead, a review of the anesthetic record and System II thinking would be needed.

Rule-based decisions are *feed-forward* in nature (see Table 7.1). They are made in the expectation of a particular result, such as an increase in blood pressure or amelioration of nausea and vomiting, for example. This expectation arises from a combination of learned theoretical knowledge and past experience. If the expected effect is obtained, this success is stored in memory, somewhat automatically, in the manner characteristic of predominantly System I thinking, and the rule will be strengthened. If the expected effect is not obtained, then this feedback may call System II thinking into play to decide on further actions and may also serve to weaken the rule. Thus, although rule-based decisions are feed-forward, the result of the decision often does provide feedback, and this feedback leads to learning. Rules may also be supplemented or refined through reading and participation in other educational activities, such as lectures, discussions, and simulation training.

A substantial part of clinical expertise lies in being able to recognize a wide variety of situations and apply appropriate rules to each of these. As noted, it is the key features of each situation that matter, and an expert is able to separate these from relevant and background features to form a conceptual schema that can be compared with previously stored schemata. Rule-based mistakes arise from misinterpretation of a situation (a faulty mental model), from the application of a poor rule to a correctly interpreted situation, or some combination of both of these processes.

The process of pattern recognition and subsequent application of a rule is largely, if not entirely, subconscious. It is emotive in nature, and Boolean logic, which reduces key items of information to true or false in the mental model, is not involved. As discussed in Chapter 6, both conscious and unconscious prejudice and bias may influence the interpretation and framing of a situation and, therefore, the choice of a rule (9,15,16). Bias may have temporal and emotional origins: Past experiences with strong emotional associations may bring associated rules to mind more readily than neutral ones and recent experiences more readily than older ones. Some stored rules may be less robust than others.

7.4.2 System II Decisions and Mistakes

In explaining the difference between the cognitive processes underlying rule-based and knowledge-based errors, Reason refers to context-specific *symptom rules*, which can be retrieved and applied quickly and effortlessly, and to more abstract *topographical rules*, which reduce problems to their fundamental elements and are therefore more universal in nature but also more laborious to locate and use (6). He also explains that although mistakes can be made through a lack of understanding of the principles of logic or through simple errors in reasoning or calculation, the primary reason for failure in knowledge-based decisions is most commonly found in deficiencies or inaccuracies in the knowledge base (6). As we have just noted, the same reason can often explain rule-based errors. In the context of medication management, the key

features of System II thinking are that it is slow and effortful and tends to use induction or deduction rather than pattern recognition. A medical student asked to review a patient and write a short case history illustrating the use of a particular medication for a particular clinical problem will probably do this almost entirely on the basis of System II thinking. With time and experience, System I thinking develops, and an expert faced with the same problem might well be able to reach effortlessly into memory for the required pharmacological response without much active thought at all – but not always. Notably, it will often be necessary to look up the pharmacology of relevant medications. This is true even for experts, but an expert is at least likely to know where to find all the required facts and then how to balance the importance of different pieces of information acquired in this laborious way. An expert will also be able to draw upon personal experience to formulate a balanced and contextual interpretation of any complex situation. Errors can easily occur through a lack of familiarity with a particular clinical scenario or a particular medication. Even something relatively basic, such as a 10-fold error in the dose of a medication, is less likely in the hands of a clinician familiar with managing medications in general, especially if familiar with the medication in question. It is difficult to know what one does not know, so a novice may be uncertain about how far to go with seeking and checking information. A list of any medication's potential interactions, side effects, and contraindications can be long and arcane, and it may not be at all obvious which ones really matter and which ones are inconsequential or rare.

An expert anesthesiologist seldom resorts to the laborious cognitive process of System II thinking during the administration of an anesthetic. Instead, an anesthesiologist will typically use System II thinking to monitor and revise decisions made using System I thinking. However, System II thinking must be called upon when rules run out because a situation has not been seen before. For routine patient care on the ward, this may not create any particular difficulty. During an anesthetic, however, things may rapidly become very problematic. One definition of a crisis is that it is an emergency in which the standard rules have failed and there is inadequate time to solve the problem using System II thinking (17).

As discussed in Chapter 6, naturalistic decision-making is typical of an expert managing a crisis. This combines implicit and explicit pattern recognition while moving rapidly between System I and System II thinking and simultaneously maintaining situational awareness. *Satisficing* decisions (see Chapter 6) are sought rather than perfect ones (17,18). It may be easy to characterize the mistake of a novice but more difficult to identify the exact source of an error made by an expert fully engaged in managing a dynamic and complex situation.

System II thinking is described as being feedback in nature. A decision is made and implemented, and then feedback is obtained from its effects and used to reassess evolving situations and guide further decisions. Administering successive intravenous boluses of a vasoactive agent to a patient with arterial monitoring in place illustrates this notion: Each successive dose is informed by the response to those previously given. In a sense, it is necessary to make progress through "trial and error." This point shows, once again, how blurred the boundaries can be between good decisions and decisions that are characterized as faulty. In the context of entrepreneurial business activities, it is sometimes said that there is virtue in "failing early." The implication is that it is essential to take risk if progress (and a large fortune) is to be made and that the only way to tell whether some decisions are sound or not is to test them, and thus recognize quickly when to limit losses and move on. As illustrated by the first of the two cases involving dopamine outlined at the beginning of this chapter, rapid feedback (in this case in the form of an unexpected massive increase in blood pressure) can often allow the consequences of an error to be mitigated. However, as illustrated by the second of these two cases, it may not always be possible to recover from a medication error. In effect, there are tight boundaries to the effective use of feedback in making decisions about medications. Even when System II thinking is used to select a medication, the decision will usually incorporate many learned rules about the pharmacology of the medication in question.

It may be thought that, whatever other limitations it might have, System II thinking would at least tend to be highly objective, strictly rational, and Boolean in nature. The reality turns out to be quite different. We have already noted that humans are simply not natural Boolean thinkers and that rule-based decisions are subject to numerous unconscious influences. System II decisions are similarly affected by conscious and unconscious biases and prejudices. Both Kahneman (9) and Stiegler (16) give many examples of such biases, some of which have been touched on in Chapter 6.

7.4.3 Mistakes More Generally

Mistakes arise either from a deficiency in the mental model on which a decision is based or from a failure in the formulation of a plan on the basis of a correct mental model, or sometimes from a mixture of the two. The process by which a plan is formulated may involve System I or System II thinking, or (most commonly) a combination of both, and can be undermined in a wide variety of ways (Table 7.3).

Table 7.3 Some of the possible causes of a mistake during the management of a patient's medications

Deficiencies in the mental model about a patient's situation and needs because of	• Deficiencies in the practitioner's own knowledge (e.g., of pharmacology) • Failure to read the patient's medical record • Deficiencies in the patient's medical record • Deficiencies in communication with the patient, the patient's family, or other members of staff • Faulty information in textbooks, journal articles, or online sources or in what one has been taught • Deficiencies in patient monitoring
Deficiencies in formulating a plan for a patient's medication from the available information because of	• Inadequate experience or training, resulting in too few or poorly formulated schemata to use in System I thinking • Poor application of logic (including Boolean logic) in System II thinking • The influence of subconscious biases (e.g., arising from recent experiences, exposure to marketing material, or deeply held prejudice) • Simple technical mistakes (e.g., in arithmetic) • Personality traits of the anesthesiologist (hubris, overconfidence, unwillingness to communicate or engage in teamwork)

7.4.4 Judgment and Uncertainty in Decisions

We have seen in Chapters 2 and 3 that considerable uncertainty pervades the science and art of managing patients' medications in the perioperative period. In managing patients, one is not just solving simple arithmetic exercises to which *the* correct answer can be found at the back of the textbook that contains illustrative exercises. On the contrary, each patient is unique; is undergoing the considerable physiologic challenges associated with pathology, surgery, and anesthesia; and is endowed with personal belief systems, wishes, and circumstances that may be very different from those of the patient in the next bed. There are also differences between anesthesiologists. Ideally, every anesthesiologist would have the same combination of perfect knowledge and skills, but this, of course, is simply not the case. Good clinicians will take into account their own strengths and limitations in managing patients, factoring in the support and advice of colleagues to the extent that they are available. A good decision for a particular patient at a particular place and time may not be the same as a good decision for another patient with essentially similar problems but in a different place and time, and therefore a different context. Furthermore, there may be more than one good (or acceptable) decision in any particular situation. We have also explained (in Chapter 6 and earlier in the present chapter) that decisions often need to be satisficing rather than perfect. It follows that *judgment* is often required when making decisions about patients' medications. If these decisions turn out well, it may be said that "good judgment" has been shown. If they turn out badly, it is often said that an "error of judgment" has been made. These terms capture the sense of uncertainty inherent in complex, evolving clinical situations.

Of course, some decisions are uncontroversial. For example, little judgment is involved in the understanding by an anesthesiologist that a response is necessary to a rapidly falling arterial oxygen saturation. The concept of judgment can only reasonably be applied to decisions made when "right" is not sharply demarked from "wrong." It turns out that there are many situations in which some difference of opinion exists, even among highly proficient experts. Unfortunately, uncertainty does not prevent individual practitioners from holding strong opinions. Rather, it may simply mean that the strong opinions held by one group of practitioners differ from those held by another (Box 7.2). There is a reasonable likelihood that if a practitioner deviates from the norms accepted in his or her department, and a patient suffers some form of adverse event that could possibly be attributed to that particular practice, criticism will follow. This may well be in the form of suggesting that the practitioner has shown "poor judgment."

One reasonable approach to managing uncertainty of this type is to establish formal policies. This may be done at international, national, or departmental levels. If an agreed or mandated policy is in place, then failure to follow this would usually constitute a violation (see Chapter 8). However, such policies are often absent, and even when present, they may change over time (e.g., policies for managing unexpected difficult airways have changed over the last few decades and may well continue to do so; Box 7.3). There may also be conflicts between policies on the same issue at the same time. Indeed, the language used in many policies is deliberately chosen to leave room for variation in practice. This may be partly because policymakers wish to avoid creating unreasonable levels of medicolegal liability for practitioners and partly in recognition that the level of evidence supporting many aspects of clinical practice, even those that are well established, is often no higher than that of expert consensus (Box 7.4).

Thus, it can be quite difficult to know whether or not a particular decision constitutes a mistake. This difficulty was illustrated in a study using highly realistic simulated scenarios in which anesthesiologists were observed (25). The investigators included one of the authors of this book (AM). They reported a mean (standard deviation [SD]) of 9.7 (3.4) errors per scenario. This result must obviously have depended on what was considered to be an error. During the design of the study, there was considerable discussion over whether failure to conform to an established guideline would constitute an error, and for the reasons outlined earlier, it was decided that such a failure would not, on its own, be sufficient. A five-stage process was finally used in the identification of these errors, the first two of which are relevant to the present discussion. The first step was to establish an agreed account of

Box 7.2 The way we do things here, and a matter of judgment

When one of the authors of this book (AM) was a resident, he returned to Auckland after a year spent in Edinburgh. Soon after this, he was reprimanded by a senior colleague for allowing a patient undergoing hand surgery to breathe spontaneously under general anesthesia. When he asked for a reason why he should ventilate this particular patient, he was told: "That is the way we do things here." At that time, many seniors in the department in Edinburgh strongly advocated spontaneous ventilation when practicable, believing among other reasons that there was a safety advantage in avoiding the use of neuromuscular blocking agents if possible. Members of this department had undertaken several studies that provided support for their practice. Spontaneous ventilation, when possible, was "The way we do things here" in Edinburgh at that time, but this clearly was not the way things were done in Auckland.

This particular story preceded the adoption of capnography into routine anesthetic practice, although the Edinburgh research had included arterial blood gas measurements in the evaluation of spontaneous ventilation in adults. The advent of routine capnography has subsequently made it obvious that many patients who are allowed to breathe spontaneously (typically through a laryngeal mask in modern practice) have elevated end-tidal carbon dioxide levels. The question arises of how high a level of carbon dioxide can or should be tolerated. It turns out that the answer to this question is somewhat elusive. In a recent publication using prolonged apnea facilitated by high-flow, humidified nasal oxygenation, levels of $PaCO_2$ up to 15 kPa were reported, without adverse consequences (19). Various case reports have been published in which patients experienced levels above 10 kPa without harm. Furthermore, permissive hypercapnia is now seen as acceptable in certain ventilated patients in intensive care. However, the assessment of safety does not hinge on small numbers of case reports, and the level of $PaCO_2$ that is safe in one patient under one set of circumstances may not be safe in another. Again, it would seem that the decision to use spontaneous ventilation and tolerate or not tolerate any particular level of end-tidal carbon dioxide in any individual patient could be construed as a matter of judgment for the anesthesiologist concerned. Unfortunately, if something were to go wrong, a $PaCO_2$ higher than that thought acceptable by other members of a department of anesthesiology might well invoke criticism.

It can be seen that there is a strong normative element in clinical practice, and practitioners stray from "the norm" somewhat at their peril, whether their decisions are well founded or not.

Box 7.3 Guidelines for managing an unexpected difficult airway

The optimal management of a difficult airway after the administration of agents to induce anesthesia, with or without the addition of neuromuscular blocking agents, is relevant to the safe management of patients' perioperative medications.

In 2015, the Difficult Airway Society (DAS) released revised guidelines (20), informed in part by evidence from the Fourth National Audit Project of the Royal College of Anaesthetists and the Difficult Airway Society study in the United Kingdom (21). These guidelines state in their abstract that if a decision is made to proceed to a surgical airway, "Scalpel cricothyroidotomy is recommended as the preferred rescue technique and should be practised by all anaesthetists." This clear (and we would say sensible) position is a substantial change in emphasis from previous guidelines that gave equal prominence to the place of cannula cricothyroidotomy (22).

However, in the body of the text, the following somewhat contradictory sentences can be found: "A simple plan to rescue the airway using familiar equipment and rehearsed techniques is likely to increase the chance of a successful outcome. Current evidence indicates that a surgical technique best meets these criteria." And then: "A cricothyroidotomy may be performed using either a scalpel or a cannula technique." The last sentence is followed by a substantial discussion of cannula-based techniques. To add to uncertainty for anesthesiologists wanting to know how best to manage a "can't intubate, can't oxygenate" crisis, the American Society of Anesthesiologists Task Force on Management of the Difficult Airway has this to say on the topic: "Invasive airway access includes surgical or percutaneous airway, jet ventilation, and retrograde intubation" (23).

One could be forgiven for concluding that the optimal approach to the management of a "can't intubate, can't ventilate" crisis is still an open question in the minds of many experienced anesthesiologists and even societies (although the authors of this book believe that the data provide reasonably strong support for standardizing on surgical cricothyrotomy).

Box 7.4 The role of epinephrine in cardiac arrest

Epinephrine has long been advocated in many authoritative guidelines for the management of cardiac arrest. Surprisingly, the evidence for its use in this context was so limited that until recently one could have argued that equipoise existed. In response to this uncertainty, the International Liaison Committee on Resuscitation called for a placebo-controlled trial. The PARAMEDIC2 trial has now demonstrated better survival in out of hospital cardiac arrest with epinephrine, but no difference in the rate of favorable neurological outcome (24).

---

the facts. This is standard practice in root-cause analysis – it is important to agree on what actually happened (26). The second step involved asking each participant, during debriefing, whether or not he or she agreed that the facts in question amounted to an error. There were instances in which the researchers believed that a guideline had not been followed or a medication error had been made, but the participant said that he or she had acted intentionally and provided a plausible reason for this. These events were not counted as errors. In effect, allowance was made for the participant to exercise judgment.

As already pointed out, people are often credited with good judgment when things turn out well and criticized for poor judgment, or an error of judgment, if the outcome is bad. Earlier in this chapter, we stressed that the soundness or otherwise of a decision should not be judged on its outcome. This point is particularly relevant to judgments based on an assessment of risk when outcome is uncertain. An example can be found in gambling. If one accepts that it is reasonable to bet on games of chance, then it would be sound to take a bet for which the odds are favorable. For example, one might accept the chance of losing $1 if the throw of a die returns a six or winning $1 if any other number is returned. These odds favor the person placing the bet because five out of every six of a large number of throws can be won. Thus, this decision would be statistically justifiable whatever the actual outcome of a particular throw, but this might be hard to recall if a six is actually thrown and one has been allowed only a single throw of the die.

In the end, the determination that an "error of judgment" has been made is often normative. It hinges on the view that an individual has made a decision that differs from the one that the person evaluating the situation would have made. In fact, this might sometimes amount to little more than a difference in opinion, influenced by outcome bias (27). Greater weight could be placed on the opinion of a group of practitioners, rather than on that of just one individual; the corollary of this is that a decision made by two or more people in consultation would be more difficult to criticize than one made by a single individual, even though the facts, the logic, and the outcome may be identical. One of the principles of safe medication practice is to consult when in doubt.

7.4.5 More on Mental Models

Consider an anesthesiologist called to the ward to assess a patient postoperatively. In Table 7.4, we listed some of the factors that might contribute to the anesthesiologist's mental model of the situation. The list is illustrative – no attempt has been made to make it comprehensive. We simply sought to illustrate the wide range of factors that might influence the decision that needs to be made.

Some of the items listed may seem surprising, such as the social factors. In fact, even if a conscientious doctor intends to set aside all personal considerations and concentrate on doing the right thing for a particular patient, factors such as being late for a dinner engagement can subconsciously add stress to an already difficult situation and increase the doctor's blood pressure, pulse rate, and sense of anxiety. This is the real world in which clinical decisions are made. Furthermore, it is the various elements that make up the individual practitioner's personal mental model of the wider situation that inform the decision, whether or not these perceptions are correct, reasonable, or edifying.

In Chapter 6, we discussed sources of information. It is often difficult to access the key facts about a patient. Furthermore, one practitioner's personal knowledge of pharmacology may be very different from another's. This itself may influence the number of medications actually available for use by a particular practitioner – people understandably tend to confine their choice of medications to those with which they are familiar.

Table 7.4 Some of the perceived factors that might contribute to the mental model of an anesthesiologist asked to see a postoperative patient (a 35-year-old woman who had a laparoscopic appendectomy)

The problems to be treated	• High blood pressure • Nausea and vomiting • Pain
Sources of relevant information	• The patient's medical record (and how long it will take to find it) • The likelihood that the nurse or junior doctor will know anything
The range of possible therapeutic options	• Inactivity – no treatment at all • Nonpharmacological therapy (heat, reassurance, massage, acupuncture) • Further diagnostic testing • Medication
Facts about medications	• Range of available medications • The pharmacology of these medications
Facts about the patient	• Her statement of her perceived pain and other symptoms • Medication history, including history of allergies • Comorbidities • Physiologic status (vital signs, laboratory results, etc.) • Belief system (faith, culture, language, view of medications, etc.) • Financial status (insured, not able to pay, etc.) • Her ethnicity • The presence or absence of tattoos • Body habitus (normal versus obese body mass index)
Facts about the setting	• Availability and collegiality (or otherwise) of the surgeon • Availability and quality of nursing staff and junior doctors • Availability and willingness to help of colleagues • Available technology (access to the Internet for information, access to monitors, etc.)
Subconscious biases	• Race based • Gender based • Appearance based • About the surgery (e.g., a belief that laparoscopic surgery is not painful) • The recent presentation from a pharmaceutical company about a new antiemetic
Social factors	• Time of day (7:30 p.m. – it has been a long day) • Expectations of family and friends (spouse's anniversary, already late for dinner at restaurant)
Distracting factors	• The other patients in the ward (delirious and noisy, quiet and critical looking) • The presence of a raging headache • The belief that the surgeon should really be dealing with this problem • A deep and growing sense that life is not fair

A similar exercise could be undertaken for a decision on what to do about a low blood pressure during an anesthetic. On the face of things, this may seem to be a simple System I problem involving recognition of a pattern and applying a rule of the type outlined earlier in this chapter: in effect, if blood pressure is low, then give a bolus of intravenous metaraminol (for example). Imagine, though, a free flap case with a difficult surgeon who wants to know exactly what "anesthesiology" is doing and does not like vasopressors to be given to his patients. Modify the picture a little and consider a situation in which the anesthesiologist is a resident who has been warned about this surgeon but is also nervous about his own attending who will expect the hypotension to be treated. All of these distracting factors may prevent the anesthesiology resident from asking the obvious question: But why is this blood pressure low?

So perhaps the situation is not as simple as it initially seems. Clearly, the starting point would be to improve the *knowledge base* on which the decision is to be made. This will involve observation (looking at the drains, looking at what the surgeon is doing to the heart), review of the case so far, analysis of the vital signs, and communication (e.g., asking the surgeon whether this patient could be bleeding). Simply giving metaraminol would have been a rule-based response to low blood pressure; it may, however, also be viewed as "misapplying a good rule in the wrong situation" by the surgeon, whose rule is "never give vasopressors in the setting of a free flap." After clarifying the facts, it may still be the appropriate response. The cognitive work required to this point is work directed at clarifying the situation and making sure the mental model is adequate and accurate. After this has been done, it may still be that all that is needed is a dose of metaraminol. This decision may still be made using System I thinking – using a rule-based response to solve a familiar problem. On the other hand, if the evolving problem requires a more individualized response, perhaps involving a combination of medications, fluid, and further evaluation, then System II thinking directed at the solution may now be required. For most experienced anesthesiologists, the key to a good decision will lie in clarifying the mental model. Once the situation is clear, it will usually be relatively straightforward to decide what to do.

7.4.5.1 Shared Mental Models

Anesthesiologists seldom work in isolation: They are part of a team that includes surgeons, residents, interns, nurses, other ward staff, and the patients themselves. The responsibility for decision-making typically shifts dynamically during the perioperative period and in the operating room. Even if the responsibility for a particular decision lies firmly with the anesthesiologist (e.g., on whether to give a vasopressor or administer fluid or start an inotropic infusion), it may well have relevance for other members of the team. The converse also applies. It should not be necessary to ask a surgeon whether bleeding is becoming excessive: information of this sort should be shared. In fact, many decisions in healthcare generally and during the perioperative period more particularly are best taken collaboratively. The direction of progress needs to be consistent, with everyone working toward the same goal. This requires a shared understanding of the situation or at least of the key elements of the situation. It also requires some consensus over what to do about the situation.

The degree to which information is shared varies considerably. It is likely that all three people whose mental models of a surgical situation are represented in Figure 7.1 would have the same view of where they were, who the patient was, and what

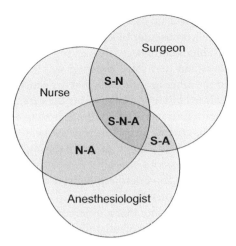

Figure 7.1 Venn diagram depicting the mental models of an anesthesiologist, a surgeon, and a nurse for an operation in progress. Only a relatively small subset of information is shared by all three – that depicted by the space S-N-A. Some information is shared by just the nurse and the anesthesiologist (N-A), some by the surgeon and the anesthesiologist (S-A), and some by the surgeon and the nurse (S-N). Errors may arise because individuals have different understandings of certain important facts or because key aspects of the situation known to one member of the team are not shared with the others.

the procedure was in general. It is unlikely that the nurse or surgeon would know all the medications used by the anesthesiologist or that the anesthesiologist would know that the nurse was concerned about a swab that he could not find but had not yet announced this fact. It may be thought that practical information directly relevant to the technicalities of the patient's care is what really needs to be shared, but other types of information may also be relevant to the effective functioning of the team. For example, if the surgeon were hard of hearing, it might be helpful for both the nurse and the anesthesiologist to know this.

Not all information needs to be shared. In Chapter 6, we discussed the problem of information overload. It is easy to see that the need to filter information may apply to the facts that need to be shared as well as to all the sensory input that each member of the team, as an individual, has to filter and analyze. In fact, in the context of healthcare, much information can often be assumed. Trained and experienced professionals can be expected to know the basic facts about their colleagues' tasks, and the detail often does not matter. For example, there is no reason why an anesthesiologist should know which particular suture a surgeon has chosen to use or why a surgeon should know which particular neuromuscular blocking agent an anesthesiologist has administered. It is enough for the one to understand that some suturing will take place and for the other to appreciate that the patient may be paralyzed but not need to know the details. On the other hand, there are circumstances in which the detail is critical. Some surgeons use nerve stimulators to identify the facial nerve during operations on the mastoid bone, but this practice is not universal. Thus, an anesthesiologist used to working with a surgeon who did not use this monitoring might not appreciate that a different surgeon was relying upon it. The potential for this second surgeon to be completely misled by a lack of twitching from a stimulated (but paralyzed) nerve would be substantial if the two parties failed to understand which details each team member needs or does not need to know.

As another example, known to one of the authors, code blue or rapid response intubating teams had changed from predominantly using succinylcholine to using the longer-acting rocuronium. The responsible team, not aware of this change, based the sedation on whether or not the patient was moving, which led to the patient being paralyzed but awake. Failures in the sharing of mental models may manifest as simple absences of key information, but they can also manifest as incorrect perceptions, so that two individual's beliefs on an overlapping point (e.g., lying in segment S-A in Figure 7.1) may be different, in which case at least one of these must be wrong. Interestingly, this particular type of error would have some of the appearances of a lapse – in our example involving nerve stimulation, it would be quite possible that both clinicians simply forgot to check with each other about their expectations. On the other hand, this might reflect an inadequate appreciation of the importance of communication in healthcare. Many errors, including many medication errors, originate from failures in the accuracy and concordance of mental models, and the key to effective countermeasures lies in effective communication. This may often mean repeating what everyone thinks everyone else already knows just to be sure that they actually do.

Advice is often given about the risks of assumption (the trivial joke is that "assume makes an ass out of u and me"). In the context of patient man-

agement, it is usually better to share too much information than too little. With this in mind, a key objective in the development of the World Health Organization's Surgical Safety Checklist was to promote the exchange of critical information and encourage an environment in which people feel able to speak up (28). Introductions done in an encouraging way serve to activate people to speak up when concerned, often by asking a question. This, in turn, serves to test, align, and correct mental models (Box 7.5). The Checklist also includes some checks that are both typical of checklists in general and relevant to medication safety – notably checking (or rechecking) the patient's allergies during "Sign In" and a reminder during "Time Out" to avoid forgetting prophylactic antibiotics when indicated.

Box 7.5 A medication error, a false mental model, and the value of communication

Some years ago, an anesthesiologist known to the authors induced a patient for mitral valve surgery, administering (among other medications) the contents of what he thought were three ampules containing 4 mg each of pancuronium. The case progressed rapidly, and just after the sternotomy had been made, the surgeon said, "The patient is moving." The anesthesiologist responded that this was impossible. The surgeon said something to the effect that it might be impossible, but that it seemed likely, nevertheless, that the patient would shortly leave the room.

It was this particular anesthesiologist's practice to retain used ampules. He inspected these and discovered that the medication administered was actually suxamethonium, which is short acting. The small plastic ampules containing suxamethonium were similar in appearance to those used for pancuronium. Someone, when stocking the medication trolley, had placed suxamethonium in the section designated for pancuronium. The problem was easily solved, and no harm occurred to the patient. The anesthesiologist's belief that the patient had received a large dose of a long-acting neuromuscular blocking agent had been quite profound, and it was only clear communication from the surgeon, reinforced by accessing information physically available "in the world," that enabled him to identify that his belief was wrong.

7.5 Skill-Based Errors

Some of the medication errors that have gained the most prominence in recent years have probably been skill-based errors (i.e., slips or lapses). The two cases of inadvertent administration of dopamine instead of doxapram (in one case) (29) and magnesium (in the other) described in Chapter 6 were presumably of this type. Skill-based errors involve failures in the execution of a sound decision or plan (4). They are characteristic of experts, in that they typically occur during the conduct of task sequences that have become familiar to the person concerned, such that they are conducted almost, or entirely, automatically. The intravenous administration of routinely used medications is a prime example of such a task sequence. Most anesthesiologists administer several hundred thousand intravenous boluses over a working lifetime. At the outset of their career, considerable attention to detail is required to select the right medication, choose the correct sized syringe, aspirate the particular medication from an ampule or vial into the syringe, label the syringe, place the syringe in a suitable tray, retain it there among several other syringes until needed, and then finally identify it again and inject its contents into the intravenous line of a patient. Over time this process becomes increasingly routine and requires less and less mental effort. The scene has been set. Something distracts the anesthesiologist at a critical point, or *decision node*, in this sequence of tasks, and a slip occurs. The slip might involve selecting the wrong vial or ampule, or the wrong syringe. A medication administration error follows, sometimes with disastrous results. Alternatively, again because of distraction ("attentional capture") at the critical moment, a lapse occurs, and a medication is forgotten. Failure to administer an indicated prophylactic antibiotic or a subsequent redose of an antibiotic are classic examples of a lapse.

To the lay public, slips and lapses often have the appearance of carelessness. In fact, they are not usually associated with a lack of care or of caring. There have been a series of reports involving parents who have forgotten their babies, typically strapped into baby seats in the back of their family vehicles, only to find, sometime later, that the child has succumbed to the effects of excessive heat (4). The idea that a parent would not care about her baby is, in general, inconceivable, yet a sufficient number of these lapses have occurred for them to

have been given the name "the forgotten baby syndrome" (although, technically, this phenomenon is not a syndrome) (30).

Many prosaic examples of slips and lapses can be found in everyday life. A common one is for a person who has decided to give up sugar after many years of using it to find that he or she has inadvertently added sugar to a cup of tea.

The primary difference between a slip or lapse and a rule-based error lies in the extent to which the former errors are completely unconscious. It is usually said that they are simply action failures, rather than failures in a plan or decision. On the other hand, they are not reflex actions. They originate from the subconscious mind. Thus, they could be seen as reflecting a temporary return to a formerly correct plan that is now wrong. Framing them in this way supports the idea that slips and lapses occupy an extreme end of the spectrum of decision-making from fast to slow, described earlier in this chapter.

Typically, slips and lapses are only discovered after the event by virtue of some consequence, such as the unexpectedly sweet taste of the tea or a dramatic hemodynamic response to an unintended medication (the unintended dopamine in the two examples in Chapter 6). In fact, it is very likely that many medication administration errors are never identified, particularly those that involve the omission of medications whose missing effects would not be obvious at that time. Omitting a prophylactic antibiotic is an example of this kind of lapse. Slips that involve syringe or vial swaps are made more likely by factors such as the similarity of labels on ampules and the colocation or mislocation of ampules that look alike but have different contents. In a series of cases, tranexamic acid has been administered intrathecally with disastrous results, due in large part to the similarity of the ampules involved (31) (Figure 7.2 [32]). As explained in Chapter 6, people tend to see what they expect to see. In the example described in Box 7.5, the plan to administer pancuronium was sound, but its execution failed for precisely these reasons.

7.6 Technical Errors

Technical errors are a category of medication event that is not captured by the Reason–Rasmussen GEMS (6), or by most phenomenological classifications. They reflect the balance between the skill of any individual and the difficulty of any particular task (33).

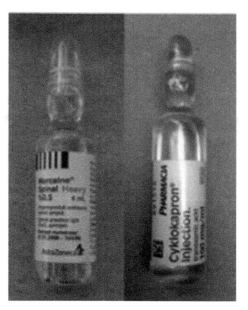

Figure 7.2 Ampules of tranexamic acid (TXA) and bupivacaine. Reprinted with permission from Hatch et al. 2016 (32).

Many procedures in medicine have an inherent failure rate. For example, undertaking an epidural is associated with a certain rate of dural puncture. The rate is increased in patients who are more difficult than normal "technically," for various anatomical reasons. It is also increased when epidurals are inserted by clinicians who are less skilled than their peers. In a technical error, the decision is appropriate, no slip or lapse occurs, there is no suggestion of a violation or of sabotage, but there is an unintended failure to carry out an intended action successfully.

Other examples of technical errors are easy to identify. Epidural catheters may run anteriorly to the spinal cord or even emerge from the epidural space having passed through it. This misplacement of the catheter will result in a failed block. It may be thought that this reflects the influence of chance, but an alternative view is that the problem lies in underspecification of the task. In this example, the specification could be improved by the use of image intensification,[2] which is routine in the epidural placement of spinal cord stimulators where it greatly increases the reliability with which electrical leads can be accurately sited in the epidural space. We are not arguing that image intensification and radiopaque catheters *should* be used rou-

tinely for the placement of epidural catheters, only that they *could* be. We accept that these failures are attributable to chance to the extent that anatomy varies, and chance determines whether a particular patient has difficult or easy anatomy. However, the effect of this type of variation could be mitigated through improvements in techniques and technology, in a way that would not be possible for true chance, such as that associated with the throw of dice. Similar comments can be made about the insertion of central venous lines. Variations in anatomy can be managed more reliably using ultrasound imaging than by relying only on anatomical landmarks. There is a balance between the skill of the operator (supported or enhanced by technology) and the difficulty of the procedure. When the challenge presented by a particular patient exceeds the capability of a particular operator on a particular day with the technology available at the time, a technical error occurs.

Technical errors can be understood intuitively in examples from sport, such as cricket in which success depends on the balance of the varying skill manifest at any moment by the bowler, the batsman, and the fielders, modified by the condition of the pitch at the time. For example, a dropped catch that was within reach of a fielder should be considered a technical error. Some possible catches are harder than others, some people are better at catching balls than others, and even good fielders have bad days.

7.7 Humans, System Complexity, and the Predictability of Error

It can be seen from the discussion in this and the previous chapter that the way in which humans make decisions and act on them is complex. It can also be seen that the opportunities for failure in medication management during anesthesia and the perioperative period are legion.

It should also be apparent by now that certain conditions or factors will predispose to certain types of error (see Table 2.3). Thus, particular types of error can be predicted under particular circumstances. For example, a syringe swap (a slip) is more likely in the presence of look-alike, sound-alike medications (see Figure 7.2). The distractions involved in administering an anesthetic make forgetting to give a prophylactic antibiotic at the right moment very likely unless specific reminders are

---

[2] Radiopaque catheters would also be needed.

built into the process. Mistakes will occur if there are deficiencies in the knowledge base on which a decision is made. In the context of anesthesia, such deficiencies are much more likely in the absence of a thorough preoperative assessment carried out at a time and in a place that facilitates acquisition of all necessary information. Similarly, the absence of medication reconciliation at transitions of care can be expected to result in deficiencies in information critical to medication safety. Failures in communication will almost certainly occur if individuals who have had no shared training in communication and have never worked together before are brought together at the last minute to undertake a difficult task (as happens in some operating rooms and many resuscitations on the ward). A similar likelihood of poor communication may apply even to anesthesia residents and attendings working together in the absence of explicit relevant effort and training. For example, if one gives a medication without recording the details in the anesthesia record or the other fails to look at the record before administering the same medication, a repetition error will occur, particularly if the two also fail to tell each other what has been done.

It follows that much can be done to reduce the rate of error in the management of medications during anesthesia and the perioperative period. A multifaceted system based on addressing at least some of the obvious latent factors in the system by which medications are administered during anesthesia has been shown in a large, observational randomized controlled trial (RCT) to be modestly effective in this regard (3). However, the case in which dopamine was administered instead of magnesium illustrates the potential for failure even when a system of this type is in place. In part, this illustrates the requirement for practitioners to engage in safety initiatives and to use support systems when they are provided. Furthermore, solutions of this type are predicated on linear approaches to improving safety, and these may not be well suited to the complexities of medication management. The use of linear solutions in this way is not entirely unreasonable. In Chapter 6, we pointed out that some aspects of the system by which medications are manufactured and then used in clinical medicine are linear, and it is well worth making these parts of the system safer. However, it is naive to lose sight of the fact that the system overall is complex.

In particular, humans are complex, and the engagement of humans in safety initiatives is therefore likely to be variable. It is not enough to simply install a barcode system and expect that it will be used. This was shown in the results of the RCT that demonstrated modest efficacy of the system in reducing medication error. There was an inverse relationship between compliance with the system principles and the rate of error in the administration and recording of medication administration errors. However, many participants did not comply with these principles (3). Other authors have found the same human inclination to not use barcode scanning even when available (34). Still more examples can be found to support the point that considerable effort informed by implementation science is key to the success of any large-scale initiative to improve patient safety (35).

Auckland City Hospital (ACH), the institution in which the RCT of the multifaceted barcode system was carried out, has an excellent track record in supporting and engaging with safety initiatives, including (among many others) the Surgical Safety Checklist (36–38). In fact the willingness to invest in the system in question and to support its investigation alongside many other studies into medication safety, and the fact that many anesthesiologists did comply with the system's principles during the study, all provide evidence of that commitment. Furthermore, there is every reason to believe that the work put into improving medication safety at ACH has made a worthwhile difference (3,39), and the same can be said for somewhat similar initiatives in other institutions, notably the University of Washington (40). This is a story of a glass half-full, but it shows that the effort required to substantially eliminate medication error is considerable. This effort also needs to be sustained and based on sound principles of implementation science (35).

7.8 A New Framework for Classifying Medication Errors

When one considers the advantages and disadvantages of the different approaches traditionally used for the classification of failures in medication management, it seems that each has merit and that some form of matrix is called for to combine them. The framework in Table 7.5 is intended to

Table 7.5 A framework for the classification of human failures in medication management incorporating the intent, mental model, and reasoning involved with the phenomenological categories of each event. Sabotage, which is rare in healthcare, has not been included. Violations are not errors and are further categorized in Table 8.2). Contributing factors should also be listed separately (see Table 2.3). Examples: A – a slip (inadvertently omitting to give a medication); B – a failure to give atropine before repeating suxamethonium because of lack of knowledge (a rule-based error); C – incorrectly repeating the administration of a medication because of failure to communicate between an attending and a resident; D – a substitution caused by misreading the label on an ampule; E – wrong dose because of an error in calculating the concentration of a medication diluted with saline (a knowledge-based error due to failure in arithmetical reasoning); F – a wrong dose because of an error in the recorded weight of a patient used in calculating the concentration of a medication diluted with saline (a knowledge-based error due to failure in the "knowledge base"); G – an inadvertent puncture of the dura during epidural placement (a technical error); H – a deliberate failure to label a syringe (a violation); I – a wrong-sided arm block because of the mistaken belief that the patient was in fact another patient on the same list. "?" = not known (no example given, but this column is provided because it may often be impossible to determine what the mental model was in a particular case).

Phenomenological description of the event	Predominant type of thinking	Intent to do the "right thing"?								
		Yes							No	
		Failure in mental model (the "knowledge base")							Technical error	Violation
		No	Individual knowledge	Information acquisition	Communication	Other	?			
Omission	UC	A								
	Fast		B							
	Slow									
	?									
Repetition	UC									
	Fast				C					
	Slow									
	?									
Substitution	UC									
	Fast			D						
	Slow									
	?									
Insertion	UC									
	Fast									
	Slow									
	?									
Incorrect dose	UC									
	Fast									
	Slow	E			F					
	?									
Incorrect route	UC								G	
	Fast									
	Slow									
	?									
Incorrect timing	UC									
	Fast									
	Slow									
	?									
Other	UC									H
	Fast					I				
	Slow									
	?									

Abbreviation: UC, unconscious.

facilitate thinking about medication errors in a way that integrates their phenomenological aspects (e.g., a syringe swap) with the cognitive processes involved in their generation. The primary objective of analyzing medication errors in this way is to facilitate the identification of effective countermeasures to them. For example, the framework starts by separating violations from errors because violations often lend themselves to different types of countermeasures from those needed to prevent errors.

In this framework, it is assumed that failures in the mental model can be the primary cause of any type of error. The mental model has been given prominence because understanding mental models is often very helpful in identifying countermeasures. For example, communication errors are a common cause of faulty mental models, and communication can be improved by training and the use of certain devices, tools, and techniques (e.g., the World Health Organization Surgical Safety Checklist). By contrast, a deficiency in an anesthesiologist's personal understanding of the properties of a particular medication would require more training in pharmacology. A failure in arithmetic is interesting: In Table 7.5, we have shown an error in slow thinking with no fault in the mental model (E). This is a possibility, but for many anesthesiologists it is more likely that an error in calculating the concentration of a diluted medication would involve fast thinking and an inadvertent mistake. For people who have a strong facility for mental arithmetic, a mistake of the latter type may have much in common with a slip. Again, the required countermeasures would probably be different in these two scenarios, although some solutions (prefilled syringes, for example) might address both types of cognitive failure.

As discussed earlier, the methods used in many studies of medication error do not lend themselves to the identification of the cognitive processes involved with each individual event. Ultimately, this information can only be obtained from the honest testimony of the practitioners who made the errors. Nevertheless, when a physician, a nurse, or a pharmacist makes an error, it is often possible to make a good guess about the processes involved. For example, if an anesthesiologist who is known to be conscientious in the careful administration of medications gives an incorrect medication while

under the pressure of time and the incident involves an ampule or vial that has a similar appearance to that of the intended medication, it is likely that this will have been a slip.

7.9 Conclusions

Medication errors are not random events, nor are they necessarily evidence of a lack of carefulness on the part of the practitioner concerned. To a substantial degree, the particular type of medication error that is likely to occur in a particular set of circumstances is predictable. Furthermore, each of these types of error will continue to occur at their current rate if we continue with current approaches to the management of medications in the perioperative period. Errors will not be reduced by ongoing calls for greater carefulness on behalf of individual practitioners. Instead, the need is for fundamental changes in the ways in which medications are presented, selected, and administered to patients. Greater investment in systems-based initiatives to improve medication management is essential if medication safety is to improve. However, it is also essential for clinicians to engage with such initiatives if they are to be effective. Achieving this requires sustained effort by departments and institutions, informed by the principles of implementation science.

References

1. Leape LL. Error in medicine. *JAMA*. 1994;272(23):1851–7.

2. Merry AF, Webster CS, Mathew DJ. A new, safety-oriented, integrated drug administration and automated anesthesia record system. *Anesth Analg*. 2001;93(2):385–90.

3. Merry AF, Webster CS, Hannam J, et al. Multimodal system designed to reduce errors in recording and administration of drugs in anaesthesia: prospective randomised clinical evaluation. *BMJ*. 2011;343:d5543.

4. Merry AF, Brookbanks W. *Merry and McCall Smith's Errors, Medicine and the Law*. 2nd ed. Cambridge, UK: Cambridge University Press; 2017.

5. Blumenthal D. Making medical errors into "medical treasures". *JAMA*. 1994;272(23):1867–8.

6. Reason J. *Human Error*. New York, NY: Cambridge University Press; 1990.

7. Leslie K, Culwick MD, Reynolds H, Hannam JA, Merry AF. Awareness during general anaesthesia

in the first 4,000 incidents reported to webAIRS. *Anaesth Intensive Care*. 2017;45(4):441–7.

8. Rouse W. Models of human problem solving: detection, diagnosis and compensation for system failures. In: Johannsen G, Rijnsdorp JE, eds. *Proceedings of IFAC/IFIP/IFORS/IEA Conference on Analysis, Design and Evaluation of Man-Machine Systems, Baden-Baden, Federal Republic of Germany*. Vol 15. Issue 6. Oxford, UK: IFAC/Elsevier; 1982:167–84.

9. Kahneman D. *Thinking, Fast and Slow*. London: Penguin Books; 2011.

10. Thaler R, Sunstein C. *Nudge: Improving Decisions about Health, Wealth and Happiness*. New Haven, CT: Yale University Press; 2008.

11. Stanovich KE, West RF. Discrepancies between normative and descriptive models of decision making and the understanding/acceptance principle. *Cogn Psychol*. 1999;38(3):349–85.

12. Stanovich KE, West RF. Individual differences in reasoning: implications for the rationality debate? *Behav Brain Sci*. 2000;23(5):645–65; discussion 665–726.

13. Reason J. *Managing the Risks of Organizational Accidents*. London: Routledge; 1997.

14. Reason J. Human error: models and management. *Br Med J*. 2000;320:768–70.

15. Gladwell M. *Blink. The Power of Thinking Without Thinking*. New York, NY: Little, Brown; 2005.

16. Stiegler MP, Tung A. Cognitive processes in anesthesiology decision making. *Anesthesiology*. 2014;120(1):204–17.

17. Merry AF. To do or not to do? How people make decisions. *J Extra Corpor Technol*. 2011;43(1): P39–43.

18. Endsley M. The role of situation awareness in naturalistic decision making. In: Zsambok CE, Klein G, eds. *Expertise: Research and Applications. Naturalistic Decision Making*, Mahwah, NJ: Lawrence Erlbaum Associates; 1997:269–83.

19. Patel A, Nouraei SA. Transnasal Humidified Rapid-Insufflation Ventilatory Exchange (THRIVE): a physiological method of increasing apnoea time in patients with difficult airways. *Anaesthesia*. 2015;70(3):323–9.

20. Frerk C, Mitchell VS, McNarry AF, et al. Difficult Airway Society 2015 guidelines for management of unanticipated difficult intubation in adults. *Br J Anaesth*. 2015;115(6):827–48.

21. Cook TM, Woodall N, Frerk C. Major complications of airway management in the UK: Results of the Fourth National Audit Project of the Royal College of Anaesthetists and the Difficult Airway Society. Part 1: Anaesthesia. *Br J Anaesth*. 2011;106(5):617–31.

22. Henderson JJ, Popat MT, Latto IP, Pearce AC. Difficult Airway Society guidelines for management of the unanticipated difficult intubation. *Anaesthesia*. 2004;59(7):675–94.

23. Apfelbaum JL, Hagberg CA, Caplan RA, et al. Practice guidelines for management of the difficult airway: an updated report by the American Society of Anesthesiologists Task Force on Management of the Difficult Airway. *Anesthesiology*. 2013;118(2):251–70.

24. Perkins GD, Ji C, Deakin CD, et al. A randomized trial of epinephrine in out-of-hospital cardiac arrest. *N Engl J Med*. 2018;1(8):711–21.

25. Merry AF, Weller JM, Robinson BJ, et al. A simulation design for research evaluating safety innovations in anaesthesia. *Anaesthesia*. 2008;63(12):1349–57.

26. Bagian JP, Gosbee J, Lee CZ, et al. The Veterans Affairs root cause analysis system in action. *Jt Comm J Qual Improv*. 2002;28(10):531–45.

27. Caplan RA, Posner KL, Cheney FW. Effect of outcome on physician judgments of appropriateness of care. *JAMA*. 1991;265(15):1957–60.

28. Weiser TG, Haynes AB, Lashoher A, et al. Perspectives in quality: designing the WHO Surgical Safety Checklist. *Int J Qual Health Care*. 2010;22(5):365–70.

29. R v Yogasakaran [1990] 1 NZLR 399.

30. Anonymous. Forgotten baby syndrome explained by neuroscientist. DailyMail Online Videos; 2015 Accessed January 3, 2020. https://www.dailymail.co.uk/video/news/video-1107664/Forgotten-baby-syndrome-explained-neuroscientist.html

31. Veisi F, Salimi B, Mohseni G, Golfam P, Kolyaei A. Accidental intrathecal injection of tranexamic acid in cesarean section: A fatal medication error. *APSF Newsletter*. 2010;25(1):9. Accessed January 3, 2020. https://www.apsf.org/article/apsf-hosts-medication-safety-conference/

32. Hatch DM, Atito-Narh E, Herschmiller EJ, Olufolabi AJ, Owen MD. Refractory status epilepticus after inadvertent intrathecal injection of tranexamic acid treated by magnesium sulfate. *Int J Obstet Anesth*. 2016;26:71–5.

33. Runciman B, Merry A, Walton M. *Safety and Ethics in Healthcare: A Guide to Getting It Right*. Aldershot, UK: Ashgate Publishing; 2007.

34. Jelacic S, Bowdle A, Nair BG, et al. A system for anesthesia drug administration using barcode technology: The Codonics Safe Label System and Smart Anesthesia Manager. *Anesth Analg*. 2015;121(2):410–21.

35. Dixon-Woods M, Leslie M, Tarrant C, Bion J. Explaining Matching Michigan: an ethnographic

study of a patient safety program. *Implement Sci.* 2013;8:70.

36. Martis WR, Hannam JA, Lee T, Merry AF, Mitchell SJ. Improved compliance with the World Health Organization Surgical Safety Checklist is associated with reduced surgical specimen labelling errors. *N Z Med J.* 2016;129(1441):63–7.

37. Haynes AB, Weiser TG, Berry WR, et al. A surgical safety checklist to reduce morbidity and mortality in a global population. *N Engl J Med.* 2009;360(5):491–9.

38. Hannam JA, Glass L, Kwon J, et al. A prospective, observational study of the effects of implementation strategy on compliance with a surgical safety checklist. *BMJ Qual Saf.* 2013;22(11):940–7.

39. Webster CS, Larsson L, Frampton CM, et al. Clinical assessment of a new anaesthetic drug administration system: a prospective, controlled, longitudinal incident monitoring study. *Anaesthesia.* 2010;65(5):490–9.

40. Bowdle TA, Jelacic S, Nair B, et al. Facilitated self-reported anaesthetic medication errors before and after implementation of a safety bundle and barcode-based safety system. *Br J Anaesth.* 2018;121(6):1338–45

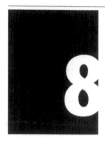

Violations and Medication Safety

The role of human error in the generation of adverse medication events (and adverse events in healthcare more generally) has received considerable attention in the literature in recent years. There has been much less written about violations. In this chapter, we discuss violations and argue that minor violations are at least as important as errors in the context of failures in medication safety.

8.1 Definition of a Violation

As explained in Chapter 7, the distinguishing feature between an error and a violation is that in an error *one tries to do the right thing but actually does the wrong thing*, whereas in a violation, *one deliberately does the wrong thing* (although, as we explain, *without malevolent intent*) (1). This raises the question of how one determines that an action is "the wrong thing." The following, more formal, definition of a violation addresses that question:

A violation is an intentional – but not malevolent *and* not necessarily reprehensible *– deviation from those practices deemed necessary (by designers, managers,* or *regulatory agencies) or appreciated* by the individual as advisable *to maintain the safe operation of a potentially hazardous system* (1).

As with our definition of an error in Chapter 7, this definition and its justification have been discussed in detail elsewhere (1).

We believe that various types of minor violation are endemic to healthcare. However, we also believe that most practitioners genuinely wish to provide good care for their patients and to avoid harming them. At the heart of this conundrum lies a fundamental point: People who violate usually do so in the belief that the violation will do no harm. Either they believe that there is no justification for the rule that is being broken or they believe that they can get away with breaking it, at least on a particular occasion. Failing to label a syringe used to administer a dose of atropine to a patient who has developed bradycardia and hypotension during

an anesthetic would be an example of this, and it is true that the risks associated with a minor violation of this sort are often negligible. The anesthesiologist might even believe that the saving of the time that would be required to label the syringe was a justification for not applying a label in these circumstances.

As indicated in Chapter 7, an actual intent to cause harm is quite different and should be labeled as *sabotage* (2). The classic example of sabotage related to the management of medications was provided by the English general practitioner, Harold Shipman, who was convicted of murdering over 200 of his patients by deliberately administering overdoses of opioids to elderly people (3,4). More recently, a French anesthesiologist, Frederic Pechier, has been charged with putting lethal doses of potassium chloride into perfusion bags during surgeries in a ploy to induce a crisis and then appear to be a hero for recognizing and managing the event (5). He has pleaded not guilty, but if proven, the story has parallels with the known phenomenon of arsonist firefighters (6). Sabotage appears to be very rare in healthcare: Shipman is apparently the only British doctor to have been found guilty of murdering his patients (7).

The story of a Canadian anesthesiologist who left his anesthetized patient unattended while he was out of the operating room (8) illustrates these differences quite nicely. He presumably believed that this could be done safely enough, even though he was breaking the widely accepted rule that the continuous presence of a trained provider is a fundamental requirement for safe anesthesia (9,10). One can be reasonably certain that a disconnection of the anesthetic circuit leading to failure to administer oxygen and severe brain damage for his patient was not something that this anesthesiologist was hoping to achieve. However, in contrast to an error, his violation was a clear deviation from practices "deemed necessary" for safety (including by those who set international standards [9,10]). Importantly, there is nothing controversial about this rule. It is obviously sensible, and most anesthesiologists appreciate its importance. As we discuss later, there are rules that are widely disputed and occasions on which it may be appropriate to break a rule, but this was not one of those rules nor one of those occasions.

8.2 Risk, Violations, and Mental Models

Many, probably most, decisions in healthcare involve some balancing of risks and benefits for patients. A large part of anesthesiologists' work lies in managing and mitigating the risks inherent in anesthesia. Even the induction of anesthesia is inherently risky, but that does not mean that administering propofol or a neuromuscular blocking agent to a patient is a violation, provided this is done by a properly qualified practitioner in the context of proper practice. The characteristic of a violation is that it creates an *unnecessary* risk for patients, equipment, or the system.

8.2.1 Not All Violations Are Equal

Minor deviations from accepted rules are common in all walks of life. For example, it is not uncommon for people to exceed speed limits by a small amount when driving. If inadvertent, this would be an error; if done knowingly, it would be a violation. Either way, the associated risk would be small, and it would be reasonable for the individual concerned to believe that there was little likelihood of consequential harm. Greater excesses of speed would carry greater risk, and there would be a certain point at which the belief that no harm is likely to occur would become implausible. At this point, the violation would constitute recklessness. These ideas are reflected by laws in many countries that specify progressively severe penalties for progressive thresholds of excess speed. The question of where to draw the line between a minor violation and recklessness is quite difficult and has been analyzed in detail elsewhere (1). It could be argued that Frederic Pechier's alleged actions were reckless. Perhaps he did not intend for the patients to die as Harold Shipman did. He "merely" wished to create events where he could play the hero, but in doing so (if indeed he did), he was putting them to serious and completely unnecessary risk. Suffice it

to say that we believe that recklessness is relatively uncommon in the context of the management of perioperative medications, whereas we believe that minor violations play a substantial role in the generation of avoidable adverse medication events.

From the perspective of the traffic police, the motivation for exceeding the speed limit is of little relevance: Even a small excess is a violation of the law, and a large excess is a more serious violation of the same law. Strict liability is a legal concept that captures the sense that a rule is a rule and breaking it is a violation, whatever the moral state of mind that underpinned this decision. For practical purposes, this is a reasonable approach to take for most minor traffic offenses, but for more serious crimes, the state of mind that led a person to commit a crime is highly relevant. In the law, this is captured in the concept of *mens rea*, Latin for "guilty mind."

8.2.1.1 Anesthesia Records and the Omission and Smoothing of Data

An example of minor violation in relation to anesthesia can be found in the attention often paid to accurately and comprehensively recording the details of every anesthetic. These details include the medications administered during the anesthetic and the patient's physiological state before and after these administrations. The anesthesia record is an important document that may be used to inform the subsequent clinical management of the patient, for audit, for medicolegal purposes, and for research (11). In one study, anesthetic records made by anesthesiologists were compared with those made by a researcher who observed the case and had no responsibilities other than correctly documenting the anesthetic. Many omissions and inaccuracies were identified (12). In a more recent study, participants were randomized to produce handwritten anesthesia records or to use an electronic anesthesia information management system (AIMS). The manually made records were found to have more missing information than the electronic records in relation to selected items from a clinical guideline (13). In a further study, when anesthesia records made manually by some anesthesiologists were digitized and redisplayed to different anesthesiologists in comparison with electronically collected (and therefore presumably accurate) physiologic data from the same anesthetics records, there was sufficient alteration of the recorded physiologic data to result in different clinical decisions (14). The authors of the first of these three studies speculated that failures to make comprehensive and reliable anesthetic records were possibly attributable to a degree of skepticism about the value of these records. A further point made was that possible deficiencies in the design of the form used for this purpose may also have contributed to these failures. We return to the roles of skepticism and design in the genesis of violations later in this chapter.

It requires considerable attention to detail to make a comprehensive and accurate anesthesia record manually, and some errors are likely in this process. Minor omissions and inaccuracies may well arise as simple errors, but for some of these there may also be an element of violation reflecting a sense that the effort required for work as prescribed (see Figure 6.1) is just not worth the trouble. Some smoothing of the recorded data might also occur for the same reason – it may simply be seen as easier to show a more or less constant set of measures over time than to try to capture each fluctuation in pulse rate and blood pressure as it occurs. On the other hand, it seems that, at times, smoothing of this sort probably does involve a deliberate attempt to represent certain imperfections in the conduct of an anesthetic in a more favorable light. This may reflect a desire to minimize medicolegal risks. Again, this example illustrates that not all violations are morally equal and also that it may be impossible to unravel the motivations for a violation other than through the testimony of the person concerned, which may or may not be completely truthful. This raises the question of whether violations should be judged on absolute grounds against established rules or whether an attempt should be made to understand the cognitive processes involved in their generation.

8.2.1.2 Rules, Fines, and Violations

In one view, breaking any rule constitutes a violation, and the absence of a formal rule implies that no violation has occurred. An alternative argument, which we endorse, places greater weight on the actor's intent and on his or her appreciation of the implications of the decision or act in question. From this perspective, the breaking of an established rule is best called exactly that – *the breaking of a rule* – and recognizes that rules may be broken in error or in violation. Furthermore, we would support the view that the deliberate taking of an unwarranted risk should be seen as a violation even if no formal rule covers the situation (1).

Again, the example of exceeding the speed limit is informative in this regard. The maximum speed limit on a particular type of road, such as a freeway, varies from country to country and sometimes even within a particular country. In Germany, some sections of road have no formal speed limit at all. This does not mean that one should have no regard to safety in the speed at which one drives, and it is even recognized within many road codes that speed should be adjusted according to the conditions of weather and traffic that pertain at any point in time. Deliberately exceeding a legal limit will constitute a violation whether the driver perceives this as safe to do or not. Choosing to break a law is a violation, even if that law is considered inappropriate (we return later to situations in which such violations may be justified). However, the point here is that it is also a violation to deliberately exceed a safe speed whether or not this speed happens to exceed a formal limit.

These nuances may make the precise interpretation of some decisions and actions quite difficult. It can be difficult to ascertain a person's state of mind. Questions of judgment may be involved – for example, the upper limit of safe speeds may be a matter of opinion. Nevertheless, these nuances are important, both from the perspective of determining the blameworthiness of an action and from that of designing a penalty for a violation that will be effective in preventing it in the future.

For example, the active implementation of police traps to catch and penalize speeding drivers does seem to be effective in reducing speed, presumably because many examples of excessive speed do reflect violation rather than error and can be avoided by an active intent to stay within the speed limit. Also, changing the legal limit for certain roads in combination with enforcement of this type can have an impact on accidents and hence the road toll. Interestingly, it seems that drivers are likely to be more concerned about the possibility of a fine, and perhaps a black mark on their record, than about the chance of an accident in which either themselves or someone else might be injured. This is partly because, if someone really believed that a serious accident was likely to result from a minor violation of this type, he or she probably would not commit that violation. It is also because high-frequency, low-impact events (such as fines arising from active policing) appear to be more likely to change behavior than low-frequency, high-impact events (such as deaths or injuries in serious car crashes). Thus, well-founded rules or laws that are enforced can be very effective in changing behavior and improving safety. This point has untapped potential in relation to medication errors, and we will return to it.

8.2.1.3 Distinguishing between Violations and Errors: The "Decision Test"

As we have seen, some violations can be quite similar to some mistakes, in that both involve a decision. One test to distinguish a violation from an error involves the following thought experiment.

Consider a practice that meets the second half of our formal definition of a violation (i.e., it is a "*deviation from those practices deemed necessary* or appreciated by the individual as advisable *to maintain the safe operation of a potentially hazardous system*"). If a practice of this sort can be ended simply on the strength of a decision to do so, then that deviation is a violation. In our example of the patient left unattended during an anesthetic, an anesthesiologist who decides *never* to leave an anesthetized patient unattended can reasonably expect to achieve this objective. Thus, to do so would always be a violation unless truly exceptional circumstances applied (we do not digress here into a discussion of what these might or might not be). By contrast, simply deciding never to draw up and administer the wrong medication during an anesthetic is highly unlikely to be completely successful – the empirical data reviewed in earlier chapters are testimony to this. Thus, giving the wrong medication during an anesthetic is likely to represent an error. This distinction is relatively straightforward when evaluating practices that are clearly safe or unsafe but much more difficult to make at the boundaries between these categories of behaviour.

8.3 Blurred Boundaries between Violation and Error: Fatigue as an Example

The relationship between fatigue and performance has received much attention in recent years. On closer evaluation, this relationship turns out to be rather complicated and dependent on context. This topic is worth discussing in some depth because it illustrates how blurred the boundaries may be between violation and appropriate practice, and also how decisions to take certain risks (such as working while fatigued) can be both necessary and well-motivated.

8.3.1 Fatigue and Alcohol

It would not be controversial to assert that giving an anesthetic or managing patients perioperatively while under the influence of alcohol would be a violation. In 1997, Dawson and Reid, in the Scientific Correspondence section of the highly prestigious journal *Nature*, published data from 40 subjects who had participated in two experiments. In one they were kept awake for 28 hours, and in the other they consumed 10–15 g alcohol at 30-minute intervals until their mean blood alcohol concentration reached 0.10%. Both experiments were begun at 8:00 a.m. Cognitive psychomotor performance was assessed at half-hourly intervals using a computer-administered test of hand-eye coordination. The results showed a striking similarity between the relationship of blood alcohol and performance and that of increasing hours of wakefulness and performance (Figure 8.1). Famously, the authors commented that 17 hours of sustained wakefulness produced a decrease in cognitive psychomotor performance equivalent to that seen at a blood alcohol concentration of 0.05%, which is the legal limit for driving in many Western industrialized countries. In many such countries, a conviction for driving above this limit would result in the suspension of one's license and might also be associated with significant reputational damage. After 24 hours without sleep, performance had decreased to a level equivalent to that seen at a blood alcohol concentration of approximately 0.10%, which considerably exceeds even the more liberal limits for legal driving in some such jurisdictions (15). There is, furthermore, plenty of other evidence to support the general concept that inadequate sleep is associated with performance impairment, some of which has been summarized in a more recent paper from Ferguson et al. (16). On face value then, it seems that in a book on reducing medication errors in anesthesia and perioperative medicine, it would be reasonable to suggest that participating in either activity

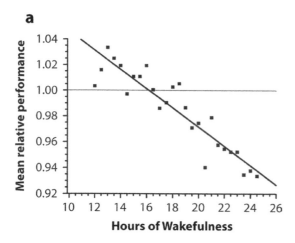

a

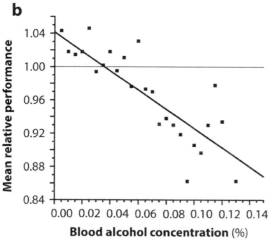

b

Figure 8.1 Scatter plot and linear regression of the mean relative performance levels of 40 subjects against **a**, time, between the 10th and 26th hour of sustained wakefulness ($F1,24 = 132.9$, $P*0.05$, $R2 = 0.92$); and **b**, blood alcohol concentrations up to 0.13% ($F1,24 = 54.4$, $P*0.05$, $R2 = 0.69$). Reproduced with permission from Dawson and Reid 1997 (15).

after a maximum of 17 hours of wakefulness should be considered a violation of safe practice and prohibited except in true emergencies.

8.3.2 Tired Doctors

The idea that it is unsafe to work while fatigued has driven reform of approaches to maximum acceptable hours of work for junior doctors in many countries over recent years. The case of Libby Zion, outlined in Chapter 3 (see Box 3.1), served to bring this issue into sharp focus in 1984. Libby Zion, who was 18 years old, died after having been admitted to the emergency department of a New York hospital (17). The junior doctors who managed her care had been on duty for more than 18

hours continuously. Recommendations for reform that followed a review of this case included limits of 12 hours for emergency room shifts, 80 work hours a week averaged over 4 weeks for residents in acute care specialties, and 24 consecutive work hours in total. Moonlighting was prohibited. Many other countries have subsequently implemented reforms to limit the working hours of junior doctors (18). Perhaps most interesting about the reforms that followed Libby Zion's death is that *new* limits were clearly excessive in relation to the evidence from Dawson and Reid, although this had not been published at that time. Furthermore, even these proposed changes provoked controversy with opponents pointing to the need to acquire adequate experience and to the risks of an increased number of handovers, among other matters (19,20). "War stories" abound about the excessive hours worked by junior doctors in the "bad old days" (see, for example, Box 8.1), and there is no doubt that the culture of medicine at the time cultivated an approach to training based on a "hero" model for doctors.

Since then reforms to limit junior doctors' hours of work have continued apace, but regulated limits have not been prominent in relation to senior doctors' hours of work. For example, in New Zealand, a 16-hour limit on single shifts was introduced for junior doctors in 1985. It is intriguing that a 16-hour limit was chosen 12 years before the data supporting this as a reasonable safe upper limit were published by Dawson and Reid (see Figure 8.1). The reasons were apparently pragmatic and reflected a recognition that more restrictive limits to work hours were unlikely to be embraced by senior doctors, as well as a desire to make the imposition of work-arounds more difficult.[1] In a subsequent survey of New Zealand anesthesiologists, both junior doctors and senior doctors in New Zealand still perceived themselves as working for longer periods than they considered safe for patients or for themselves (22). Legal limits to work hours for senior doctors are still unusual, and even today we can attest to many examples of individual senior surgeons and anesthesiologists working continuously for periods of 24 hours or longer in New Zealand, the United States, and many other countries.

---

[1] Personal communication, Dr. Jeremy Cooper.

Box 8.1 A traditional start to the career of a junior doctor

One of the authors of this book, AM, began his first job as a resident (or "houseman") in Harare Central Hospital, Harare, Zimbabwe, on Saturday, January 1, 1977. At that time and place, there was an absolute shortage of junior doctors in the country, and long work hours were the norm. As it happened, AM was rostered off duty for this particular weekend and was due to start work on Monday, January 3. He went out on Friday night to celebrate New Year's Eve in traditional fashion and got to bed at about 4 a.m.

At 6:30 a.m. the telephone rang. The attending (or "consultant") of the day had telephoned to say that the resident assigned for the weekend had called in unwell, and it would be appreciated if AM could cover the weekend. Instead of inquiring as to the nature of the resident's illness and its potential similarity with his own already fatigued condition, AM agreed, and headed in for work. He managed to get some 4 or 5 hours of interrupted sleep on each of the Saturday and Sunday nights, but worked essentially without stop for the rest of the weekend.

On Monday, January 3, he presented to work as assigned, and at the end of a busy day was expected to do the Monday night on-call as well, which he did. On the Tuesday morning, work continued as normal.

At around 11 a.m. his attending noticed that he was looking decidedly unwell and sent him home to sleep.

This story is not out of the ordinary for that period in time, and indeed is probably quite modest in comparison with some tales that could be told. The only unusual aspect of the story is probably the sympathy shown by the attending on Tuesday.

Interestingly, no harmful mistakes seem to have been made during this initiation to life as a junior doctor, which continued in much the same vein for the next 2 years and beyond. So far as we know, no audit was ever undertaken of the appropriateness or accuracy of medications prescribed or administered by AM during that weekend. If no errors were made, that was probably a matter of good fortune. By contrast, fortune did not favor Dr. Teoh, a junior doctor who inadvertently administered penicillin through the wrong line after working for 120 hours in 1 week in Belfast, Ireland. This error led to the death of her patient and to the (unsuccessful) prosecution of Dr. Teoh for manslaughter (21). This provides a striking illustration of the role of luck in determining the consequences of both errors and violations.

8.3.3 Working while Fatigued as an Example of a Necessary, Appropriate, or Correct Violation

Given the evidence summarized so far, the argument that undertaking clinical work while fatigued should be seen as a violation appears to be quite strong. It has also been suggested that driving while fatigued is comparable to drinking and driving (23). On the grounds of safety, the aviation industry has severely curtailed the hours to be worked by any pilot. In fact, some commercial pilots spend fewer hours flying per month than some doctors work per week.

On the other hand, working excessive hours does not have connotations of egregiousness. On the contrary, many doctors who work excessively long hours are well motivated and feel themselves to be caught in what Reason has described as a "system double-bind" (2). They are virtually compelled to do so on account of their rosters or their dedication to serving patients, or both. The terms "necessary violation" or "appropriate violation" would

seem to apply, and when no harm ensues, these violations can also be categorized as "correct" (see section 8.5.3). However, as with Drs. Bawa-Gaba and Teoh, when a patient dies, a different view may be taken of the circumstances that contributed to that death.

If the requirement to work excessively long hours arises from unreasonable terms of employment, reinforced by the unrealistic culture of the institution in which one works, then surely those responsible for administering the particular service are primarily accountable for this violation of safe practice. However, if the requirement arises out of a fundamental necessity to care for sick patients under circumstances of limited resources (as in the example described in Box 8.1), the situation is a little different. In many countries entire healthcare systems are underresourced. Even in highly resourced countries, it can be difficult to adequately staff hospitals for fluctuations in demand for highly specialized healthcare services. Thus, a cardiac surgeon in a small practice may have a reasonable routine workload but may be compelled to work excessive hours when several patients in need of urgent surgery present over a short period of time. Situations of this general type are quite common in healthcare, particularly in smaller centers. In a well-known case in which bupivacaine intended for epidural analgesia in a laboring parturient was administered intravenously, the nurse in question had completed back-to-back 8-hour shifts (covering for an ill coworker), then slept for about 6 hours, and was beginning her third 8-hour shift in 24 hours at 7 a.m. (24). Even in large centers with reasonable numbers of staff, patients requiring urgent major surgery may present late in the day. This may leave no alternative other than for surgeons and anesthesiologists who have been working all day to continue working throughout the entire night and beyond.

On the other hand, willingness to work excessively long hours may not always be entirely altruistic. Financial considerations may play a part. Many people make substantial financial gains by working long hours. In fact, financial drivers in both directions may well enter into negotiations around doctors' hours of work. If the total cost of remunerating the workforce could be held constant, administrators and funders would presumably have little reason to oppose employing more staff to reduce the work hours of each individual. However, a request for reduced hours without a concomitant reduction in pay would be more difficult to meet. Contracts that pay a set salary to doctors irrespective of hours worked are certainly open to abuse by employers, but enticing overtime rates may drive doctors to take on cases after working hours that could reasonably be deferred until the next day. The rhetoric about safety and hours worked is not always entirely unbiased under these two contrasting scenarios.

8.3.4 A Deeper Dive into Fatigue and Safety

Context is central to the relationship between fatigue and patient safety. At the extreme limit it is clear that all animals, including humans, need sleep, and if continuously deprived of sleep will eventually die. However, the extent of deprivation of sleep that can be tolerated without impacting on safe medical care is less clear and may vary depending on an individual's ability to tolerate such deprivation. Furthermore, the impact of regulation

of working hours of groups of doctors (typically interns and residents) on patient safety is very difficult to predict. Such regulation impacts not only on the hours worked by the regulated group (e.g., residents) but also potentially on the hours worked by other groups (senior doctors may have to take up some of the gaps created by the reduced work hours of their junior staff), on the frequency of patient handoffs, and hence on continuity of care, and on the opportunity for doctors in training to gain or maintain experience. If shift work is adopted as a solution, this will have implications related to circadian physiology, which also need to be considered. There may also be an impact on the health budget of institutions or even whole countries, with consequent opportunity costs. Money spent on salaries cannot be spent on other things, such as much-needed but expensive medications. Furthermore, it is not only work hours that contribute to fatigue and to degradation of performance. Domestic responsibilities (notably childcare), domestic stresses, social activities, and secondary employment are all relevant. (It is noteworthy that the reforms following the Libby Zion case included a prohibition on moonlighting.) The data published by Dawson and Reid relate to hours of continuous wakefulness rather than hours of work. Staff assigned to an evening shift may well arrive at work after a day's wakefulness, particularly at the beginning of a series of such shifts. Furthermore, ill health, including acute viral infections, mental health problems, and the morning hangover effects of excess alcohol consumption the night before may all impact on performance as much or more than fatigue and may also compound the effect of fatigue if it is present.

Excessive work hours and continuous loss of sleep may also impact on practitioners' personal health and well-being, creating the potential for vicious cycles to develop. The need for doctors to look after their own health in order to be able to look after their patients properly has been reflected in a recent amendment to the World Medical Association's Declaration of Geneva, which now includes the following clause (25,26):

I WILL ATTEND TO my own health, well-being, and abilities in order to provide care of the highest standard.

All of these factors have been discussed at length over the years, notably in relation to the regulatory changes that followed the Libby Zion case (17) and those that followed the implementation of European Union limitations on hours to doctors in the United Kingdom (27,28). They do not imply that no action was or is needed to address excessive hours of work – we consider that the hours worked by junior doctors at the time of Libby Zion and the example in Box 8.1 were often clearly excessive. They do imply that a sophisticated approach to the management of fatigue is required to achieve the best outcomes for both patients and staff (18).

An easily overlooked aspect of this problem is that very little of the research into fatigue has been relevant to the context of clinical practice in general or safe medication management more specifically. Most studies of the impact of wakefulness or fatigue have primarily used highly sensitive instruments to detect decrements in generic performance rather than measures of clinical performance or patient outcomes. Performance on a psychomotor vigilance task (for example), which in essence involves responding to a repetitive presentation on the screen of an electronic device, has little obvious validity as a measure of how accurately one might administer a medication to a patient during an anesthetic in the middle of the night. Giving an anesthetic is also quite different from driving a car or truck. In the latter situation, even a brief period of inattention is likely to have catastrophic results, whereas actual microsleeps may be without consequence if they occur at a stable time during an anesthetic. Similarly, while half of perfusionists in a survey of fatigue and performance during cardiopulmonary bypass reported that they had experienced microsleeps during a pump run, none reported serious errors or accidents occurring during those times (29). Also, as with most things in nature, individuals vary in their capacity to work after various lengths of wakefulness. Within-individual variation also occurs, influenced by other factors such as the nature and context of the work that needs to be done. The task of monitoring a routine anesthetic at 3 a.m. may well be soporific, but an exciting acute case may produce the adrenaline needed to enhance performance. Thus, in a simulation-based study comparing the performance of 12 residents when sleep deprived or actively rested, Howard et al. were able to show differences in responses to a vigilance probe but not in clinical performance (30). In two studies in

the setting of a medical intensive care unit, interns made substantially more serious medical errors when they worked frequent shifts of 24 hours or more than when they worked shorter shifts. Eliminating extended work shifts significantly increased sleep and decreased attentional failures during night work hours (31,32). However, three relatively large, real-world studies in cardiac surgery found no effect of surgeons' sleep deprivation on serious complications or mortality among patients (33–35). These studies did not examine the rate of errors, serious or otherwise, and may indicate an ability of the team to compensate and correct errors rather than a lack of errors. Furthermore, findings of no difference in patient outcomes may not rule out an actual impact. Rather, they may reflect the fact that much larger studies would be needed to show a difference that might only manifest when a failure in attention coincided with a critical moment in the surgery or anesthetic (30).

Circadian rhythms may also have a profound effect on performance. The Howard study was conducted in the morning during normal work hours. If it were to be repeated at the circadian trough (i.e., the hours following midnight), the differences between the residents' fatigued and rested states might have been more marked. There is also the question of the chronicity of fatigue. Howard et al. explored these factors further in another study of anesthesia residents. Three states were compared: (1) during a normal (baseline) work schedule, (2) after an in-hospital 24-hour on-call period, and (3) following a period of extended sleep. The key findings were that sleep latency at baseline (condition 1) was as abnormal as after a 24-hour period on call (condition 2), indicating serious chronic fatigue. The sleep latency test involves measuring the time taken for a subject to fall asleep in a quiet and darkened room with eyes closed. The results in these first two conditions (5–6 minutes) were similar to those seen in patients with narcolepsy but very different from the 12 minutes seen after active resting (condition 3). Time of day also had a significant effect on sleep latency (36).

The association of fatigue with medication error has been commented on in various studies (37,38). For example, multiple studies have shown that nurses working longer hours or atypical shifts are at increased risk for medication errors (39,40).

However, simply asking survey respondents or those submitting incident reports to indicate whether they were fatigued or not, or whether they thought fatigue was a contributory factor to the error, is not particularly informative because many errors also occur in the absence of fatigue. Factors such as the additive effects of aging may also need to be considered (41). Thus, the relevant question is whether fatigue increases the rate of error, and answering this requires a more sophisticated analysis or, ideally, a different type of study altogether. In a large study that used facilitated incident reporting to investigate medication administration errors in anesthesia, diarized sleep histories showed no significant relationship to subjective comments that fatigue had been a contributory factor to the reported errors (42).

In an effort to improve the relevance of a psychomotor vigilance task to medication administration, Cheeseman et al. designed a medication recognition and confirmation test (MRCT) (43). In essence, the test involves displaying several photographs of medication ampules or user-applied labels for syringes of medication on the touch screen of a computer and asking participants to select a particular one by touching the screen. Either the touched photograph or (randomly) another photograph is then displayed, and the participant is asked to confirm that this is indeed the intended choice, or to indicate that it is not. In this way it is possible to run hundreds of tests with any individual participant over quite short periods of time (such as 20 minutes) and to do this with particular groups of people (such as anesthesiologists) at various times of day and night after varying lengths of time spent working. Cheeseman et al. conducted two experiments, each during an 8- to 12-hour day shift and an 8- to 12-hour night shift. Among other findings, they found that participants obtained about an hour less sleep while working night shifts than while working day shifts (mean difference 57 minutes, 95% confidence interval [CI] 0:15–1:39 hours; $P = 0.013$), which illustrates the complexity of trying to manage fatigue through various approaches to rostering. They also found that mean confirmation reaction times were a little slower during night shifts than during day shifts. However, no differences in error rates were observed between shifts.

Griffiths et al. took a different approach to exploring the effect of fatigue on activities relevant to anesthesia. In this Australian study, investigators used a standard computerized battery of cognitive tests (Cogstate [44]) to investigate the performance of anesthetic registrars (in effect, residents) before and after a series of seven consecutive day shifts and seven consecutive night shifts. As the week progressed, a small but significant decline was detected in the speed of detection and identification tasks at the end of night shifts, but without any loss of accuracy (45). These studies suggest that although it may well be harder and slower to carry out cognitive tasks when one is tired, it is usually still possible to work accurately (46).

This discussion shows once again the elements of complexity and uncertainty that pervade healthcare. We have summarized only a small portion of the evidence on the effects of fatigue on performance. Although it is difficult to find data that unequivocally demonstrate a greater risk of medication error in the presence of fatigue, there is enough indirect evidence to conclude that working while fatigued should be avoided to the extent practicable. Conversely, there is also enough evidence to suggest that safe management of medications (and provision of anesthesia) is at least possible even in the presence of quite severe fatigue. Fatigue should probably be seen as a form of acute ill health, and its implications for continuing to work should be assessed on the circumstances of each particular situation. Common sense would dictate that undertaking potentially dangerous work when unfit should be avoided except in truly necessary circumstances. In those truly necessary circumstances, it would be wise to explicitly name the issue during any time out or briefing and state the need for increased team monitoring and backup of the fatigued member(s) of the team.

8.3.5 Fatigue as a Violation

The fact that airlines, and now many healthcare institutions, have engaged effectively in minimizing the fatigue of staff indicates that this is something that can be done if the will is there to do it. Therefore, we think that a failure to adopt a responsible approach to managing fatigue should be viewed as a violation, and the responsibility for this may well lie as much with those who manage hospitals as with those who work in them. At the same time, the management of fatigue needs to be thoughtful and pragmatic. Notwithstanding the complexities that we have discussed, it seems clear that working longer than 16 (and certainly 24) hours is likely to be associated with at least some deterioration in performance. There is no simple formula for addressing this problem. Those responsible for rosters need to consider circadian factors as well as hours worked. Various fatigue countermeasures can be very helpful, including the provision for staff working at night to take short "power naps" and the use of caffeine (and possibly other stimulants) (46,47). The core requirement is for a safe culture in which both junior and senior doctors (and other staff as well) are expected to declare themselves unfit to work if they have been up all night or have an acute illness and expect to be relieved of their duties without being penalized for speaking up. In well-staffed departments, this may be possible without disrupting services, but from time to time service disruption may be preferable to subjecting patients undergoing elective procedures to unnecessary risk.

A useful test is to ask patients (or perhaps just consider if one were oneself a patient in the same situation) whether they would like their elective surgery to proceed with an anesthesiologist or a surgeon who had no sleep in the last 24 hours (for example). Working when fatigued is an issue that provides a very illuminating illustration of the blurred boundaries that often exist, notably in healthcare, between violation and appropriately pragmatic and dedicated practice.

8.4 Human Factors and Violation

It may be quite difficult to avoid certain violations. There are many barriers between practitioners and good practice. The inadequate provision of dispensers of alcohol solution on wards and in operating rooms is a classic example of a barrier to hand hygiene. Even after such dispensers have been installed, they need to be kept full and functioning. Furthermore, they are more likely to be used if they are designed to be easy to use. The book *The Psychology of Everyday Things* (48) (later renamed *The Design of Everyday Things*) by Norman provides an excellent overview of the role of design in making things intuitive to use and therefore more likely to be used as intended. For example, an upright bellows intuitively informs an anesthesiologist of the state of an anesthetic circuit in a way that a hanging bellows does not (Box 8.2). Norman describes certain things as having *affordances*, meaning that they lend themselves to certain uses. Thus, a bat lends itself to hitting a ball, for example, and a hat almost draws itself to the top of one's head. Jaywalking is common in New Zealand (as it is in many countries) (49). It is not necessarily illegal, and laws on jaywalking vary between countries. Nevertheless, it seems likely to be safer to use a controlled pedestrian crossing if one is available than to jaywalk; most of us, however, will prefer to jaywalk than to walk extra blocks out of our way to reach a controlled crossing. Figure 8.2 shows three footpaths designed to facilitate the flow of pedestrians between two major buildings separated by a road. The buildings are both used by many of the same people because one belongs to a university and the other is a hospital in which the university's staff contribute to the training of health professionals and conduct clinical research. It seems that

---

Box 8.2 Hanging bellows

An excellent example of a good human factors design is to be found in the elimination of the hanging bellows from automatic ventilators. The problem with the hanging bellows is that, in expiration, it defaults to a "full" position because of gravity, even when the anesthetic circuit is disconnected. Therefore, a disconnect of the circuit is not obvious. By contrast, a bellows that is upright collapses and cannot fill when a substantial leak is present in the circuit. A disconnected circuit is immediately visible to anyone in the operating room, and even the sound of the ventilator may change.

It might be thought that a vigilant anesthesiologist ought to be able to detect a circuit disconnect with either type of bellows, particularly from the perspective of a clinician using modern monitoring and the disconnect alarms that are integrated into nearly all anesthesia machines today. However, this monitoring and these alarms have not always been present or reliable. From a human factors perspective, an upright bellows simply makes it easier for this potentially lethal problem to be detected.

the primary purpose of the paths is to reduce the number of people walking directly across a pleasant area of grass, and casual observation suggests that they are reasonably successful in promoting this objective.

One of the paths leads to a pedestrian crossing controlled by traffic lights. The other two lead to points in the road that lack pedestrian crossings. The distance to be walked to go from one building to the other appears to be a little shorter if the latter footpaths are used. At any rate, two of these three paths (i.e., paths 2 and 3 in Figure 8.2) seem to draw people away from the controlled crossing, and one can see jaywalkers using the uncontrolled parts of the road at most times of the day, despite quite heavy traffic. From a human factors perspective, people will tend to choose the easiest way to achieve a goal. The layout of these paths actively promotes this minor violation. The example is also relevant to the discussion later in this chapter of the blurred boundaries between some violations and acceptable practice and the earlier discussion of nuances around the need for a formal rule to determine whether or not a violation has occurred.

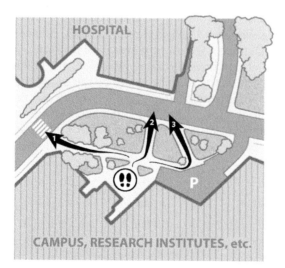

Figure 8.2 Plan of a real situation. A pedestrian (shown by two footprints) wishing to walk from the main entrance of a university healthcare campus (with research institutes and other facilities) to a hospital across the road (in which the university's medical students receive some of their clinical training and much clinical research is undertaken) has three choices; path 1 will take him to a pedestrian crossing controlled with traffic lights, but paths 2 and 3 are a little more direct so many people choose these (particularly path 2) even though these routes require jaywalking to reach the hospital.

To our knowledge, there have been no accidents to date from this jaywalking, and it is not illegal in the country in question. One could argue, therefore, that the practice is reasonable and that no violation is involved. On the other hand, we think most people would accept that there is an increased risk in choosing to cross the road at an uncontrolled point rather than an available pedestrian crossing. Furthermore, if an accident were to occur, we think it is likely that action would be taken to prohibit and prevent jaywalking at this particular location.

8.4.1 Hard and Soft Engineering

As indicated in Chapter 6, a classic illustration of the successful use of improved engineering in medication management in anesthesia is to be found in the pin-indexing systems to prevent incorrect connections of gases to anesthetic machines. Various other forms of physical indexing are now used to ensure that vaporizer fillers fit only into the correct containers for the relevant volatile agents. Antihypoxic devices on anesthetic machines provide another example of successful engineering to eliminate the potential for human error, and so does the decision to simply remove carbon dioxide cylinders from all anesthetic machines after several disasters in which carbon dioxide was administered instead of oxygen. Norman, in a subsequent book, *Things That Make Us Smart: Defending Human Attributes in the Age of the Machine* (50), pointed out that machines lend themselves to certain activities (such as automatically recording physiologic data during an anesthetic), whereas humans are better at other things, such as deciding which medication to administer to a particular patient. In this book, he introduced the idea of design that plays to the strength of both humans and machines, which he called *soft engineering* in contrast to *hard engineering*, in which the aim is to find solutions that eliminate humans altogether. Successes like pin-indexing contributed to the notion that human error can be "engineered out of the system." The dynamic and complex nature of medication management in anesthesia and the perioperative period make it very difficult to find more than isolated opportunities to do this. Unfortunately, many initiatives to improve medication safety today depend on the engagement of clinicians. In effect, clinicians are often asked to take extra care and introduce extra steps into the process of medication management. As with the example of the paths and the jaywalkers, humans have a strong preference for the easiest way to get a job done, and initiatives to improve medication safety that increase workload will usually be difficult to embed in practice.

8.4.1.1 Facilitating Compliance: Oxygen Monitoring and Informed Consent

Pulse oximetry and capnography have had a profound impact on the safety of medication management in anesthesia, specifically in relation to the use of oxygen and the many other powerful medications with which the triad of anesthesia, analgesia, and muscle relaxation are provided. When they were first introduced, their adoption involved a relatively substantial change in practice and considerable advocacy on the part of anesthesiologists. This change was facilitated by the introduction of formal practice standards at Harvard (51), followed either by the wide adoption of these standards or the promulgation of similar local standards in other parts of the world. The introduction of standards was a commendable example of efforts to advance the safety of anesthesia care. The standards not only served to inform practitioners, they also created pressure on funders and institutions to provide the necessary monitoring equipment and to promote its use locally. Another change relevant to the management of medications (again, particularly those inherent in administering anesthesia) that has occurred over the last 30 years or so is to be found in the expectation for so-called "fully informed consent." This change in practice has also been supported by various standards and, in some countries at least, by explicit provision in the law of the land (52). However, the adoption of these two changes in practice has been notably different.

To the extent that it could be afforded (i.e., in effect, throughout the well-resourced parts of the world), monitoring with pulse oximetry and capnography has been enthusiastically and consistently adopted by practitioners. In high-income countries, the use of this monitoring is remarkably uniform, and violations of the relevant standards are virtually unknown. By contrast, within Australia and New Zealand, the law and the formal expectations of the Australian and New Zealand College of Anaesthetists on informed consent are

both clear (52), yet acceptance of the need to provide informed consent has been somewhat slower than that of oximetry and capnography, and there is considerable variation in practice. For example, responses to a survey showed that some anesthesiologists never tell patients that they might die during anesthesia for a laparotomy, whereas others always do – and similar variation occurred in relation to many other key elements of information (53). It is interesting to speculate on the reasons for this difference in adoption (Table 8.1). It is intuitively likely that the factors that led to the rapid adoption of oximetry and capnography include their high face validity, their ease of use, and also the markedly positive messaging they provide about an early adopter. Today everyone uses these monitors, but the first anesthesiologists to do so would have been seen as pioneers and innovators. The use of these monitors is also binary – either one is monitoring the patient with oximetry and capnography or one is not. By contrast, there is a blurring between acceptable and unacceptable ways of obtaining informed consent. Furthermore, it is not a particularly visible activity to one's colleagues, and the fact that an anesthesiologist takes the time to obtain informed consent really well may be invisible to anesthetic colleagues and (particularly during earlier days) may even be a source of irritation to surgical colleagues who may see this as contributing to unnecessary delays.

At some point, failure to properly inform a patient about proposed treatments (including anesthesia) constitutes a violation, but this point is not precisely defined. We can see then that violation may be a binary matter, or it may be a matter of degree and opinion. Furthermore, the likelihood that compliance will be achieved in relation to a particular practice depends on many factors including the design of the system, the face validity of the practice, and the amount of difficulty involved.

One could extend this discussion into many areas of medicine: It seems that providers in general and physicians in particular are much quicker to adopt technical solutions or mechanical advances than the "softer" solutions. As noted, things like capnography, pulse oximetry, pin-indexing, and the elimination of the hanging bellows were all relatively rapidly implemented, while teamwork skills, such as speak-back communication or use

Table 8.1 A comparison of some characteristics of two aspects in which practice has changed over the last 30 years: the routine adoption of pulse oximetry and capnography to monitor anesthetized patients and the practice of obtaining "fully" informed consent from patients for anesthesia (as well as surgery)

	Pulse oximetry and capnography	Informed consent
Required by practice guidelines or standards	Yes	Yes – in some countries
Required by the law of the land	Not explicitly	Variable – but required in many jurisdictions
Compliance or noncompliance is binary	Yes	No – there is a spectrum of practice from poor to excellent
Extra work involved	Hardly any	Considerable
Provides direct, obvious, and immediate assistance to anesthesiologist	Considerable	Minimal
Early adoption benefits practitioners' reputations	Considerable	Variable
Risk of litigation if not adopted and harm occurs	High	High
Visibility of violation	Immediate and obvious	Delayed and less obvious
Cost	Moderate (in purchase and maintenance of equipment)	Moderate (in anesthesiologists' time)
Fun to use or do	Yes, particularly when novel	Neither fun nor comfortable to discuss risk of death or serious adverse events with patients
Makes clinicians' work easier	Yes	No
Supported by level I evidence or expert consensus	Expert consensus (see Box 8.3)	Expert consensus
Clear path of responsibility	Yes, anesthesiologists' "own" pulse oximetry and capnography	Less so – there may be overlap and disagreement between surgeon and anesthesiologist over who should be responsible for covering particular risks, including that of dying after major surgery

of protocols for handoffs, have had inconsistent and difficult uptake. Despite years of evidence and large-scale studies demonstrating the benefit of improved teamwork skills (54) (e.g., for the Surgical Safety Checklist, improved medication reconciliation at each transfer, etc.), we seem to resist improvement in this area. On the other hand, even some highly technical advances, such as barcode scanning in the operating room, have also been met with resistance. The point at which individual resistance to adoption of a new "advance" becomes a violation rather than sensible conservatism is difficult to determine precisely.

8.4.1.2 Process Design and Medication Safety

The disparate elements of the process by which medications are typically prescribed and administered to patients during anesthesia and on the ward provide an impressive example of failure to design safety into the system. With some exceptions, it almost seems as if the science of human factors has been deliberately eschewed. The repeated injunctions from various authorities to "read the label" without a parallel effort to ensure that labels on ampules are legible and easily distinguishable from each other are but one example of this. In earlier chapters we discussed this issue in relation to errors. It is interesting to examine it under a lens focused on violation. Almost every step of the traditional process by which medications are administered according to the "rights" involves extra effort on the part of the practitioner. This effort is not particularly visible, and compliance does not typically translate into enhanced reputation for the clinician in a culture that celebrates heroism and innovation, although it might in a culture that values safety. Safety innovations such as the use of prefilled, prelabeled syringes carry a cost, and the need for that investment is not completely apparent to hospital managers. Standards

---

Box 8.3 The evidence supporting pulse oximetry

A Cochrane review on pulse oximetry (55) reached the following conclusion:

"The studies confirmed that pulse oximetry can detect hypoxaemia and related events. However, we have found no evidence that pulse oximetry affects the outcome of anaesthesia. The conflicting subjective and objective results of the studies, despite an intense, methodical collection of data from a relatively large population, indicate that the value of perioperative monitoring with pulse oximetry is questionable in relation to improved reliable outcomes, effectiveness, and efficiency."

This conclusion has been challenged (56). However, it is correct to say that the mandated use of pulse oximetry is not supported by primary outcome data from one or more randomized controlled trials. Instead, it reflects expert consensus. Yet a decision not to use this monitoring during anesthesia would undoubtedly be seen as a serious violation in any country not constrained by serious economic limitations.

---

and guidelines do exist but have less prominence than those related to monitoring, for example, and also less specificity. In addition, much of the weight behind these standards is expert opinion rather than hard outcome data from randomized controlled trials and thus can be discounted more easily. Conversely, the same could be said about the evidence supporting the standards that mandate the use of pulse oximetry (Box 8.3). Later we return to an analysis of the nature and extent of violation in medication management, but the point here is that the system by which medications are administered perioperatively does seem to be designed not only to produce error, but also to encourage violation. No doubt the real issue is that the processes by which we manage medications in anesthesia and perioperative measurement have not really been subject to an overall process of design – they have mostly just developed over time, with the whole system just growing up like Topsy, as it were.

8.5 Types of Violation

Reason has provided a useful outline of the different types of violation (Table 8.2) (2). In Chapter 7,

Table 8.2 Types of decisions and their corresponding actions. More than one term may apply: for example, something that appears to be an optimizing violation (speeding) may have a satisfactory outcome (reaching the destination earlier) and also fit into the categories of appropriate and correct violations (e.g., with wife in labor, about to deliver[a])

Type of decision or action	Comment
Good practice	Appropriate decisions executed as intended
Error	Completely unintentional
Violation	Intentional (but without intent to cause harm)
Necessary violation	Forced by the system
Appropriate violation	Breaks a rule but for justifiable reasons
Correct violation	Justifiable and with a satisfactory outcome[b]
Routine violation	Characteristic of an individual or an entire population and repeatedly seen in an individual's everyday practice, or widespread within a community (as normalized deviance)
Exceptional violation	Uncharacteristic of an individual and seldom seen in his or her everyday practice
Optimizing violation	Made in pursuit of thrills or gratification
Sabotage	Intentional (and with intent to cause harm)

[a] The appropriateness of this example is debatable and (arguably) depends on the extent of risk taken, noting that the driver is putting other people at risk to serve his own family's interests. A classic example of an appropriate violation is the historical one of lying to the Nazi Secret Service about the fact that one is hiding a Jewish person in one's cellar. However, few things are that straightforward, and we think a judicious use of a mild excess of speed would at least be understandable under the stated circumstances.
[b] Many violations achieve their desired outcome and could arguably be considered "correct": we think this fact alone is insufficient to justify the implications of the name.

we discussed the point that most studies of adverse medication events categorize events on a phenomenological basis. We made the point that few of these studies even attempt to make the basic distinction between errors and violations. Nevertheless, there is value in this distinction and in understanding the different types of violation that might occur. For completeness, it is also worth clearly distinguishing violation from sabotage (see Table 8.2), although the latter is rare in healthcare.

8.5.1 Routine Violations

There are many minor violations in healthcare that have come to be part of everyday practice for individuals or for whole groups of people. Failure to comply with hand hygiene guidelines is an excellent example of a routine violation, and we discuss this important topic in considerable depth later in the chapter. The fact that violations of this kind happen repeatedly every day in most hospitals of the world characterizes them as *routine*. It is typical of routine violations that few people appear to be concerned about them. The widespread tolerance of poor practices is known as *normalized deviance.* If everyone (or almost everyone) does something, it implies a level of acceptance that has its origins in social constructs rather than in science. In fact, bad habits in medical practice are often learned from seniors and simply passed from generation to generation without much active thought. Normalized deviance around any particular violation may be widespread or it may be characteristic of a particular institution, but virtually no institution is altogether free of this problem.

8.5.2 Optimizing Violations and the "Hero" Culture in Healthcare

Optimizing violations gratify the individual concerned. The name is not entirely intuitive, and it would be easy to confuse this category with *necessary* or *appropriate* violations (see our discussion of fatigue for examples of these). A commonly given example of an optimizing violation is that of driving too fast for the thrill of doing so.

Perhaps one of the most difficult human traits to understand and manage is the "powerfulness" construct. It is a joy to accomplish a task with skill and efficiency; for some, seeking this "joy"

becomes thrill seeking, where more and more risks are taken in the belief that "it won't happen to me" (57,58). This may have been what led the captain of the *Costa Concordia* to steer the ocean liner close to the rocks off Isola del Giglio, a significant diversion from the planned course, resulting in a shipwreck and loss of 32 lives (59).

Inherent in some violations is the concept of risk compensation: As a task becomes safer (e.g., as with antilock brakes and seat belts), people take greater risks (e.g., following other cars more closely and changing lanes rapidly); therefore, the overall accident rate does not change (60,61). "Risk tolerance" implies that there is a certain level of risk that humans are comfortable with and that, as safety increases because of better technology, we are willing to take more extreme risks and likely are willing to violate, thinking the rules are unnecessary with the technology in place. An easily recognized example is drivers who would previously have crept cautiously along snowy and iced roadways but drive at normal speeds once their cars are equipped with all-wheel drive and antilock braking technologies.

It is interesting to reflect on the massive cultural and marketing influences that support the notion that an excessive capability for speed is a virtue in the design of motorcars today. Many cars are even designed to *look* fast, and the vast majority of modern cars are capable of speeds far higher than legal limits and of accelerating to such speeds increasingly quickly. Motorcar manufacturers actually market these potentially law-breaking capabilities as virtues. There is a strong argument that at least some responsibility for widespread speeding and the need for considerable investment in patrolling the roads can be placed at the feet of those whose marketing promotes fast driving – although manufacturers are simply catering to a common human preference for thrills rather than safety. Similarly, healthcare management that emphasizes production over safety should be held accountable for doing so. Culture is also important. Imagine a society in which people would be embarrassed to own a car that even looked as if it could go too fast. Then change context and imagine an institution in which both management and staff truly placed the safety of patients at the center of everything they did. By contrast, reflect on the status quo. For many of us, even in well-resourced institutions, the status quo involves working without the full benefit of the numerous technological and organizational supports that could now be put in place to support safe medication practice. There may be many reasons for the continued toleration of this fact, but among these reasons is an element of pride in coping under such circumstances. After all, it is easy to think that a good practitioner should not need technical assistance simply to avoid making errors. This perception of ourselves is part and parcel of the notion of the physician as hero. An anesthesiologist may well take pride in a reputation for being fast and able to manage difficult cases without "fussing" about investigations or tests or demanding extra monitoring or the help of colleagues. A "can-do" attitude can certainly be virtuous in appropriate circumstances, but taking shortcuts or compromising standards primarily in order to gain the respect of certain surgical or other colleagues could reflect the same attitude that underpins optimizing violations.

Although it is quite natural to say that we should simply choose to not drive fast, or to cope heroically without safety advances, thrill seeking in general and the "hero mentality" in particular may be driven as much by genetic polymorphisms as by conscious choices. As early as 1996, the number of repeated exon III alleles on the D4 dopamine receptor was thought to be associated with novelty seeking in males (62). Over the subsequent 20 years, similar polymorphism of the D4 region has been associated with cognitive empathy in females (but not in males) (63,64), with impulsiveness in males with adverse life events (65), and with decreased conscientiousness in male medical students (63). A thorough review of the genetic polymorphism associated with violation behavior is beyond the scope of this book, but it is important to recognize that some of these behaviors are driven as much by nature (perhaps determined by the number of repetitions of a single D4DR) as by nurture and experience (notably of adverse life events). Furthermore, as we noted in Chapter 5 (see Box 5.2), there may well be a place for at least some degree of "heroism" in healthcare, particularly in relation to certain very challenging disciplines.

8.5.3 Exceptional, Appropriate, Necessary, and Correct Violations

Exceptional violations usually arise from circumstances that are themselves exceptional. Health practitioners working in a complex system frequently have to deal with situations that are unique. However many rules one has learned and however much experience one has gained, situations arise from time to time in which problems can only be solved from first principles using System II thinking. Sometimes in such situations a rule may need to be broken, particularly in an emergency. Later in this chapter, we make the point that an anesthesiologist may sometimes think that securing a patient's airway takes precedence over meticulous aseptic practice, and there are certainly circumstances in which this view would be absolutely justifiable. In the words attributed by Paul Brickhill to Harry Day (a fighter pilot in the First World War), *Rules are for the guidance of wise men and the obedience of fools* (66).

Our example (in Table 8.2) of exceeding the speed limit to reach the hospital in an obstetric emergency might be thought of in this way. On the other hand (as noted there), at least some of the increased risk taken in the interests of the pregnant passenger is borne by others – motorists and pedestrians who have nothing to gain from the violation. In a similar way, in healthcare, violations rarely increase the risk of harm to the violator, but only to someone else (needlesticks are an exception to this rule) (57). In this respect, violations are quite different from accepting one risk for a patient in the knowledge that the same patient thereby stands to avoid another more serious risk or to gain in other worthwhile ways. Decisions of this latter type are particularly supportable if made by a patient and a practitioner together, but they may be supportable even if taken by a practitioner for a patient, particularly in circumstances in which the patient cannot be consulted, such as during an anesthetic. For example, it is usually appropriate to turn off the anesthetic vapor while managing serious hypotension during an anesthetic despite the risk of awareness associated with this.

One of the difficulties with breaking a rule or taking a risk in the belief that this is the appropriate thing to do under the circumstances is the tendency for decisions to be judged on their outcomes. If all goes well, the person involved may be commended for a cool head and good sense. Reason uses the term *correct violations* to describe this sort of situation (67), which essentially implies that things worked out well. However, an outcome of this type may simply reflect good luck. If the decision goes wrong, the person may be described as hot-headed and reckless, but it is equally true that the outcome may have more to do with chance than with the quality of the decision. These considerations have much overlap with those discussed in Chapter 7, in relation to so-called "*errors of judgment.*"

One of the best examples of necessary or appropriate violations is that of individuals or groups working while fatigued, where the alternative is for sick patients not to be treated at all.

8.5.4 Routine Violations, Normalized Deviance, and Changes in Practice over Time

In Chapter 6, we discussed the different types of work (see Figure 6.1). It turns out that *work as done* is frequently characterized by routine violations when judged against *work as imagined* or *work as prescribed*. In this section, we explore the reasons for routine violations in greater depth.

8.5.4.1 Why Minor Violations Are Common: Speeding Anesthesiologists and Poor Hand Hygiene

Many minor violations are motivated by understandable objectives. For example, an anesthesiologist exceeding the speed limit may be motivated by the desire to get to the hospital as quickly as possible to deal with an emergency. As with our obstetric example, this violation involves more than simply balancing risk with benefit for one individual, because the burden of risk is shared more widely than the potential benefit. Not only the driver, but other people as well are put to increased risk by the speeding, but for many of these people there is no potential benefit, and they have not had input into the decision to create this risk. Furthermore, the need for urgency could have been anticipated (in a general sense) and addressed by having the appropriate staff on call in hospital rather than at home. This again raises the issue of the responsibility of those who organize healthcare as well as those who deliver it at the sharp end of patient care.

Many violations in healthcare are like this. They occur for understandable reasons, but they are violations nonetheless. Investigation into self-reported violations during medication administration in two pediatric hospitals found that the percentage of nurses reporting their own violations varied from 33.3% to as many as 90.8%, and that violations differed between the unit, the step of the process, and the situation in which the violation occurred (68). Among other factors, these authors concluded that when the work as done on the front lines does not match up with the work as imagined by the designers of the policies or protocols, violations will occur. Busy clinicians often feel that they need to work around aspects of a system that they see as underresourced, overregulated, and poorly designed to support their responsibility to care for patients. Their decisions may appear to be well motivated, but it is unusual for patients to be asked about them, except perhaps in a general way at times of industrial dispute, when unreasonable working conditions are sometimes evoked as justification for various demands or actions.

Interpreting a decision to work around a rule is made more difficult by the fact that hospitals often have an excessive number of policies and rules, many of which appear to have been created and imposed by remote authorities with little clinical experience or understanding of the conditions under which healthcare is delivered. Sensitivity to operations and deference to expertise (see Chapter 9) (69) often seem conspicuous by their absence. This problem is not unique to healthcare, as can be seen from the admonition quoted by Iszatt-White: "Do not slip and maintain control of your vehicle at all times" (57). Another illuminating example was the creation of a policy requiring road repair crews to wear ear protectors to prevent hearing loss, which may have been well meaning but possibly created a greater risk (i.e., that of death) through the repair workers' consequent inability to hear approaching traffic when wearing the protectors (57). Actually, the promulgation of such policies may not even be well meaning. Reason has pointed out that the principal driver for many policies is protection of those responsible for the organization – the directors or the senior managers (2). From that perspective, a view that certain expectations are impracticable and that violation is both reasonable and unlikely to result in material harm to anyone is understandable. A classic example of this is to be found with hand hygiene in the context of anesthesia.

8.5.4.2 Hand Hygiene and Anesthesia

Across the globe, hospital-acquired infections are a serious cause of harm to patients (70,71). Among other aseptic practices, good hand hygiene contributes to the prevention of these infections

> **Box 8.4 The World Health Organization's "My five moments of hand hygiene"**
>
> 1. Before touching a patient
> 2. Before clean/aseptic procedure
> 3. After body fluid exposure risk
> 4. After touching a patient
> 5. After touching patient surroundings
>
> *Source*: From World Health Organization 2009 (77). See www.who.int/infection-prevention/campaigns/clean-hands/5moments/en/, accessed July 18, 2020.

> **Box 8.5 Consensus recommendations on how to perform hand hygiene with category of evidence in brackets. Evidence category IA: Strongly recommended for implementation and strongly supported by well-designed experimental, clinical, or epidemiological studies. Evidence category IB: Strongly recommended for implementation and supported by some experimental, clinical, or epidemiological studies and a strong theoretical rationale. Evidence category II: Suggested for implementation and supported by suggestive clinical or epidemiological studies or a theoretical rationale or a consensus by a panel of experts**
>
> - Wash hands with soap and water when visibly dirty or visibly soiled with blood or other body fluids (IB) or after using the toilet (II).
> - If exposure to potential spore-forming pathogens is strongly suspected or proven, including outbreaks of *Clostridium difficile*, handwashing with soap and water is the preferred means (IB).
> - Use an alcohol-based hand rub as the preferred means for routine hand antisepsis in all other clinical situations if hands are not visibly soiled (IA). If alcohol-based hand rub is not obtainable, wash hands with soap and water (IB).
>
> *Source*: Adapted from World Health Organization 2009 (77), in which each of these approaches is supported by numerous references.

(72–74). In response to widespread failures in hand hygiene, the World Health Organization (WHO) initiated the first global challenge of the WHO World Alliance for Patient Safety, "Clean Care is Safer Care" (75). A key element of this challenge was the development of the WHO Guidelines on Hand Hygiene in Healthcare, which included five defined moments for hand hygiene (Box 8.4 and 8.5) (72,76–78). The Society for Healthcare Epidemiology of America recently published expert guidance on infection prevention in the operating room anesthesia area, beginning with adherence to the WHO five moments (79). Despite widespread promulgation of this guidance, audits of hand hygiene practices routinely show quite substantial proportions of "failed moments" (80). This implies that many healthcare professionals (including anesthesiologists [81]) are commonly violating the requirement for appropriate hand hygiene and thereby exposing patients to an increased risk of infection. Understandably, laypeople are often shocked to learn this, and much effort has been put into initiatives to improve compliance with the rules of hand hygiene in recent times (73,82).

The question arises of why this extra effort should be necessary – why would highly trained professionals like anesthesiologists be so uncaring as to routinely violate hand hygiene requirements? The first step to understanding the answer to this question lies in noting that the same anesthesiologists typically pay close attention to sterility when inserting central venous lines and epidural catheters (for example). This is presumably because these are procedures for which the importance of sterility is more obvious. On the other hand, they may not observe sterility quite so meticulously when placing arterial catheters, per-

haps because central line infections are common and potentially fatal, while arterial line infections are much less common and likely to be less serious if they do occur. Even in respect of central venous lines, it turns out that until recently there has been widespread room for improvement. Interestingly, campaigns to achieve this improvement have met with considerable success (83,84). Thus, it seems likely that poor aseptic technique is more about a lack of conviction that this matters in the particular context than about a lack of concern for patients. Furthermore, some anesthesiologists might argue that failure to comply with the WHO five moments does not in fact equate with poor aseptic technique. They might plausibly believe that they do have adequate aseptic technique, that adequate technique is not equivalent to compliance with the five moments, and that some balance is needed between attention paid to hand hygiene and attention paid to other aspects of anesthesia care. Once again, they might well argue that the guidelines show a lack of sensitivity to operations and deference to expertise (69).

The context of anesthesia is very different than the context of the hospital ward, for which the five moments were designed. The work of anesthesiologists is often very demanding and includes undertaking various tasks (some of which may be difficult), including the administration of a surprisingly high number of intravenous medications, often under considerable time pressure (11). In the period immediately following the induction of anesthesia, the primary responsibility of an anesthetist is to secure the patient's airway. This usually involves contaminating the laryngoscope (and perhaps other instruments) and the anesthesiologists' gloved hands with the patient's saliva and occasionally some blood. Ideally, used instruments should be placed into a specified receptacle to avoid spreading potential infected contaminants to working surfaces in the operating room. Also, the anesthesiologist should remove contaminated gloves before adjusting the flowmeters and other controls on the anesthesia machine to set the rate of administration of gases and vapors to the patient and before reaching for the next syringe of intravenous medication and administering this to the patient. However, we suspect that the image occupying the front of the typical anesthesiologist's mind at such a moment is not one of either the present patient or the next one on the list returning 6 weeks later with an infected postsurgical wound acquired through a sequence of events that began with these failures in aseptic technique. After all, anesthesiologists seldom even see patients who return to hospital because of infection, except for the minority who are brought back for surgical management of that infection. Failures in aseptic technique by an anesthesiologist in the operating room are very loosely coupled to subsequent postoperative infections (see Chapter 6 for a discussion of coupling). Furthermore, it must be rare in practice that a postoperative infection is linked back to such a failure, even where a direct causal relationship actually does exist.

We suspect that a rather different type of image occupies anesthesiologists' minds at times like this. We think their preoccupation is likely to be with avoiding awareness, hypoxia, brain damage, and hemodynamic instability, as well as with positioning their patient safely for surgery. Put simply, an anesthesiologist's primary concern would be the *immediate* safety of the patient. In consequence, anecdotal observation (supported by observations in simulated anesthesia cases [85]) suggests that quite serious failures in aseptic technique are common during the early stages of an anesthetic. In simulation studies, a marker dye placed in a mannequin's oral cavity can be found widely spread across the operating room within 20 minutes of tracheal intubation (see Figure 2.2 [86]). Furthermore, there is a growing body of evidence that failures of asepsis by the anesthesiology team may lead to postoperative infections in some patients (87,88).

During an anesthetic, multiple contacts are typically made with the same patient over quite prolonged periods. Under these circumstances, the risk of spreading microorganisms from one patient to another *during* the anesthetic may appear remote, and it could be argued that the most important time for hand hygiene is *between* patients – at the time between leaving one patient in the postanesthetic care unit (PACU) and beginning to interact with the next one on the operating list. From the perspective of an anesthesiologist, then, the five moments are likely to be perceived as an example of an impracticable guideline of little clinical relevance originating from a remote authority whose knowledge of the clinical context of anesthesia is sparse. It could even be argued that obsessive engagement in the five moments might be a distraction that would increase the net risk to a patient (rather like the ear protector example presented earlier).

Even in the context of hospital wards, the situation in relation to hand hygiene may not be quite as straightforward as it at first seems. To begin with, a strong case can be made that the individual moments are not of equal importance (80). Among the five moments, moment 2 (before clean/aseptic procedure) and moment 3 (after body fluid exposure risk) would seem (intuitively) to create the greatest opportunities for infection for patients. A health professional might well respect these two moments but perhaps not moment 5 (after touching patient surroundings). There is no doubt that the surfaces surrounding a patient may harbor microorganisms, but the risk of transmission of infection to or from a patient through contact with these is probably lower than that associated with changing the dressings of a surgical wound. At the very least, a perception to this effect would be understandable. We are not suggesting that moment 5 is unimportant, simply that a violation related to moment 5 may be perceived as less serious, on average, than one related to moments 2 and 3. Furthermore, it is a substantial burden to insist that all members of a retinue of six or eight people on a busy ward round perform hand hygiene between each patient whether they have had direct contact with that patient or not. This is in marked contrast with insisting that a single person perform hand hygiene before and after dressing a patient's wound.

8.5.4.3 Autonomy and Variation in Healthcare

In the previous examples, we have tried to show how and why an apparently well-motivated practitioner may fall into the habit of making what, on the face of things, look like uncaring violations. We have shown that there may be reasons for choosing to exceed the speed limit or deciding that the benefit of complying with the five moments repeatedly throughout a long case is simply not worth the effort. In Chapter 11, we deal with the belief held by many doctors that it is their right to make autonomous decisions about the care of their patients, on the basis of authority arising from being an attending (or "consultant") physician, with all that implies. There is an appropriate place for the exercise of this autonomy, but violating the five moments is not one of them. They are part of a carefully researched and constructed WHO guideline, well supported by careful analysis of published research and developed through a process of wide consultation. This does not in itself mean that this guideline is perfect in all respects (indeed, we have already suggested that it might not be), but the authority behind it and the process used in its development do place an onus of proof on those who wish to ignore or modify it. It is one thing for a group of skeptical practitioners to provide a careful critique of the guideline's weaknesses in the context of the operating room, supported by their own analysis of the evidence, and then advance and adopt an approach that they collectively agree is better. It is quite another for an individual practitioner to simply ignore a guideline of this type, particularly if it has been endorsed by his or her own institution.

Ideally, collective efforts to improve on a guideline of this sort should include formal adoption of the proposed modification by these practitioners' institution or department. In a perfect world, the change would be audited and the results of the audit published so that others could learn from this experience. The same could be said of other standards and guidelines related to medication management and clinical practice more generally.

The general view of violation developed in this chapter has support from other commentators. In 1997, James Reason advanced the view that "a no-blame" culture is "neither feasible nor desirable." He wrote:

A small proportion of human and unsafe acts are egregious … and warrant sanctions, severe ones in some cases. A blanket amnesty on all unsafe acts lacks credibility in the eyes of the workforce. More importantly, it would be seen to oppose natural justice. What is needed is a just culture, an atmosphere of trust in which people are encouraged, even rewarded, for providing essential safety related information – but in which they are also clear about where the line must be drawn between acceptable and unacceptable behaviour. (67)

More recently, Wachter and Pronovost argued that a "no blame" approach to failures in patient care must be balanced by accountability (89). The existence of substantial levels of normalized deviance in relation to a particular guideline should be seen as an indication for institutional review to understand the underlying reasons and address both the barriers to compliance and the cultural change required to improve that practice. We discuss these matters further in Chapters 11 and 12. The Keystone ICU project (see Box 11.4), led by Pronovost, provides a case study for how leadership within an institution can overcome the problems of unjustified practice variation and minor violation in the name of clinical autonomy.

8.5.4.4 Changes in Practice over Time

Practice typically changes over time. Many practices that were acceptable 30 years ago would not be acceptable today – developments in monitoring anesthetized patients provide an excellent example of this. Today it is unthinkable that practitioners in countries and institutions that have adopted the bundle of measures for reducing central line–associated bloodstream infection (CLABSI) would revert to former idiosyncratic practices. However, such change typically occurs progressively, as in the case of the WHO Surgical Safety Checklist. It is thus possible for a practitioner who fails to change with the times to move from being a role model of best practice to being in violation of emerging standards of care.

As another example, it used to be common for anesthesiologists to use unlabeled syringes for administering intravenous medications. They coded their syringes by size and location to keep track of their contents. At that time, labeling syringes was neither *deemed necessary* nor *appreciated by the individual as advisable*, so failing to label a syringe would not have been a violation. Trainees taught by these practitioners would have correctly believed that they were following standard practice, and they would have mostly continued to practice as they had been taught. Gradually, individual anesthesiologists realized that this approach was unreliable. This realization would have arisen in various ways, including through experience of adverse events due to syringe swaps, logic, talking with colleagues, attending lectures, and reading emerging papers, book chapters, and guidelines. At some point in this evolution of the standard of care, the requirement for syringes (and various lines used in the administration of medications) to be labeled began to be included in formal guidelines (90,91). It became progressively more difficult for individuals to continue in their old ways. Each person would at some point have had to make an active decision and some effort to break established habits and adopt the new and improved practice of labeling syringes.

As practices change, some individuals are early adopters and, for a while, become positive outliers. Over time, as more and more people adopt the new practice, the early adopters are absorbed into the masses, and those who persisted in their old habits become negative outliers. At a certain point in time, a failure to adopt the new standard of practice becomes a violation.

Failing to be an early adopter of a change in practice does not necessarily mean that one is guilty of violation. Not all changes in practice turn out to be justified. A certain threshold of evidence or expert consensus is required before one can reasonably expect most people to adopt a new way of doing things. Even if it is asking too much to expect the substantial commitment of resource associated with initiatives such as the Keystone ICU project to justify every change in practice, it is reasonable to expect a period of education and promotion to get the message across that change is required. Nevertheless, at some point in time, it becomes clear that a change has taken place in the standard of care and that failing to recognize this has become a vio-

lation. However, the exact point in time at which one can say that a practice should be considered unacceptable may be difficult to pinpoint. Unfortunately, it has been estimated that it takes 17 years for new evidence to become the standard of care, and this must be seen as too long (92,93).

It is even more difficult to evaluate the onus on those with overall responsibility for practice within an institution to recognize that change is needed and to do something about it. The nature of normalized deviance is that it is normalized and thus easily overlooked. Until at least some people have pointed out that there is a problem about which something needs to be done, it is probably unreasonable to criticize any group or individual for failing to be the first person to notice this. But once many people have pointed out a problem, there must be some responsibility on institutional leaders to at least evaluate the situation and make a formal decision on whether or not a response is both required and practicable. Again, this is a situation in which reasonable expectations change over time, but a time must come when it is reasonable to say that failing to engage in a problem constitutes a violation.

8.6 Medication Management, Systems, Practitioners, and Violation

We are long past the first of many calls for the persistent and substantial problem of medication safety to be addressed, during anesthesia and more generally within our hospitals and in primary care settings. Furthermore, several worthwhile initiatives have long since been identified that have the potential to improve the design of the system by which medications are administered intravenously to patients during anesthesia and by other routes on hospital wards. We discuss possible approaches to improving medication safety in Chapter 9 and barriers to implementing some or all of these in Chapter 13. Anesthesia colleges and societies have produced guidelines for the administration of medications during anesthesia (91), and the Anesthesia Patient Safety Foundation (APSF) has produced consensus recommendations for improving medication safety in the operating room (see Figure 9.2) (94). Few institutions could claim to be even nearly compliant with any of these guidelines. The question at this point is why hospitals that could afford to take these recommended steps have not done so. Has enough evidence and expert consensus been generated to justify stating that continuing with traditional approaches to medication management is not only a form of normalized deviance but now constitutes a violation? It is not our position that any particular system or device should be adopted. Rather, we are asking whether it is reasonable to expect, as a minimum, that institutions will by now have formally reviewed their current systems of medication management and made formal decisions about what aspects to improve or accept. We return to this theme in Chapter 14.

8.7 Conclusions

The literature has traditionally emphasized error as the primary problem in the genesis of adverse medication events. In this chapter, we have argued that violation is also very important. In the context of medication safety, violation may vary from an individual practitioner's failure to label a syringe to an organization's failure to consider and properly evaluate the wider opportunities to invest in medication safety that exist today. Perhaps the most compelling challenge in this regard is lack of engagement by practitioners in the safety initiatives that are funded within their organizations.

On the basis of research involving operators and supervisors working on oil rigs in the North Sea, Hudson et al. (95,96) describe four main reasons for violations, which neatly summarize the main points we have made in this chapter:

- An expectation that the rules must be violated in order for the work to be done
- A sense of powerfulness, or the feeling that one can skillfully complete the job without needing to follow the rules
- Seeing opportunities for shortcuts that allow the work to be done better or faster
- Inadequate work planning, which results in having to invent the work process as one goes and solve problems as they arise

Hudson et al. offer approaches to reducing violations that are based on understanding *and fixing* the basic reasons why people violate. They comment: "*Do not expect that punishment will be an effective solution; most of the violators in this study were trying to get the job done, on time or faster, in the face of procedures that seem to them to be impossible to follow in the real world*" (95).

An understanding of violation in all its shades, and a greater willingness to name this problem and to expect accountability for it within the context of a just culture, may well be the key to improving medication safety in the future.

References

1. Merry AF, Brookbanks W. *Merry and McCall Smith's Errors, Medicine and the Law*. 2nd ed. Cambridge, UK: Cambridge University Press; 2017.

2. Reason J. *Human Error*. New York, NY: Cambridge University Press; 1990.

3. Baker R, Hurwitz B. Intentionally harmful violations and patient safety: the example of Harold Shipman. *J R Soc Med*. 2009;102(6):223–7.

4. Haines D. The legacy of Dr. Harold Shipman. *Med Leg J*. 2015;83(3):115.

5. Stubbley P. *Frederic Pechier: doctor charged with killing nine patients by "poisoning them during surgery*." London: Independent; 2019. Accessed January 17, 2020. https://www.independent.co.uk/news/world/europe/frederic-pechier-doctor-poison-patients-france-surgery-besancon-a8917811.html

6. Wikipedia contributors. Firefighter arson. Wikipedia, The Free Encyclopedia; 2019. Accessed January 18, 2020. https://en.wikipedia.org/wiki/Firefighter_arson

7. Wikipedia contributors. Harold Shipman. Wikipedia, The Free Encyclopedia; 2018. Accessed January 18, 2020. https://en.wikipedia.org/w/index.php?title=Harold_Shipman&oldid=848386767

8. Williams LS. Anesthetist receives jail sentence after patient left in vegetative state. *CMAJ*. 1995;153:619–20.

9. International Taskforce on Anaesthesia Safety. International standards for a safe practice of anaesthesia. *Eur J Anaesthesiol*. 1993;10(suppl 7):12–15.

10. Gelb AW, Morriss WW, Johnson W, Merry AF, International Standards for a Safe Practice of Anesthesia Workgroup. World Health Organization-World Federation of Societies of Anaesthesiologists (WHO-WFSA) International Standards for a Safe Practice of Anesthesia. *Anesth Analg*. 2018;126(6):2047–55.

11. Merry AF, Webster CS, Hannam J, et al. Multimodal system designed to reduce errors in recording and administration of drugs in anaesthesia: prospective randomised clinical evaluation. *BMJ*. 2011;343:d5543.

12. Rowe L, Galletly DC, Henderson RS. Accuracy of text entries within a manually compiled anaesthetic record. *Br J Anaesth*. 1992;68:381–7.

13. Edwards KE, Hagen SM, Hannam J, et al. A randomized comparison between records made with an anesthesia information management system and by hand, and evaluation of the Hawthorne effect. *Can J Anaesth*. 2013;60(10):990–7.

14. Van Schalkwyk JM, Lowes D, Frampton C, Merry AF. Does manual anaesthetic record capture remove clinically important data? *Br J Anaesth*. 2011;107(4):546–52.

15. Dawson D, Reid K. Fatigue, alcohol and performance impairment. *Nature*. 1997;388:235.

16. Ferguson SA, Thomas MJ, Dorrian J, et al. Work hours and sleep/wake behavior of Australian hospital doctors. *Chronobiol Int*. 2010;27(5):997–1012.

17. Asch DA, Parker RM. The Libby Zion case. One step forward or two steps backward? *N Engl J Med*. 1988;318(12):771–5.

18. Bhananker SM, Cullen BF. Resident work hours. *Curr Opin Anaesthesiol*. 2003;16(6):603–9.

19. Spritz N. Oversight of physicians' conduct by state licensing agencies. Lessons from New York's Libby Zion case. *Ann Intern Med*. 1991;115(3):219–22.

20. Patel N. Learning lessons: the Libby Zion case revisited. *J Am Coll Cardiol*. 2014;64(25):2802–4.

21. Savill R. Tired doctor cleared over patient's death. *The Daily Telegraph*. May 20, 1995.

22. Gander PH, Merry A, Millar MM, Weller J. Hours of work and fatigue-related error: a survey of New Zealand anaesthetists. *Anaesth Intensive Care*. 2000;28(2):178–83.

23. Dement WC. The perils of drowsy driving [editorial]. *N Engl J Med*. 1997;337(11):783–4.

24. Smetzer J, Baker C, Byrne FD, Cohen MR. Shaping systems for better behavioral choices: lessons learned from a fatal medication error. *Jt Comm J Qual Patient Saf*. 2010;36(4):152–63.

25. Parsa-Parsi RW. The revised declaration of Geneva: a modern-day physician's pledge. *JAMA*. 2017;318(20):1971–2.

26. WMA Declaration of Geneva. *Ferney-Voltaire, France*: World Medical Association; 2017. Accessed January 18, 2020. https://www.wma.net/policies-post/wma-declaration-of-geneva/

27. Maisonneuve JJ, Lambert TW, Goldacre MJ. UK doctors' views on the implementation of the European Working Time Directive as applied to medical practice: a quantitative analysis. *BMJ Open*. 2014;4(2):e004391.

28. Clarke RT, Pitcher A, Lambert TW, Goldacre MJ. UK doctors' views on the implementation of the European Working Time Directive as applied to medical practice: a qualitative analysis. *BMJ Open*. 2014;4(2):e004390.

29. Trew A, Searles B, Smith T, Darling EM. Fatigue and extended work hours among cardiovascular perfusionists: 2010 Survey. *Perfusion*. 2011;26(5):361–70.

30. Howard SK, Gaba DM, Smith BE, et al. Simulation study of rested versus sleep-deprived anesthesiologists. *Anesthesiology*. 2003;98(6):1345–55.

31. Landrigan CP, Rothschild JM, Cronin JW, et al. Effect of reducing interns' work hours on serious medical errors in intensive care units. *N Engl J Med*. 2004;351(18):1838–48.

32. Lockley SW, Cronin JW, Evans EE, et al. Effect of reducing interns' weekly work hours on sleep and attentional failures. *N Engl J Med*. 2004;351(18):1829–37.

33. Chu MW, Stitt LW, Fox SA, et al. Prospective evaluation of consultant surgeon sleep deprivation and outcomes in more than 4000 consecutive cardiac surgical procedures. *Arch Surg*. 2011;146(9):1080–5.

34. Ellman PI, Kron IL, Alvis JS, et al. Acute sleep deprivation in the thoracic surgical resident does not affect operative outcomes. *Ann Thorac Surg*. 2005;80(1):60–4.

35. Ellman PI, Law MG, Tache-Leon C, et al. Sleep deprivation does not affect operative results in cardiac surgery. *Ann Thorac Surg*. 2004;78(3):906–11.

36. Howard SK, Gaba DM, Rosekind MR, Zarcone VP. The risks and implications of excessive daytime sleepiness in resident physicians. *Acad Med*. 2002;77(10):1019–25.

37. Gander P, Millar M, Webster C, Merry A. Sleep loss and performance of anaesthesia trainees and specialists. *Chronobiol Int*. 2008;25(6):1077–91.

38. Garden AL, Currie M, Gander PH. Sleep loss, performance and the safe conduct of anaesthesia. In: Keneally J, Jones M, eds. *Australasian Anaesthesia*. Melbourne: Australian and New Zealand College of Anaesthetists; 1996:43–51.

39. Saleh A, Awadalla N, El-masri Y, Sleem W. Impacts of nurses' circadian rhythm sleep disorders, fatigue, and depression on medication administration errors. *Egypt J Chest Dis Tuberc*. 2014;63:145–53.

40. Valentin A, Capuzzo M, Guidet B, et al. Errors in administration of parenteral drugs in intensive

care units: multinational prospective study. *BMJ*. 2009;338:b814.

41. Zhao J, Warman GR, Cheeseman JF. The functional changes of the circadian system organization in aging. *Ageing Res Rev.* 2019;52:64–71.

42. Webster CS, Merry AF, Larsson L, McGrath KA, Weller J. The frequency and nature of drug administration error during anaesthesia. *Anaesth Intensive Care.* 2001;29(5):494–500.

43. Cheeseman JF, Webster CS, Pawley MDM, et al. Use of a new task-relevant test to assess the effects of shift work and drug labelling formats on anesthesia trainees' drug recognition and confirmation. *Can J Anaesth.* 2011;58(1):38–47.

44. Silbert BS, Maruff P, Evered LA, et al. Detection of cognitive decline after coronary surgery: a comparison of computerized and conventional tests. *Br J Anaesth.* 2004;92(6):814–20.

45. Griffiths JD, McCutcheon C, Silbert BS, Maruff P. A prospective observational study of the effect of night duty on the cognitive function of anaesthetic registrars. *Anaesth Intensive Care.* 2006;34(5):621–8.

46. Merry AF, Warman GR. Fatigue and the anaesthetist. *Anaesth Intensive Care.* 2006;34(5):577–8.

47. Huffmyer JL, Kleiman AM, Moncrief M, et al. Impact of caffeine ingestion on the driving performance of anesthesiology residents after 6 consecutive overnight work shifts. *Anesth Analg.* 2020;130(1):66–75.

48. Norman DA. *The Psychology of Everyday Things.* New York, NY: Basic Books; 1998.

49. Shadwell T. Jaywalk and you could be in court. *Dominion Post.* February 10, 2014.

50. Norman D. *Things That Make Us Smart: Defending Human Attributes in the Age of the Machine.* Reading, MA: Perseus; 1993.

51. Eichhorn JH, Cooper JB, Cullen DJ, et al. Standards for patient monitoring during anesthesia at Harvard Medical School. *JAMA.* 1986;256(8):1017–20.

52. Braun AR, Skene L, Merry AF. Informed consent for anaesthesia in Australia and New Zealand. *Anaesth Intensive Care.* 2010;38(5):809–22.

53. Braun AR, Leslie K, Merry AF, Story D. What are we telling our patients? A survey of risk disclosure for anaesthesia in Australia and New Zealand. *Anaesth Intensive Care.* 2010;38(5):935–8.

54. Wahr JA, Prager RL, Abernathy JH 3rd, et al. Patient safety in the cardiac operating room: human factors and teamwork: a scientific statement from the American Heart Association. *Circulation.* 2013;128(10):1139–69.

55. Pedersen T, Nicholson A, Hovhannisyan K, et al. Pulse oximetry for perioperative monitoring. *Cochrane Database Syst Rev.* 2014;(3):CD002013.

56. Merry AF, Eichhorn JH, Wilson IH. Extending the WHO "Safe Surgery Saves Lives" project through global oximetry. *Anaesthesia.* 2009;64(10):1045–8.

57. Iszatt-White M. Catching them at it: an ethnography of rule violation. *Ethnography.* 2007;8(4):445–65.

58. Reason J. *The Human Contribution: Unsafe Acts, Accidents and Heroic Recoveries.* Burlington, VT: Ashgate Publishing; 2008.

59. Anonymous. *Costa Concordia: Captain Schettino tried to "impress."* BBC News. December 2, 2014. Accessed January 18, 2020. https://www.bbc.com/news/world-europe-30297395

60. Janssen W. Seat-belt wearing and driving behavior: an instrumented-vehicle study. *Accid Anal Prev.* 1994;26(2):249–61.

61. Sagberg F, Fosser S, Saetermo IA. An investigation of behavioural adaptation to airbags and antilock brakes among taxi drivers. *Accid Anal Prev.* 1997;29(3):293–302.

62. Ebstein RP, Novick O, Umansky R, et al. Dopamine D4 receptor (D4DR) exon III polymorphism associated with the human personality trait of Novelty Seeking. *Nat Genet.* 1996;12(1):78–80.

63. Ham BJ, Lee YM, Kim MK, et al. Personality, dopamine receptor D4 exon III polymorphisms, and academic achievement in medical students. *Neuropsychobiology.* 2006;53(4):203–9.

64. Uzefovsky F, Shalev I, Israel S, et al. The dopamine D4 receptor gene shows a gender-sensitive association with cognitive empathy: evidence from two independent samples. *Emotion.* 2014;14(4):712–21.

65. Reiner I, Spangler G. Dopamine D4 receptor exon III polymorphism, adverse life events and personality traits in a nonclinical German adult sample. *Neuropsychobiology.* 2011;63(1):52–8.

66. Brickhill P. *Reach for the Sky: The Story of Douglas Bader DSO, DFC.* London: Odhams Press Ltd; 1954.

67. Reason J. *Managing the Risks of Organizational Accidents.* London: Routledge; 1997.

68. Alper SJ, Holden RJ, Scanlon MC, et al. Self-reported violations during medication administration in two paediatric hospitals: A systematic review of safety violations in industry. *BMJ Qual Saf.* 2012;21:408–15.

69. Weick KE, Sutcliffe KM. *Managing the Unexpected: Resilient Performance in an Age of Uncertainty.* 2nd ed. San Francisco, CA: Jossey-Bass; 2007.

70. Zimlichman E, Henderson D, Tamir O, et al. Health care-associated infections: a meta-analysis of costs and financial impact on the US health care system. *JAMA Intern Med.* 2013;173(22):2039-46.

71. Donaldson LJ, Panesar SS, Darzi A. Patient-safety-related hospital deaths in England: thematic analysis of incidents reported to a national database, 2010–2012. *PLoS Med.* 2014;11(6):e1001667.

72. Allegranzi B, Pittet D. Role of hand hygiene in healthcare-associated infection prevention. *J Hosp Infect.* 2009;73(4):305-15.

73. Allegranzi B, Gayet-Ageron A, Damani N, et al. Global implementation of WHO's multimodal strategy for improvement of hand hygiene: a quasi-experimental study. *Lancet Infect Dis.* 2013;13(10):843-51.

74. Huang GKL, Stewardson AJ, Grayson ML. Back to basics: hand hygiene and isolation. *Curr Opin Infect Dis.* 2014;27(4):379-89.

75. Pittet D, Allegranzi B, Storr J. The WHO Clean Care is Safer Care programme: field-testing to enhance sustainability and spread of hand hygiene improvements. *J Infect Public Health.* 2008;1(1):4-10.

76. Allegranzi B, Pittet D. Healthcare-associated infection in developing countries: simple solutions to meet complex challenges. *Infect Control Hosp Epidemiol.* 2007;28(12):1323-7.

77. Clean Care is Safer Care Team. *WHO Guidelines on Hand Hygiene in Health Care: a Summary.* Geneva: World Health Organization; 2009. Accessed January 18, 2020. https://apps.who.int/iris/bitstream/handle/10665/70126/WHO_IER_PSP_2009.07_eng.pdf;jsessionid=427B1CDF65656AAC96D50E4329449EE3?sequence=1

78. Lau T, Tang G, Mak KL, Leung G. Moment-specific compliance with hand hygiene. *Clin Teach.* 2014;11(3):159-64.

79. Munoz-Price LS, Bowdle A, Johnston BL, et al. Infection prevention in the operating room anesthesia work area. *Infect Control Hosp Epidemiol.* 2018;11:1-17.

80. Lucas NC, Hume CG, Al-Chanati A, et al. Student-led intervention to inNOvate hand hygiene practice in Auckland Region's medical students (the No HHARMS study). *N Z Med J.* 2017;130(1448):54-63.

81. Koff MD, Loftus RW, Burchman CC, et al. Reduction in intraoperative bacterial contamination of peripheral intravenous tubing through the use of a novel device. *Anesthesiology.* 2009;110(5):978-85.

82. Stone SP, Fuller C, Savage J, et al. Evaluation of the national Cleanyourhands campaign to reduce *Staphylococcus aureus* bacteraemia and *Clostridium difficile* infection in hospitals in England and Wales by improved hand hygiene: four year, prospective, ecological, interrupted time series study. *BMJ.* 2012;344:e3005.

83. Pronovost P, Needham D, Berenholtz S, et al. An intervention to decrease catheter-related bloodstream infections in the ICU. *N Engl J Med.* 2006;355(26):2725-32.

84. Gray J, Proudfoot S, Power M, et al. Target CLAB Zero: a national improvement collaborative to reduce central line-associated bacteraemia in New Zealand intensive care units. *N Z Med J.* 2015;128(1421):13-21.

85. Gargiulo DA, Sheridan J, Webster CS, et al. Anaesthetic drug administration as a potential contributor to healthcare-associated infections: a prospective simulation-based evaluation of aseptic techniques in the administration of anaesthetic drugs. *BMJ Qual Saf.* 2012;21(10):826-34.

86. Birnbach DJ, Rosen LF, Fitzpatrick M, et al. Double gloves: a randomized trial to evaluate a simple strategy to reduce contamination in the operating room. *Anesth Analg.* 2015;120(4):848-52.

87. Loftus RW, Brown JR, Koff MD, et al. Multiple reservoirs contribute to intraoperative bacterial transmission. *Anesth Analg.* 2012;114(6):1236-48.

88. Loftus RW, Koff MD, Birnbach DJ. The dynamics and implications of bacterial transmission events arising from the anesthesia work area. *Anesth Analg.* 2015;120(4):853-60.

89. Wachter RM, Pronovost PJ. Balancing "no blame" with accountability in patient safety. *N Engl J Med.* 2009;361(14):1401-6.

90. Merry AF, Shipp DH, Lowinger JS. The contribution of labelling to safe medication administration in anaesthetic practice. *Best Pract Res Clin Anaesthesiol.* 2011;25(2):145-59.

91. Australian and New Zealand College of Anaesthetists. *Guidelines for the Safe Administration of Injectable Drugs in Anaesthesia.* Melbourne: Australian and New Zealand College of Anaesthetists; 2009. *Policy document PS 51.*

92. Institute of Medicine. *Crossing the Quality Chasm: A New Health System for the 21st Century.* Washington, DC: National Academy Press; 2001.

93. Morris ZS, Wooding S, Grant J. The answer is 17 years, what is the question: understanding

time lags in translational research. *J R Soc Med.* 2011;104(12):510–20.

94. Eichhorn J. APSF hosts medication safety conference: consensus group defines challenges and opportunities for improved practice. *APSF Newsletter.* 2010;25(1):1–7. Accessed January 3, 2020. www.apsf.org/article/apsf-hosts-medication-safety-conference/

95. Hudson P, Verschuur W, Parker D, Lawton R, van der Graaf G. *Bending the rules: managing violation in the workplace.* Leiden: Centre for Safety Science, Leiden University; 1998. Accessed January 21, 2020. https://www.naris.com/wp-content/uploads/2016/10/Bending-the-rules.pdf

96. Hudson P, Verschuur W, Lawton R, Parker D, Reason J. *Bending the rules II: the violation manual.* Leiden: Centre for Safety Science, Leiden University; 1997. Accessed January 21, 2020. https://www.academia.edu/21944364/Bending_the_Rules_Managing_Violation_in_the_Workplace

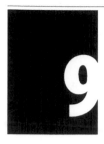

9 Interventions to Improve Medication Safety

9.1 Introduction

The extensive variability in how errors are reported from location to location and the wide variability in work processes in different locations make it difficult to define, for all locations, and for all institutions, what interventions will indisputably make the medication process safer. This view has been espoused again and again in the literature, with little change over the past 20 years (1). In addition, it is clear that local safety culture and climate vary substantially, even between units within the same hospital (2); these variations will influence which interventions are likely to improve local medication safety, and which would likely just represent extra work without benefit. Interventions can range from small improvements in workflow (e.g., always providing a sheath of appropriate size when stocking intensive care units [ICUs] with temporary pacing wires) (3) to system-wide capital expenditures on things such as electronic health records and computerized physician order entry (CPOE). Every proposed intervention should be evaluated for its strength in preventing errors (Table 9.1), as many will have little to no impact (e.g., a new policy is seldom effective in reducing error). Unfortunately, the easy and cheap interventions (e.g., admonitions to try harder, reeducation, writing a policy or procedure) are generally weak at preventing the next error. Strong interventions, such as forcing functions (e.g., pin-indexing of gas and vapor connections), CPOE and the use of barcoding, increased staffing, or increased executive involvement are more expensive. As discussed later, very often improvements in medication safety come not with a single decisive intervention but through a comprehensive bundle of interventions (4–7); the key to success lies in the aggregation of multiple marginal gains (8). Although these multifaceted approaches typically reduce medication errors, it is not possible to determine which of the component interventions was more or less responsible for the improvement.

For many of the interventions described later, recommendations can only be based on expert opinion. Randomized controlled trial (RCT) evidence would be ideal, but the challenges in accurately measuring medication errors make it difficult to perform such trials. Simulation offers an alternative approach for testing interventions (9–13), but simulation-based research into medication error is not yet widespread. For major technological solutions such as CPOE, or barcode-assisted medication administration, it has been possible to analyze error rates pre- and postimplementation, or between similar units with and without that technology. For example, Nuckols et al. conducted a meta-analysis of 16 studies comparing CPOE with paper order entry that provides relatively convincing evidence of a clinically worthwhile reduction in medication errors and in adverse medication events, but with a caveat related to weak study designs (Figure 9.1): CPOE was associated with half as many preventable adverse medication events (pooled risk ratio [RR] = 0.47, 95% confidence interval [CI] 0.31–0.71) and medication errors (RR = 0.46, 95% CI 0.35–0.60) as paper order entry (14). However, many suggested or theoretical best practices have not been tested or sometimes even precisely defined (e.g., advice to "avoid look-alikes" or "provide adequate lighting"). The fact that many individuals use the lack of evidence to defend their autonomy to practice in whatever way they prefer is discussed in Chapter 12. Jensen et al. (15) have argued that "a paucity of evidence at levels I and II does not justify such idiosyncrasy." These authors went on to state, "On the contrary, Sackett et al. state that evidence-based medicine implies 'tracking down the best external evidence with which to answer our clinical questions' (16)." This "best external evidence" would certainly start with randomized trials, but if such evidence does not exist, "we must follow the trail to the next best external evidence and work

Table 9.1 Strength of interventions to improve medication safety, with examples

Weaker actions	Intermediate actions	Stronger actions
Double checks	Checklists or other cognitive aids	Architectural or physical changes
Warnings and labels	Increased staffing or reduced workload	Tangible involvement and action by leadership in support of patient safety
New procedures, memoranda, or policies	Redundancy	Simplification of process or removal of unnecessary steps
Training and education	Enhanced communication techniques (e.g., read back)	Standardization of equipment and process of care mapping
Additional study or analysis	Software enhancements Elimination of look-alike and sound-alike medications Separation of dangerous medications (strong KCl) from routine medications Elimination or reduction of distractions	New device usability testing before purchase Forcing functions (e.g., pin-indexing of cylinders)

Source: Adapted from part of the Agency for Healthcare Research and Quality's Learn from Defects Tool (3) (and see www.ahrq.gov/hai/cusp/toolkit/learn-defects.html, accessed January 10, 2020).

from there" (16). Such evidence would come from clinical experience, expert consensus, thoughtful deliberations about how and why errors have occurred, and even Delphi processes to formulate recommendations for safe medication processes.

There are several systematic reviews of medication error reduction strategies; recommendations from two are presented in Table 9.2. The first, from Wahr et al. (17), updated an earlier review of strategies for use in anesthesia by Jensen and colleagues (15); the second by Miller and colleagues concerned strategies specific to pediatric care (1). Nearly all of the recommendations in both settings are based on expert opinion, but it is remarkable how similar the recommendations are. The list of recommendations for the operating room is more detailed than that for pediatrics, but there are many common themes that are applicable in all settings. The Institute for Safe Medication Practices (ISMP) has published a toolkit for institutions to use in evaluating their medication error prevention strategies: this list was used in the Wahr review but was not available at the time of the Miller review. It is more detailed than either of the lists in Table 9.2 and covers virtually every possible aspect of medication safety.

The Anesthesia Patient Safety Foundation (APSF) held two expert meetings to synthesize all available evidence and opinion into "Consensus Recommendations for Improving Medication Safety in the Operating Room" (Figure 9.2) (18). What follows here is more a conceptual overview of the major strategies than an exhaustive list of every possible intervention that has been proposed. We have structured this chapter on the APSF guidelines.

9.2 Culture

The concept of "safety culture" or "safety climate" originated in industries that consistently achieve high reliability despite performing complex and often dangerous work, such as commercial aviation and the nuclear power industry. An aircraft carrier provides another example of a high-reliability organization (HRO). The traits that characterize these HROs include (1) a reluctance to oversimplify reasons for errors, (2) a preoccupation with failure, (3) a sensitivity to operations, (4) a deference to expertise, and (5) resilience in the face of errors (19). In healthcare and within the field of medication safety, preoccupation with failure begins with a nonpunitive environment where workers can report incidents and errors without fear of retaliation or discipline. The preoccupation with failure establishes a culture where each team member is continually watching for and then reporting potential system vulnerabilities that expose a patient to danger. These vulnerabilities are what Reason calls "error traps," situations that predispose any individual to make an error. Teams that are preoccupied with failure are more open to understanding their errors and are also reluctant to accept the first and easiest explanation for an error, using multidisciplinary groups to design solutions. A culture of safety also reduces the power differential between roles and works to eliminate disruptive and disrespectful behavior (20). A prospective, cross-sectional study

A

Study	CPOE Errors, N	CPOE Units, N	Paper Errors, N	Paper Units, N	Weight	Risk Ratio, D-L, Random (95%-CI)	
Bates 1998	54	11,235*	127	12,218	6.08	0.46 (0.34-0.64)	
Bates 1999	50	1,878*	242	1,704	6.12	0.19 (0.14-0.25)	
Bizovi 2002	11	1,594†	54	2,326	4.81	0.30 (0.16-0.57)	
Oliven 2005	220	5,033*	617	4,969	6.50	0.35 (0.30-0.41)	
Shulman 2005	117	2,429†	71	1,036	6.15	0.70 (0.52-0.94)	
Barron 2006	77	240,096‡	252	240,096	6.27	0.31 (0.24-0.39)	
Colpaert 2006	35	1,286†	106	1,224	5.86	0.31 (0.21-0.46)	
Aronsky 2007	73	2,567†	125	3,383	6.17	0.77 (0.58-1.03)	
Mahoney 2007	2,319	1,390,789†	4,960	1,452,346	6.62	0.49 (0.47-0.51)	
Wess 2007	57	13,105†	239	8,595	6.17	0.16 (0.12-0.21)	
Franklin 2009	127	501*	135	438	6.30	0.88 (0.65-1.05)	
van Doormal 2009	1,203	7,068†	3,971	7,106	6.61	0.31 (0.29-0.33)	
Shawnha 2011	1,142	14,064†	3,008	13,328	6.61	0.36 (0.34-0.39)	
Leung 2012	645	1,000§	550	1,000	6.56	1.17 (1.04-1.31)	
Menendez 2012	1,197	11,347§	356	7,001	6.55	2.08 (1.84-2.34)	
Westbrook 2012	1,029	629§	4,270	1,053	6.61	0.40 (0.38-0.43)	

Total Medication Errors: 8,361(CPOE); 19,083 (Paper)
Tests for Heterogeneity: I² 98%; Q statistic p < 0.0001
Overall Effect: z = -5.62, p < 0.0001

Overall 0.46 (0.35-0.60)

Intervention Design and Implementation (I), Contextual (C), and Methodological (M) Factors

I: *Type of Developer*	Homegrown (6 studies)	**0.37 (0.29-0.47)**
	Commercial (9 studies)	**0.56 (0.36-0.85)**
I: *Clinical Decision Support - Any*	Absent (4 studies)	**0.51 (0.31-0.87)**
	Present (12 studies)	**0.44 (0.32-0.62)**
I: *Clinical Decision Support - Sophistication*	Basic (4 studies)	**0.40 (0.38-0.87)**
	Moderate or Advanced (6 studies)	**0.51 (0.26-0.97)**
I: *Scope of Implementation*	Limited Number of Units (12 studies)	**0.38 (0.32-0.46)**
	Hospital-wide (4 studies)	**0.78 (0.36-1.70)**
C: *Country*	U.S. (9 studies)	**0.39 (0.27-0.57)**
	Non-U.S. (7 studies)	**0.56 (0.35-0.89)**
M: *Event Detection Methods*	Pharmacist Order Review (7 studies)	**0.38 (0.27-0.53)**
	More Comprehensive Methods (9 studies)	**0.53 (0.36-0.79)**

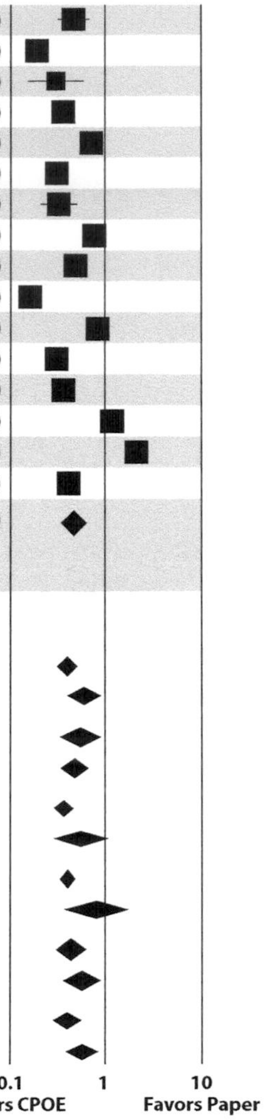

0.1   1   10
Favors CPOE   Favors Paper

B

Study	CPOE pADEs, N	CPOE Units, N	Paper pADEs, N	Paper Units, N	Weight	Risk Ratio, D-L, Random (95%-CI)	Risk Ratio, D-L, Random (95%-CI)
Bates 1998	41	11,235*	55	12,218	22.96	0.811 (0.541–1.215)	
Bates 1999	2	11,878*	55	1,704	5.19	0.363 (0.707–1.871)	
Colpaert 2006	2	80*	12	80	6.01	0.167 (0.037–0.745)	
van Doormal 2009	44	603*	92	592	24.09	0.470 (0.328–0.672)	
Leung 2012	70	1,000†	106	1,000	25.46	0.660 (0.488–0.893)	
Menendez 2012	11	11,347†	33	7,001	16.29	0.206 (0.104–0.407)	

Total pADEs: 170(CPOE); 303 (Paper)
Tests for Heterogeneity: I² 69.4%; Q statistic p = 0.0059
Overall Effect: z = –3.59, p = 0.0003

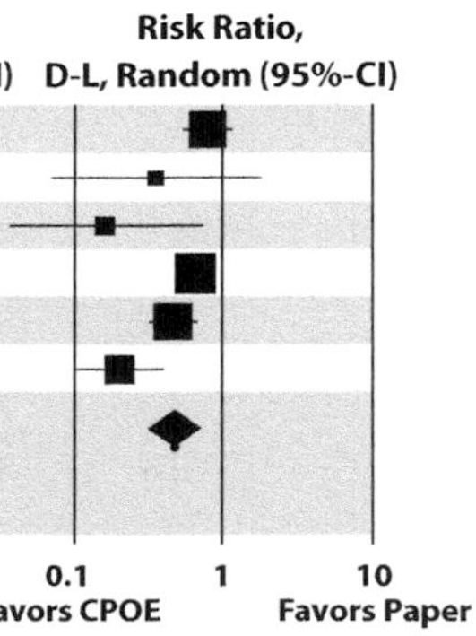

0.471 (0.312–0.710)

0.1   1   10
Favors CPOE   Favors Paper

Figure 9.1 Meta-analysis: relative risk of medication errors and adverse medication events with computerized physician order entry (CPOE) versus paper order entry (Paper) in hospital acute care settings. Units of exposure: *1000 patient days; †orders; ‡dispensed doses; §admissions. The majority of trial designs were pre/post or comparisons of similar units. With permission from Nuckols et al. 2014 (14). (A) All medication errors. (B) Adverse medication events. Units of exposure: *1000 patient days; †admissions.

158

Table 9.2 Recommended approaches to reducing medication errors in the operating room and in pediatric care

Medication safety in the operating room	Medication safety in pediatric care (focused on both the ward and the intensive care unit)
Complete medication reconciliation Medications in standard format in chart	
Single location for recording medications across surgery (pre-, intra-, postanesthetic care unit)	Accurate documentation of medication administration

Time-out includes:
  Patient identification
  Weight
  Allergies
  Medication information, such as antibiotic given
	Standardize metrics (kg, cm rather than pounds, inches)

Automated alerts within anesthesia information system:
  Dose
  Allergy
  Medication-medication interactions
	Computer alerts for potential adverse medication events
	Standardize order sheets to include allergies and weight

Establish weight-based dose limits[a]
  Infusion device has prompts regarding limits
  Computer prompted
  Paper sheet to consult
	Calculation tools for emergency medications

Cognitive aids, checklists, protocols; infusion rate charts Specialized carts have protocols	Easy access to current clinical information and references

Medication trays in anesthesia carts:
  Standardized across all locations
  Tray divisions labeled clearly
  Medications placed to minimize confusion
  Modular system
  Pharmacy manages medication trays	

Eliminate unusual medications from usual locations
  Unique location or tray
  Remove at end of case	

Single-use vials preferable If multidose vial required, discard at end of case	

Management of high-risk/dangerous medications
  No concentrated medications
  Only one standard concentration on cart
  Pharmacy provides diluted, high-risk medications (insulin, heparin)
  Alert label on concentrated or high-risk medications
  No large-volume epinephrine
	Medication standardization and appropriate storage

Separate regional cart for regional medications	
Only preservative-free local anesthetics	
Subcutaneous or topical local anesthetics clearly labeled	
Pharmacy prepares all compounded medications	
Regional anesthetic solutions clearly segregated from intravenous medications	

Table 9.2 (cont.)

Medication safety in the operating room	Medication safety in pediatric care (focused on both the ward and the intensive care unit)
Every medication labeled with name, date, concentration[a]	Clear and accurate labeling
Barcode system used	
Preprinted, color coded per ISO standards	
Avoid abbreviations and trailing zeros	
Unlabeled syringe immediately discarded	
Minimize provider-prepared syringes	
Prefilled whenever possible	
Compounded and diluted medications prepared by pharmacy	
When provider prepares dilutions of high-risk medications use two-person check or careful double check	
Verify high-risk medication and weight-based doses with two people	Special procedures and protocols for high-alert medications
Asepsis	
Cap syringes	
Sterile technique for spinal/epidural placement, injection	
Read and verify every vial, ampule, syringe label prior to administration[a]:	Barcoding for medication administration
Barcode system in use with audible and visual cues	
Use a two-person check	
Single-person check	
Smart pump used for all infusions	Standardize equipment
Smart pumps are standardized across units	
Pumps have libraries with guardrails and alerts	
Clearly identify route of administration:	
Route specific administration sets (epidural, intravenous, etc.)	
Color-coding (yellow epidural, red arterial)	
Labels on every infusion line and port	
No ports on epidural/intrathecal lines	
Sterile field medications:	
Only one medication passed to field at a time	
Checked and verified aloud by two persons	
Labeled with medication name, date, concentration	
Any unlabeled discarded	
Segregation of topical or irrigation fluids (not in parenteral syringe)	
Handovers (shift changes, relief, postanesthetic care unit/intensive care unit, nurse, doctor) have protocol-driven review of medications given and all medications on cart, field	
Verbal medication orders verified by speak back, announced when given, entered into chart (preferably recorded in anesthesia information management system)	Policies on verbal orders
Discard all syringes, containers, multidose vials at end of case unless connected to patient – clean sweep	
Nonpunitive quality assurance system for incident reporting, analysis, and intervention	Quality improvement efforts: medication use evaluation, incident reporting/review

Table 9.2 *(cont.)*

Medication safety in the operating room	Medication safety in pediatric care (focused on both the ward and the intensive care unit)
Written policies for medication safety; adequate teaching of new staff on policies	
Establish a culture of respect and collaboration that endorses patient safety and establishes compliance (just culture/compliance)	Encourage team environment for review of orders
Adequate supervision, teaching, and in-service training	Training on appropriate prescribing, labeling, dispensing, monitoring, and administration
Formulary designed to avoid purchase of look-alike medications; when unable to avoid, do not store in proximity; add alert labels to look-alike medications	
Pharmacist assigned to support operating room	Pharmacist participation in clinical care
Pharmacists available 24/7 for questions	Pharmacist on call when pharmacy closed
Pharmacists participate in educational, morbidity and mortality meetings	
Operating room pharmacists receive specialized education about operating room	
Pharmacy responsible for medication flow (ordering to discard)	Pediatric presence with formulary management
Pharmacy stocks, tracks, delivers medication trays	Appropriate pharmacy personnel and environment
Pharmacy prepares all compounded or diluted high-risk medications	Pharmaceutical software
Pharmacy prepares infusions	
Policy for return of unused or unusual medications – clean sweep	Computerized provider order entry
	Automated dispensing devices
	Unit dose distribution systems
	Reduce adverse medication events related to anticoagulants
	Patient education on medications

Source: Column one, relating to the operating room, from Wahr et al. 2017 (17); column two, relating to pediatric care, from Miller et al. 2007 (1).
[a] Recommendations listed in order of strength per Table 9.1.

done in 57 ICUs in three countries collected self-reported medical errors and assessments of safety climate. Units with a better safety climate had significantly lower risk of medication and dislodgement (i.e., of lines and tubes) errors (odds ratio [OR] per standard deviation 0.62, 95% CI 0.51–0.89) (21).

Singer and Vogus (22) provide a conceptual framework for establishing a climate of safety, recognizing three types of interventions: those that *enable* (e.g., leadership activity that promotes safety and creates an environment where frontline staff can improve safety); those that *enact* (e.g., work done by frontline staff to identify and correct system vulnerabilities); and those that *elaborate* (e.g., through continually and systematically reflecting on and improving safety efforts). It is beyond the

scope of this book to review all of the interventions that have been tested for efficacy in improving safety culture; the interested reader is directed to these authors' exhaustive review of nearly 200 studies of interventions to build a safety culture (22).

9.2.1 Leadership and a Comprehensive Medication (Patient) Safety Program

Leadership is critical to the establishment of a safety culture; without clear support from executives, no safety culture can exist. Transformational leadership, defined as providing an inspiring vision for the organization and encouraging all staff to identify with this vision, is strongly associated with improving safety culture (20). As noted earlier,

Consensus Recommendations for Improving Medication Safety in the Operating Room

Standardization

1. High alert drugs (such as phenylephrine and epinephrine) should be available in standardized concentrations/diluents prepared by pharmacy in a ready-to-use (bolus or infusion) form that is appropriate for both adult and pediatric patients.
Infusions should be delivered by an electronically-controlled smart device containing a drug library.

2. Ready-to-use syringes and infusions should have standardized fully compliant machine-readable labels.

3. *Additional Ideas:*
   a) Interdisciplinary and uniform curriculum for medication administration safety to be available to all training programs and facilities.

   b) No concentrated versions of any potentially lethal agents in the operating room.

   c) Required read-back in an environment for extremely high alert drugs such as heparin.

   d) Standardized placement of drugs within all anesthesia workstations in an institution.

   e) Convenient required method to save all used syringes and drug containers until case concluded.

   f) Standardized infusion libraries/protocols throughout an institution.

   g) Standardized route-specific connectors for tubing (IV, arterial, epidural, enteral).

Technology

1. Every anesthetizing location should have a mechanism to identify medications before drawing up or administering them (bar code reader) and a mechanism to provide feedback, decision support, and documentation (automated information system).

2. *Additional Ideas:*
   a) Technology training and device education for all users, possibly requiring formal certification.

   b) Improved and standardized user interfaces on infusion pumps.

   c) Mandatory safety checklists incorporated into all operating room systems.

Pharmacy/Prefilled/Premixed

1. Routine provider-prepared medications should be discontinued whenever possible.

2. Clinical pharmacists should be part of the perioperative/operating room team.

3. Standardized pre-prepared medication kits by case type should be used whenever possible.

4. *Additional Ideas:*
   a) Interdisciplinary and uniform curriculum for medication administration safety for all anesthesia professionals and pharmacists.

   b) Enhanced training of operating room pharmacists specifically as perioperative consultants.

   c) Deployment of ubiquitous automated dispensing machines in the operating room suite (with communication to central pharmacy and its information management system).

Culture

1. Establish a *"just culture"* for reporting errors (including near misses) and discussions of lessons learned.

2. Establish a culture of education, understanding, and accountability via a required curriculum and CME and dissemination of dramatic stories in the *APSF Newsletter* and educational videos.

3. Establish a culture of cooperation and recognition of the benefits of STPC within and between institutions, professional organizations, and accreditation agencies.

Figure 9.2 The Anesthesia Patient Safety Foundation's consensus recommendations for improving medication safety in the operating room. Reproduced from Eichhorn 2010 (18), with permission from the Anesthesia Patient Safety Foundation.

HROs have sensitivity to operations, as well as deference to expertise (19). Leaders with this mentality seek to understand the "work as done" at the frontline rather than "work as imagined" (see Chapter 6). They welcome and depend on input from the frontline staff about where errors are likely to occur (or where and why they have occurred), and they defer to the expertise of those who do the job every day when designing systems improvement. Key in the leadership activities to improve safety culture are "gemba" walks. As defined within the Toyota Production System, these occur when an executive walks "where the value is made," which, in healthcare, is on the wards, in the intensive care unit (ICU), the operating rooms, and so on. Frankel and colleagues within the Institute for Healthcare Improvement (IHI) (23) term these walks "WalkRounds" and further define three initiatives that leaders should take to improve safety culture: development and implementation of a just culture, broad application of training in teamwork skills and communication, and tools like WalkRounds, adopt-a-unit, or patient safety rounding (23,24). These initiatives lead to alignment of frontline workers with the safety vision of leadership. A leader cannot be sensitive to operations without being present from time to time; however, Frankel and colleagues stipulate that this is much more than just walking on the wards and chatting to the staff. Rather, it is a "cyclical flow of information," where issues or system vulnerabilities are identified, combined with other relevant inputs such as incident reports and root-cause analyses (RCAs), and action is taken to resolve the identified vulnerabilities (23).

In 2005, shortly after shocking the nation with an exposé of the enormity of human error in medicine, the Institute of Medicine (IOM) published a "road map for the development of these standards in the context of delivering high-quality, safe care," titled *Patient Safety: Achieving a New Standard for Care*. Recommendation 5 stated: "All health care settings should establish comprehensive patient safety programs operated by trained personnel within a culture of safety. These programs should encompass (1) case finding – identifying system failures, (2) analysis – understanding the factors that contribute to system failures, and (3) system redesign – making improvements in care processes to prevent errors in the future. Patient safety programs should invite the participation of patients and their families and be responsive to their inquiries" (25). Our knowledge of what a comprehensive safety program should include has expanded tremendously since that time, but the basic tenets of that recommendation still hold:

- Trained individuals, rather than just those who have an interest in the field, must lead the quality and safety programs. Personnel may include quality analysts, human factors engineers, data analysts, and project managers who can lead implementation efforts.
- Current processes, especially those with high levels of preventable patient harm such as hospital-acquired infections, adverse medication events, and pressure ulcers, should be examined for vulnerabilities and system failures and redesigned using proven methods. Medication process vulnerabilities can be assessed broadly using the ISMP "Medication Safety Self Assessment for Hospitals" (www .ismp.org/assessments/hospitals, accessed January 20, 2020).

- A comprehensive program to address these vulnerabilities should be designed with input from the frontline staff, and a robust implementation program developed, with ongoing monitoring and audits (7). Such an approach can reduce harm, including mortality (26). For example, one comprehensive medication safety program decreased the quarterly adverse medication event (AME) rate from 0.17 to 0.04 AME per 1000 dispensed doses ($p < 0.001$) (7).
- Incident reporting systems should be established and promoted in order to identify new or previously unrecognized vulnerabilities. Reported events should be promptly analyzed and resolved. Such systems have been shown to decrease medication errors (27).
- Each unit should have a local safety team to both drive implementation of best practices and address incidents as they are reported (28,29). Units should each be assigned an executive to provide needed guidance or resources. Comprehensive Unit-based Safety Programs (CUSPs), designed by Pronovost et al., have been shown to be effective in reducing infections (30,31) and improving the safety climate (32).
- Robust data analysis, including audits of compliance with safety interventions, is required. As stated by Deming, "you cannot manage what you do not measure" (33). Simply measuring and presenting the data, however, has not been found to be effective in changing behavior (34).

9.2.2 Incident Reporting Systems and Measurement More Generally

It is a truism of quality improvement that you cannot improve what you cannot measure. In Chapter 2, we discussed some of the approaches to measuring the rate of medication error. Doing this in a manner that could meaningfully show changes over time turns out to be very difficult, in part because observation is the only reliable method for identifying medication errors, and this is just too expensive for routine surveillance. A comprehensive quality improvement initiative to improve medication safety would include measures of structure (e.g., the technology in place, the number of pharmacists involved in perioperative medication management), process (e.g., random observations of hand hygiene and compliance with barcode technology if present), and outcome. The last of these is the most challenging, in part because attribution of harm from medication events can be very difficult. For example, how does one determine whether a postoperative infection was really attributable to the late administration of a postoperative antibiotic?

Nevertheless, some effort to measure the state of medication processes in an institution and show change over time is a key requirement of any serious attempt to improve their safety. Facilitated incident reporting (explained in Chapter 2) supplemented by occasional "biopsies" of process by observation provide a reasonable compromise. The University of Washington has provided an excellent model for adopting this pragmatic and relatively inexpensive approach to measuring progress over time as efforts are made to improve medication safety (35).

As alluded to earlier, the tremendous variability in processes and workflow across institutions and units means that, although units can learn from each other and from the published literature, each unit should have a local means by which to report and analyze errors and incidents, and to design safety defenses informed by these reports. Facilitated incident reporting (recommended in the previous paragraph) will achieve this more comprehensively than simple incident reporting. As discussed in Chapter 11, these systems must be just, where human errors that harm a patient are seen as system failures and solutions do not include firing or disciplining the reporter, but also where workers are held accountable for violations of best practices. This is often termed as having a "just culture" (36). A unit cannot hope to improve safety if it is not known where errors occur; no workers will report an error if they fear retaliation, shame and blame, or punishment. Incident reporting systems work best if they encourage reporting of all events that did affect *or could have* affected patient safety; if the reporting is contemporary; if those designing solutions defer to expertise (i.e., listen to the frontline workers with the best knowledge of the systems and work processes involved in the incident); and if analysis of the incident is detailed and

thorough (i.e., there is reluctance to oversimplify). Typical hospital incident reporting systems are separate from individual patients' electronic hospital records (EHRs), but some incident reporting systems have been integrated into the EHR, with prompts to report linked to a separate database. In anesthesia, such systems have been developed locally (e.g., at Alfred Hospital, Australia) (37) or within commercially available electronic anesthesia records (e.g., Epic, Centricity).

A combined cultural and technological intervention bundle in one ICU increased medication error reporting by 25% and reduced the rate at which errors resulted in harm by 71% (38). When well done, incident reporting systems have been shown to decrease medication error rates (39). Reporting of errors, however, is fraught with personal fears of being shamed and blamed, of retaliation, and of loss of esteem among one's colleagues (see Chapter 11). In a litigious healthcare system such as that in the United States, reporting of errors within an EHR also raises fears of "discoverability."

9.2.3 Root-Cause Analyses, Medication Event Huddles, Learning from Defects, and Medication Safety Walk-Arounds

When medication incidents are identified through critical incident reporting systems, pharmacist interventions, trigger tool analyses, or other mechanisms, they need to be addressed and resolved as quickly as possible. A system of triage is required to identify those events that should be analyzed through a formal RCA to identify underlying causes for the event, and to design system changes to ensure that no future similar events occur. Typically, serious harm is one of the criteria used in identifying the events to analyze, but clearly many patient deaths are not subjected to RCA, and it may be the *potential* for serious harm from similar events in the future that should determine whether an RCA is undertaken. There are many resources for conducting RCAs, available from the Centers for Medicare and Medicaid Services (CMS), the Joint Commission, and the Agency for Healthcare Research and Quality, so RCA is not discussed further here. The term "RCA" should not be taken as implying that a single cause should be found – often there are several factors that need to be addressed if safety is to be improved effectively (40). Also, it may be appropriate to undertake an RCA of aggregated groups of medication events rather than treating each event as unique.

As discussed in Chapters 11 and 12, less serious events, those that cause little or no harm, are often overlooked. In fact, these events do matter collectively, and they do provide substantial opportunity for learning. Every unit should have a defined process for addressing these minor events, such as the Agency for Healthcare Research and Quality (AHRQ) Learning from Defects tool (3), or medication huddles whereby a core interdisciplinary team (e.g., a nurse, a pharmacist, a provider, a quality expert) reviews the events and identifies possible interventions (41,42). Safety walk-arounds are different from huddles in that they occur on a regular basis, are not initiated by an event, and are designed to allow quality leadership to understand local processes and hear from frontline staff where potential hazards exist. Again, such programs can reduce adverse medication errors (7) as well as overall hospital mortality (26).

9.2.4 Policies and Procedures

Clearly, there are a host of policies and defined procedures that every unit, hospital, state, or country must have around various aspects of the medication process. Although policies and procedures are a relatively weak means of preventing medication errors (43), they do make expectations explicit. There is little research on the effectiveness of policies and procedures, with some studies reporting that their absence is associated with more errors and others showing no such relationship (43). Despite this, policies and procedures are useful for specifying how work should be done and which safeguards and protections should be built in. They are the mechanism by which institutions embed recommended best practices (Institute for Safe Medication Practices [ISMP] [44]) or standards (the Joint Commission [TJC]) into everyday work. For example, the *2020–21 Targeted Medication Safety Best Practices* released by the ISMP states: "BEST PRACTICE 1: Dispense vinCRIStine (and other vinca alkaloids) in a minibag of a compatible solution and not in a syringe" (44). A local institution might then embed this best practice into a corresponding pharmacy policy and make any other

changes to its systems required to implement this policy. For example, order sets would be changed to indicate the infusion rates for the administration of these medications.

Without specific and precise documents that dictate policies and procedures, employees cannot be expected to know how to perform many important aspects of their jobs. The list of policies and procedures that a hospital should have in place around medication safety is enormous and beyond the purview of this book: the ISMP, TJC, the World Health Organization, and many other societies have detailed guidelines, best practices, standards, and goals (e.g., the National Patient Safety Goals [NPSG] of TJC: Table 9.3 [45]) that are released on a regular basis and need to be translated by each institution into local policies and procedures and then into improved workflow and patient safety.

The development and implementation of policies and procedures can be challenging. Poorly written policies can be difficult to implement and will virtually guarantee violations (46). TJC offers 1-, 3-, and 5-day workshops on how to write effective policies (see www.jointcommissioninternational.org/improve/create-effective-policies/, accessed January 21, 2020). An illustration of one hospital's local processes to implement a NPSG for the use of warfarin is provided in Table 9.3 (45). Simply codifying the local policy around each element of the national policy is not sufficient. In this case, a new, mandatory order set was developed, and electronic alerts were built into the order set. A computer check that the required international normalized ratio (INR) and hemoglobin orders had been placed and a mandatory warfarin adjustment and monitoring by a pharmacist were also implemented.

Once policies and procedures have been written and corresponding order sets and software changes developed, effective implementation is necessary. Among other things, there must be robust and mandatory education around the required practice and the evidence supporting it. Internal audits need to be set up to track compliance with the policies and procedures, with specific interventions when compliance is not optimal. Even with the best policies and procedures, unanticipated challenges to safety will occur, as barcode readers fail to work or scan, medication shortages require substitution of familiar formulations with dangerous look-alike

Table 9.3 Example of the translation of Joint Commission National Patient Safety Goal (NPSG) 03.05.01 into an institution's procedures

NPSG 03.05.01 element	Institution procedure
Use only oral unit-dose products when these types of products are available.	Only prepacked unit-dose products are stocked in the automated dispensing cabinets for nursing use.
Use approved protocols for the initiation and maintenance of anticoagulant therapy.	An order set and policy were developed.
Before starting a patient on warfarin, assess the patient's baseline coagulation status; for all patients receiving warfarin therapy, use a current INR to adjust this therapy. The baseline status and current INR are documented in the medical record.	An INR within the last 72 hours[a] is required for all patients with an order for warfarin. A daily INR is required until the patient is within target range for a minimum of 4 consecutive days; then the INR may be ordered every 3 days.
Use authoritative resources to manage potential food and drug interactions for patients receiving warfarin.	Each patient is reviewed daily by a pharmacist to manage potential food and drug interactions.
A written policy addresses baseline and ongoing laboratory tests that are required for anticoagulants	INR within 72 hours[a] prior to warfarin initiation. INR daily until the target range is achieved for a minimum of 4 consecutive days; then INR every 3 days. Hgb within 72 hours[a] prior to warfarin initiation. Hgb every 7 days while on warfarin.
Provide education regarding anticoagulation therapy to prescribers, staff, patients, and families. Patient/family education includes the following: • Importance of follow-up monitoring • Compliance • Drug-food interactions • The potential for adverse drug reactions and interactions	Verbal education is to be done by a pharmacist prior to discharge. Written materials and a warfarin video are made available to patients for use.
Evaluate anticoagulation safety practices, take action to improve practices, and measure the effectiveness of those actions in a time frame determined by the organization.	Quality improvement metrics are performed and reported annually to the Anticoagulation Quality Committee.

Source: Excerpted with permission from Nisly et al. 2013 (45).
Note: Hgb, hemoglobin; INR, international normalized ratio.
[a] If the patient was admitted for an elective procedure, laboratory testing done within the previous 30 days was accepted.

agents, or short staffing leads to interruptions and distractions during nursing rounds. It also must be recognized that even highly sensible changes in the medication process (such as changing from insulin vials to insulin pens) can create their own new errors and necessitate new or changed policies (47).

The relationship between policies and violations is discussed in Chapter 8. An unmanageably large number of policies and poorly designed policies both tend to promote violation, sometimes out of the necessity to get work done and sometimes even to ensure patient safety. As discussed in Chapter 11, practitioners of all disciplines have, over the years, become adept at primary problem-solving and often manage to get around policies and procedures that they view as unworkable, outdated, or unsafe. It follows that leadership must be sensitive to operational challenges and that policies are only one element in promoting safety within complex systems.

9.3 Technology

Technology has tremendous potential to improve medication safety. In particular, well-designed "forcing functions" have the potential to decrease the likelihood that a slip or a lapse will reach the patient. Over the past 50 years, significant technological advances (often involving computers) have made the medication process much safer, but each advance represents a change, which by itself can introduce errors, albeit different errors from those seen with the prior method.

9.3.1 Electronic Management Systems (or Electronic Health Records) and Integration

Electronic health records (EHRs) have dramatically changed the landscape of medical care and patient safety. In the 1970s, when both authors trained, paper charts were the norm, with many clerical staff in the operating room tasked with nothing other than making sure that each surgical patient's paper chart made its way from the records room to the operating room on the day of surgery. Complex patients often had charts whose thickness was measured in feet and which were only loosely arranged by chronology. For most systems, there was no single location in the chart for recording current medications or allergies. Allergies were frequently missed, often with life-threatening results.

Electronic health information capture began in the late 1960s, with the earliest systems used primarily for billing purposes. In 1968, Harvard and the Massachusetts Hospital developed the Computer-Stored Ambulatory Record (COSTAR). Soon, health systems around the United States were developing their own local electronic records, recognizing the tremendous advantage of immediate availability of accurate records and of the fact that many providers could access the record at the same time (48). By the 1990s, it was apparent that EHR offered great advantages but also that there were significant hazards that needed to be recognized and addressed. In 1997, the IOM published a study analyzing these issues of EHRs and helped establish an organization to set standards for EHR systems within the United States. For example, Health Level Seven (HL7) is an international standard for the transfer of clinical and administrative data between software applications (48). EHRs offer great potential to improve the care of individual patients by enhancing care coordination and can thereby contribute to improving the health of populations. However, differences in healthcare structure between countries have led to substantial variation internationally in the form and functionality of EHRs. In the Netherlands, for example, in 2011, 99% of all primary care physicians had fully functional EHRs connected to a national network that allowed general practitioners to exchange data with hospitals, pharmacies, and other healthcare providers (49). At that time, only 46% of United States physician offices used electronic records; there was so much resistance to transitioning to EHRs that, in 2008, the United States government offered significant financial incentives to providers and institutions that implemented EHRs (49).

At the most basic level, an EHR allows instant access to the latest medication record, weight, and list of allergies of each patient. As discussed in Chapters 2 and 3, many of these medication records will be wrong, as medications frequently change, but these electronic lists facilitate reconciliation. The best EHRs not only contain the patient's clinical information but are also linked to order entry systems, laboratories, and other repositories of relevant information. This allows for significant safeguards, with weight-based dosing, allergy alerts, medication-medication alerts, and links to laboratory and radiology results. As shown in Table 9.3, effective EHR linking can enhance policy implementation: for example, when an order for warfarin is placed, an order for INR at the appropriate intervals can be automatically initiated.

Effective networking of pharmacies, ambulatory records, and hospital data can significantly improve medication reconciliation, but in the United States, at least, such networking is in its infancy. In Denmark, 100% of prescriptions are created electronically, and all prescriptions are stored in a national database that patients and physicians can access (49); in the United States, while many prescriptions are created electronically, individual medication lists are maintained, separated by each provider who writes a prescription and each pharmacy that fills a script, with no electronic sharing except for narcotic medications. It is beyond the scope of this book to explore the variations in EHRs within or across countries, but we consider some of the features of EHRs that show the most promise for medication safety.

9.3.2 Computerized Provider Order Entry

The first CPOE system in the world is believed to be one that Lockheed Martin developed for the El Camino Hospital in Mountain View, California, in 1971. In the 1980s, a few hospitals built local computer-based order entry systems; in the 1990s, multiple commercial CPOE systems became available (http://clinfowiki.org/wiki/index.php/History_of_computerized_physician_order_entry, accessed July 18, 2020). There has been a proliferation of commercial CPOE systems internationally, but, as noted earlier, implementation has varied widely across hospitals and nations (50). In 2005, the United Kingdom's National Health Service began implementing a national system for some 60 million patients; in 2009, only 10% of United States hospitals had fully functional CPOE, while Denmark had nearly 100%.

The elements of a CPOE may include the following:

- Menu-driven selection of medications.
- Display of suggested pediatric or adult dosing regimes for the selected medication, together with options for frequency and start and stop times.
- In the ambulatory setting, options presented for the number of pills to be dispensed and for refills.
- Order sets that are unique for particular disease conditions (51) such as asthma (e.g., a variety of bronchodilators, respiratory therapy visits, and pulmonary consults) or for given surgical procedures (e.g., a series of medications, diets, infusions, and ambulation instructions). These order sets provide guidance on the appropriate medications for a condition and embed appropriate laboratory testing for monitoring of the selected medication (e.g., blood levels of tacrolimus, INR for warfarin dosing, etc.).
- A varying degree of decision support (discussed later).
- In pediatric settings, weight-based dosing (this should be provided, but this does not always occur).
- Automatic electronic flow of orders to a pharmacy, whether in the ambulatory setting or within a hospital; a pharmacist can then review the order and add an expert human check of the dose and frequency and check for possible medication-medication interactions or contraindications (allergies, incorrect medication for the condition).
- A link of checked order to automated dispensing cabinets, with controls to ensure that a nurse can only withdraw medications that have been prescribed for a particular patient.

Computerized entry removes the issue of illegibility of handwritten prescriptions as well as the errors associated with inappropriate abbreviations; it can reduce but not eliminate decision errors and dosing errors. The provision of order sets has significant potential to enhance the "monitoring" aspect of medication practice.

Bates et al. published one of the first studies of the effect of CPOE in 1998, in which CPOE decreased the rate of nonintercepted serious medication errors from 10.7 per 1000 patient days to 4.9 per 1000, a 55% decrease (52). Carayon et al. found that implementation of CPOE in a community hospital was followed by an overall reduction in the rate of errors at transcription phase from 0.13 per admission to 0; error types that decreased were omitted information, error-prone abbreviations, illegible orders, and failure to renew orders (53). The evidence supporting CPOE from the systematic review of Nuckols et al. has already been noted (see Figure 9.1) (14).

CPOE opens the door for clinical decision support. Alerts can be provided for contraindicated medications (e.g., if the patient is allergic to the medication) or medication-medication interactions (e.g., enoxaparin and heparin ordered in the same patient). Ordered medications can be flagged if no correspondingly appropriate diagnosis is recorded. Dosing ranges can be suggested, based on the patient's recorded weight. Certain orders can be suggested if they are missing (e.g., for DDAVP for patients with diabetes insipidus). Decision support systems are in their infancy but hold great promise, particularly with pediatric weight-based dosing (54). One CPOE, developed for the neonatal intensive care unit (NICU), provided clinical decision support that incorporated dose rules, therapeutic protocols, and formulations; it nearly eliminated "out of range" dosing (55). A similar system in the pediatric intensive care unit (PICU) provided either "soft" or "hard" alerts for inappropriate doses. After implementation, 29% of hard alerts resulted in reduced dosing and 64% in cancellation of the order, with no alteration to the prescription in only 7% (56). Li et al. developed a set of algorithms to detect medication administration errors in the NICU and found that the algorithms identified errors that had not been found with an incident reporting system (57). A systematic review of 20 studies of CPOE that incorporated clinical decision support concluded that these systems were associated with an 85% reduction in prescribing errors and a 12% reduction in ICU mortality (58).

CPOE systems are not error free, however. The study, noted earlier, by Carayon et al., found that four error types actually increased after CPOE implementation: wrong medication, wrong start or stop time, duplicate orders, and orders with wrong information (53). In order to find a desired medication in a CPOE, the prescriber may need to be able to spell it correctly: Senger et al. found that medication spelling errors resulted in no medication being found 17% of the time in a web-based medication information system containing over 105,000 brand names and active ingredients accessible from the Heidelberg University Hospital (59). As noted earlier, CPOE systems cannot eliminate diagnostic errors or errors in the choice of medication, although formal review by a pharmacist can reduce the latter. Nevertheless, the evidence reviewed here does provide considerable support for the value of CPOE systems in improving medication safety overall, and these systems have the potential to reduce errors even further as they become more refined with greater and more sophisticated decision support.

Institutions may be reluctant to implement these systems, given perceptions of high capital costs. However, an analysis of CPOE versus paper prescribing found the costs to be relatively similar: US$13.79 per patient per day for paper and US$16.62 for CPOE (60). A study using a decision-analytical model found that, despite some sensitivity to implementation costs (which can vary substantially), CPOE had, on average, greater than 99% probability of improving health and yielding lifetime savings to society. Estimated savings ranged from US$11.6 million for hospitals with 25–72 beds to US$170 million for hospitals with fewer than 250 beds, and the estimated gain in quality adjusted life-years gained ranged from 19.9 for small hospitals to 249 years for the largest (61).

Unfortunately, CPOE systems have not made substantial inroads into the operating room; although automated dispensing cabinets are quite common, they are not typically linked to decision support tools, to laboratory results, or to the pharmacy. Medications administered by the anesthesia staff are simply entered into the anesthesia record, without being linked to the central pharmacy and without any review. Some electronic anesthesia records do link to patients' allergy lists, but few, if any, provide alerts for medication-medication interactions.

9.3.3 Electronic Medication Reconciliation

As detailed in Chapter 2, medication reconciliation is a significant source of error for patients at every transition of care. Despite widespread implementation of EHRs and CPOE systems, few institutions have taken the next logical step of electronic reconciliation. Two different groups have developed local software programs that present the admitting physician with a list drawn from the ambulatory medication record, after which the physician must chose an action: continue, substitute, suspend, or discontinue (62,63). In one setting, physicians were not permitted to enter new medication orders until the reconciliation process had been completed (this was a forcing function). Another electronic reconciliation algorithm linked the inpatient medication record to electronic pharmacy claims data; this aspect of electronic reconciliation could have prevented 61% of inpatient order errors (64). In New Zealand, the Health Quality and Safety Commission has promoted medication reconciliation over recent years, with some success in reducing errors (65). Use of these systems decreases the number of unintended discrepancies (66), but few data are available on reduction in patient harm by this means. In addition, the studies in the literature to date focus primarily on electronic reconciliation at admission but not at discharge, where the potential for harm is also high, notably if interrupted medications are not restarted (e.g., warfarin, aspirin). Clearly, there is an opportunity to improve medication reconciliation by linking inpatient and ambulatory medication lists both at admission and at discharge.

9.3.4 Automated Dispensing Cabinets

Once orders are received in the pharmacy and verified, the pharmacy must deliver the medication to the ward for administration by the nurses. There is wide variability in how this occurs, ranging from unlocked, open medication cabinets on the ward from which a nurse withdraws medication for administration to fully automated dispensing cabinets (ADCs) that are electronically integrated with pharmacy, such that a medication drawer will open only when a nurse has entered the patient's name and the medication requested has been ordered and approved by a pharmacist. If barcode administration is also in place, the loop can be closed electronically from order entry to administration to the patient. The benefits of ADCs include the following: medications are locked up but nurses can access them in a timely way; stocking, distribution, and inventory control occur electronically and contemporaneously; and ADCs can interface with other databases, across admission, transfer of care, discharge, and potentially even to billing (67). One study reported a reduction in overall medication errors with ADCs (68), but harmful errors were not reduced. A recent systematic review found little or no reduction in medication administration errors (69). Many of the earlier studies were performed with first-generation ADCs, which permitted errors when filling the drawers and when withdrawing medications. These errors typically involve sound-alike (and spelled similarly) medications such as Fioricet versus Fiorinal, hydromorphone instead of morphine, and diazepam instead of diltiazem. More sophisticated cabinets include barcoding or even automated filling, which may reduce these errors. Even without a significant reduction in medication errors, ADCs consistently improve the efficiency of pharmacy and nursing staff (70). The ISMP has detailed guidance for safe use of ADCs (71).

9.3.5 Barcode Technology

Barcode technology is used in virtually all aspects of modern life, from package tracking to checkout in stores and processing airline tickets. Barcode scanners are dramatically more accurate than humans: highly trained data entry personnel make errors at a rate of 1:300 keystrokes, while the ubiquitous Universal Product Code (UPC) systems have an error rate of 1 in 294,000. More sophisticated coding formats, such as dot matrix, are estimated to have an error rate of 1 in 10.5 million. As discussed in Chapters 6 and 7, as human beings we tend to "see" the medication or patient name that we are expecting, instead of what is actually written on the vial or name band, even when double checking with a second person. Barcode readers, by contrast, read what is actually there.

9.3.5.1 Inpatient Settings

In the best implementations, barcode scanning systems are used throughout the hospital, for all processes, and are integrated into all of the electronic databases. When a patient is admitted, a wristband is printed with a unique barcode that identifies the patient, as well as the current admission. Whenever blood is drawn, imaging performed, or medication given, the wristband is scanned. This opens a link to that patient's chart, verifies that an order exists for the planned intervention, and automatically records the intervention. With modern hospital pharmacy inventory systems, every medication is labeled when it enters the pharmacy stock with a sophisticated barcode that includes information about manufacturer, concentration, dosage, formulation, intended route of administration, expiration date, and so on. When ADCs are filled, barcodes are scanned to ensure the correct medication is in the correct drawer, and to enable inventory control. At the time of administration, the nurse retrieves the correct medication from the ADC (which automatically verifies that an order has been placed, and is intended to be given at the time the nurse is retrieving it), then uses a barcode scanner at the bedside to check the patient's wristband and then the medication label. This final scan electronically records the administration in the patient's medication administration record (MAR). In a quasi-scientific study of medication errors before and after implementation of barcoding and an electronic MAR, nontiming errors in medical administration were reduced from 11.5% to 6.8%, and the rate of potential adverse medication events fell from 3.1% to 1.9% (Figure 9.3) (53,72–74).

A recent systematic review and meta-analysis found five studies that reported the error rate when barcode medication administration (BCMA) is used with CPOE and ADCs (75). BCMA significantly reduced both timing and nontiming administration errors and virtually eliminated transcription errors (75). Although medication administration errors are significantly reduced, some errors remain. Barcode scanners can be defective or low on battery power, and patient wristbands can be difficult to scan because of the curved nature of the band, smudging during the printing process, or degradation through exposure to water or alcohol. It is difficult to achieve 100% BCMA compliance. Nonetheless, use of this technology is a key strategy for medication safety.

9.3.5.2 Operating Room Settings

Implementation of barcode technology in the operating room has lagged significantly behind its use in other settings. In 2001, Merry et al. reported a safety-oriented, integrated medication administration and automated anesthesia recording system (now marketed as SAFERsleep).[1] This system

---

[1] Disclosure: Dr Merry is the Chair of the Board of Directors of Safer Sleep LLC, and has financial interests in this product.

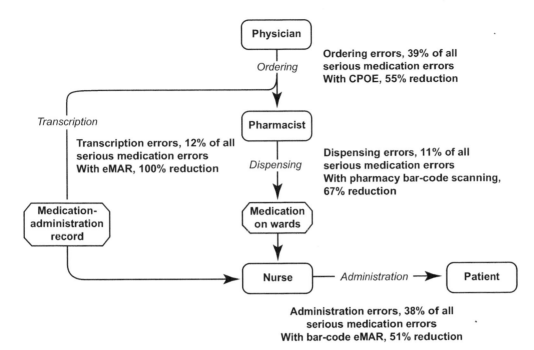

Figure 9.3 Effect of health information technology at key stages in the process of medication use, with permission from Poon et al. (72). Data on errors during the four phases of medication use came from Leape et al. (73). The percent reduction in ordering errors with the use of computerized physician order entry (CPOE) was calculated from Bates et al. (53). The percent reduction in dispensing errors with barcode scanning in the pharmacy was from Poon et al. (74). The percentage reduction in medication administration errors with the barcode electronic medication administration record (eMAR) technology and the percentage reduction in transcribing errors were from Poon et al. (72).

includes barcode technology to scan medication syringes prior to administration, with attendant visual and auditory displays of the medication's name and electronic recording of the administration in an electronic anesthesia record (76). The system is multifaceted, with several other elements to improve medication safety (Table 9.4). In both the real world and in simulation, the use of the SAFERsleep system versus conventional anesthesia management decreased the number of errors in medication administration and recording from 11.6 to 9.1 errors per 100 administrations (real world) (77) and 11.6 to 6.0 per 100 administrations (simulation) (11). At the University of Washington Medical School, a similar comprehensive anesthesia information management system (AIMS) was created, which went further by integrating the Codonics Safe Label System (SLS 500i: Codonics Inc., Middleburg Heights, Ohio) into a locally developed anesthesia recording system (78). With the Codonics system, a user scans the barcode on a medication vial and an appropriate syringe label is printed, which includes a barcode. This is placed

Table 9.4 Elements of a multifaceted system to improve medication safety during anesthesia

- Labels barcoded – swiping produces an auditory and visual confirmation of the medication's name
- Labels color coded by class of medication according to national and international standards
- Both class (e.g., "opioid") and name (e.g., "morphine") of medication displayed in a large font on the labels and again on the computer screen after swiping the barcode
- Organization of workspace facilitated by purpose-designed trays
- Organization of medication drawers standardized, rationalized, and facilitated by color-coding of compartments
- Process to include the retention of used ampules and vials as a physical record of administered medications and the use of full ampules or vials as prompts for medications still to be given
- Selected medications provided in prefilled syringes clearly labeled as earlier
- Other medications provided in vials and ampules with added "flag-labels" for transfer to syringes
- Pharmacist (part-time) explicitly designated to manage medications for Department of Anesthesiology

Source: Described by Merry et al. 2001 (76).

on the syringe. At the time of administration, the barcode on the syringe is scanned, visual and auditory alerts are provided, and the medication (although not the dose) is automatically entered into the anesthesia record (78). The rate of medication errors reported via a facilitated incident reporting process at the University of Washington showed progressive statistically significant reductions following the stepwise introduction of these technological initiatives to improve medication safety (35).

Nearly 20 years later, only a handful of hospitals around the world have implemented systems of this type, despite the evidence that they can reduce errors in medication administration. As with many technologies, human nature can thwart barcode technology as there is typically no forcing function. The user must choose to scan the syringe: In both Merry studies (11,77) and in the Jelacic study (78) many users resisted timely scanning (i.e., *before* administration of the medication). In the University of Washington study, although the Codonics labeling system was highly accurate, anesthesia personnel scanned syringes at time of administration only 58% of the time (78). There are some downsides to attempting to force the use of a checking system for medication administration during anesthesia. Technology can fail in many ways and sometimes at the worst possible moment. It would clearly be a problem if a system of this sort ended up impeding an anesthesiologist from administering an essential medication during a crisis. One of the principles underlying the development of SAFERsleep was that the fallback position in the event of any failure of the technology should be no worse than the status quo before the adoption of the system. Thus, no attempt was made to force users to scan medications. In the future, better technological solutions may be found that automate the detection of medication administrations without the need for active interaction with a device (like a scanner). Notwithstanding our discussion of the problem of clinician autonomy discussed elsewhere in this book, we think this would be, on balance, a better approach than trying to restrict anesthesiologists' freedom to administer medications in what they believe to be the best way at any particular point in a patient's management.

DocuSys, invented by Dr. Robert Evans, marketed an AIMS that combined barcoding with a specialized injection port that measured the volume of medication injected and hence calculated the dose given (79). The DocuSys System used a pre-barcoded syringe-loaded cartridge (SLC) that had to be dispensed with the vial of medication. This did have some implications for storage and cost. We can find very little in the peer-reviewed literature on this system (80).

Although not widely available at present, the Becton, Dickinson Intelliport Medication Management System (see www.youtube.com/watch?v=6daYmY7rxVs, accessed January 20, 2020) is a new innovation that also provides barcoded syringe labeling with a specialized injection port that scans the barcode at the time of injection, provides audible and visual prompts, and measures the volume of medication administered (and hence the dose). Importantly, injections can be made through the port using syringes with non-proprietary labels, although these of course cannot be scanned. Thus, the system allows some trade-off between forcing and versatility.

9.3.6 Smart Pumps

Virtually every hospitalized patient has an intravenous catheter in place for most of the hospital stay. The first intravenous infusion device was created by Sir Christopher Wren in 1791. It consisted of a pig's bladder and a quill that allowed him to infuse solutions into a dog. The evolution of practice from that starting point to current infusion pumps is beyond the scope of this text, so we focus on the improvements that have occurred over the past 20 years. We also exclude discussion of ambulatory, elastomeric, enteral, and large-volume pumps, although medication errors and AMEs occur with all of them. We focus primarily on medication infusion pumps, with and without smart technology, including patient-controlled analgesia systems.

Medication infusion pumps became ubiquitous in hospitals between the late 1960s and the 1980s. These pumps, despite safety features such as alarms for blockage or air in the line, have been associated with thousands of reports of error. Between 2005 and 2009, the United States Food and Drug Administration (FDA) received 56,000 reports of infusion pump errors, some resulting in injury and death (see www.fda.gov/MedicalDevices/ProductsandMedicalProcedures/GeneralHospitalDevicesandSupplies/InfusionPumps/, accessed January 20,

2020). Although many of these events were due to human error (e.g., misprogramming), many were due to deficiencies in design with resulting software problems, runaway infusions, inadvertent free flow, miscalibration of devices with erroneous rates of infusion, failed alarms, broken components, battery failure leading to no alarm, electrical shocks, or even burns. Design flaws that contribute to human error also abounded, with small fonts, failure to display medication name when paused, key bounce leading to an intended 10 becoming 100 when setting infusion rates, decimal points so small as to be invisible, and so on. In 2010, the FDA initiated a comprehensive plan to improve infusion pump safety. Again, the scope of this plan is beyond this text, but the reader can review these issues on the FDA website noted earlier.

Smart pumps were introduced in the early 2000s. These pumps have integrated software that includes medication library profiles for high-risk medications, including dosing safety limits, sometimes called "guardrails." The medication libraries are typically written by each institution's pharmacy department and can be updated remotely as needed; separate libraries can be written for neonatal, pediatric, and adult patients. In 2014, Ohashi et al. conducted a systematic review of their benefits and risks in reducing the rate of medication errors (81). They concluded that smart pumps reduce, but do not eliminate, programming errors. They emphasized the importance of ensuring comprehensive medication libraries and provided an outline of the relevant processes showing some of the vulnerabilities of smart pumps (Figure 9.4). It seems that smart pumps have considerable potential to improve patient safety, but this potential has not yet been fully realized. Also, there are certain errors that they cannot eliminate, such as two common

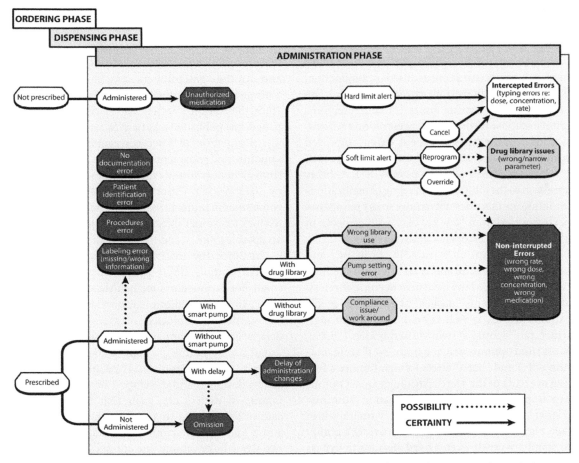

Figure 9.4 Processes of intravenous medication administration with smart pumps and potential or intercepted errors in the prescribing, dispensing, and administration phases. Redrawn with permission from Ohashi et al. 2014 (81).

errors with infusions of medications – failure to monitor or to adjust to changing conditions (82).

In conjunction with smart pumps, multiple regulatory and guidance organizations strongly encourage the use of only a few concentrations for any given medication. In 2007, a survey found that 154 critical care units had 372 different preparations for 20 specified medications (83). Although insulin was remarkably standardized (I unit/mL), there were 18 concentrations of adrenaline and 16 of noradrenaline (83). In addition, in pediatrics where infusion volumes can be a significant problem, concentrations have often been based on an infant's weight, with the result that hundreds of different concentrations would be required for the same medication (whether syringes were prepared by the pharmacy or by the users) (84). It is well recognized that many providers have difficulty calculating weight-based concentrations (66) and that inaccurate doses are frequent in pediatrics. In addition, different units within a hospital can have different preferences for concentrations or rules, requiring changing the syringe and the pump programming with every patient transfer. When smart pumps and standard medication concentrations are used in conjunction, reported medication errors are reduced (85,86). Use of standard concentrations and a computer program to choose medication concentration and infusion rate on the basis of patient weight improved continuity of care across care units. This approach can be used in lieu of smart pumps (87). Another approach to the dilution and labeling of medications for infusions that does not require smart pumps has been reported from New Zealand, with evidence of a reduced rate of errors in calculation (88).

Smart pumps are rapidly evolving and increasingly have the ability to intercept medication errors (89). Many have now become wireless, allowing for remote "pushes" of updates to medication libraries as well as analysis of event logs, which can identify system vulnerabilities (86,89). Most smart pumps provide both "soft" (information only) and "hard" alerts (which require a formal override of the alert). Although smart pumps can improve intravenous medication administration, there remain significant vulnerabilities (see Figure 9.4), including the provider's ability to simply override even a hard alert, or to bypass the medication library altogether and simply program the pump in "mL/hr." In addition, most smart pumps cannot recognize erroneous weight entry, choice of a wrong medication, or duplicate infusions, although they theoretically have the capacity to do so. The latest technologies allow a patient's EHR to communicate with both pharmacy and the smart pump assigned to a patient. This eliminates pump programming altogether, as the pump is programmed automatically when an order is written and then approved by a pharmacist, which offers a chance to intercept wrong medication choices (the patient's weight is taken directly from the EHR, into which the nurses previously entered the information) and also provides automatic recording of the infusion. Again, since anesthesiologists typically do not write orders for medications administered in the operating room, this functionality would not apply.

9.3.7 Route-Specific Small-Bore Connectors

This book began with stories of the tragic consequences of the administration of medications by the wrong route. For several decades, safety experts and frontline practitioners alike have agitated for a unique connector for each medication route. In 2009, the National Patient Safety Agency (United Kingdom) published a Patient Safety Alert requiring elimination of Luer connectors for lumbar puncture and subarachnoid injections by 2011 and from all neuraxial and regional anesthesia supplies by 2013 (90,91). Unfortunately, although several companies manufactured unique needles and connectors for spinal injections, the quality was not acceptable (90,91), and they were discontinued.

In 2016, the International Organization for Standardization (ISO) published standards for small-bore connectors for healthcare liquids and gases, including unique connections for enteral tubing, neuraxial blocks, intravenous and hypodermic injections, and limb cuff devices (see www.iso.org/search.html?q=small%20bore%20connectors, accessed January 21, 2020). This organization designed and developed novel connectors unique to each route, such that enteral tubing cannot be attached to an intravenous Luer port, and a Luer syringe cannot be attached to a neuraxial needle or tubing. The connectors for enteral feeding (ENFit) and those for neuraxial blockade (NRFit; shown in Figure 9.5) are now produced by

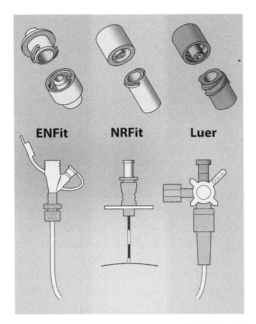

ENFit   **NRFit**   **Luer**

Figure 9.5 Unique enteral (ENFit), neuraxial (NRFit), and Luer connectors per ISO 80369.

multiple manufacturers, although production difficulties have slowed their widespread adoption. Nonetheless, adoption of these route-specific connectors will occur over time and has the potential to dramatically decrease wrong-route errors, even as agent-specific pin-indexed yoke adaptors for gas cylinders have reduced errors in the delivery of gases. Until these devices are fully implemented, and are in routine use, anesthesia providers should clearly label all lines and points of entry (e.g., stopcock, infusion hub) to indicate their route. These labels should be color coded, if possible, in line with established standards (red – arterial, blue – venous, yellow – neuraxial, green – enteral) (92).

9.4 Standardization, Storage, and Preparation

9.4.1 Equipment

The benefits of standardization have been touched on in the prior section in relation to the concentrations of infusions. The same principle extends to most aspects of medication management. For example, smart pumps should be standardized across any institution so that clinicians are not met with different (and unfamiliar) pumps in each different location. Standardization allows patients to be moved between units (e.g., emergency

department, operating room, ward, and ICU) without requiring a pump change. It reduces the amount of effort needed to keep medication libraries updated and reduces inventory control problems. Medication libraries should also be standardized, but alerts and limits should be tailored for pediatric versus adult dosing. Automated dispensing cabinets should be the same across an institution.

9.4.2 Labeling

One of the most critical requirements, often done poorly, is that every single medication, whether in a vial, an ampule, a syringe, an infusion bag, or a container on a sterile field, should be legibly labeled. At a minimum, the label should include the name and concentration of the medication, but ideally it should also include the date and time drawn up, and the initials of the person who prepared it (17). For both handwritten prescriptions and handwritten labels, the ISMP and TJC provide guidelines for abbreviations, the use of leading but not trailing zero, and the avoidance of "lingo."

9.4.2.1 Tall Man Labeling

When labels are preprinted, use of tall man lettering (e.g., DOXOrubicin versus DAUNOrubicin) has been suggested to reduce confusion in soundalike medications (17,93). The evidence for this is not compelling. A recent study in 42 pediatrics hospitals in the United States showed no reduction in medication error associated with the use of tall man letters (94), and an accompanying editorial called for more studies before adopting this technique more widely (95). Conversely, a thoughtful approach adopted in Australia has focused on identifying those medications in which the risk of confusion between names is high and the consequences of an error is also high. Adopting tall man lettering in just the 35 "extreme risk" medications identified in this project makes a great deal of sense. An Australian standard has been promulgated to this end (96).

9.4.2.2 Color-Coding

Given our propensity to recognize patterns, it seems likely that color will have an influence on our ability to recognize ampules or syringes of medication. Given this propensity, if the label color is different from that expected (e.g., red for rocuronium versus purple for neostigmine), one might be less likely to misperceive the written text. It has been suggested that the color-coding of labels by class of medication has the potential to reduce interclass errors, which are likely to be more hazardous than intraclass errors (76,97). The underlying idea is that color-coding by class of medication is likely to decrease between-class errors (e.g., giving a neuromuscular blocking agent instead of an opioid or sedative agent to an awake patient before inducing anesthesia), at the possible risk of increasing within-class errors (e.g., giving atracurium when vecuronium was intended): the former are likely to be more dangerous in most cases (98).

There are several national or international codes or standards for user-applied syringe labels for anesthesia that include color-coding by class of medication (Figure 9.6) (99–101). The idea that syringes themselves should be color coded has gained considerable traction in Australia and New Zealand, where some departments have introduced syringes with red plungers to be used exclusively and invariably for the administration of muscle relaxants (102,103).

Fasting and Gisvold prospectively recorded information from more than 55 000 cases over 36 months. After 18 months, they introduced color-coded syringe labels (104). They observed a reduced incidence of medication errors, with 40 errors in the first period and 23 errors in the second period. However, they reported this difference as not statistically significant ($P = 0.07$). They concluded that color-coding of labels did not "eliminate" syringe swaps but pointed out that the study was underpowered for this endpoint, given their low incidence of medication errors overall. In an editorial, Orser went further and argued that this trial warranted a one-sided statistical test and that, on this basis, the findings were significant and did support the use of color-coded syringe labels (105).

As outlined in Chapter 8, in relation to fatigue, Cheeseman et al. used a computer-based, task-relevant medication recognition and confirmation test to explore this issue in a rather different way and again added to the evidence supporting the use of color (106). It is interesting that no medication error associated with awareness was reported with propofol in the NAP5 study, perhaps because of this medication's striking color (107).

Experience from currency may also be of some relevance. In many countries, banknotes are color coded, but not in the United States. We know of no

	PMS [a]	ASTM [b] - RGB		ISO [c] - RGB
Induction Agents	Process Yellow C	255.255.0		255.255.0
Benzodiazepines and Tranquilizers	Orange 151	255.102.0		255.102.0
Benzodiazepine Antagonists	Orange 151 / White Diagonal Stripes	255.102.0		255.102.0
Muscle Relaxants	Florescent Red 805 [d]	255.114.118		
	Florescent Red 811 [e]			253.121.86
	Warm Red [f]			245.64.41
Muscle Relaxant Antagonists	Florescent Red / White Diagonal Stripes	255.114.118		253.121.86
Opiod/Narcotics	Blue 297	133.199.227		133.199.227
Opiod/Narcotic Antagonists	Blue 297 / White Diagonal Stripes	133.199.227		133.199.227
Major Tranquilizers and Anti-Emetics	Salmon 156	237.194.130		237.194.130
Vasopressors	Violet 256	222.191.217		222.191.217
Hypotensive Agents	Violet 256 / White Diagonal Stripes	222.191.217		222.191.217
Local Anesthetics	Gray 401	194.184.171		194.184.171
Anticholinergic Agents	Green 367	163.217.99		163.217.99
Beta Blockers	Copper 876 U	176.135.112		NA [g]
	White	255.255.255		255.255.255

Figure 9.6 Standard specifications for user-applied labels in anesthesiology (ISO 26825:2008). Reprinted with permission from the American Society of Anesthesiologists Statement on Labeling of Pharmaceuticals in Anesthesiology. Available at www.asahq.org/standards-and-guidelines/statement-on-labeling-of-pharmaceuticals-for-use-in-anesthesiology, accessed December 30, 2019.

trials comparing the propensity to make errors in selecting banknotes to pay bills, but personal experience suggests that the monochromatic United States system is not particularly more prone to such problems than the systems in the United Kingdom, Canada, Australia, and New Zealand (all of which use variable color to denote denomination).

As mentioned in Chapter 6, some commentators, notably some pharmacists, suggest that the color-coding of labels may actually promote errors (108,109). The weight placed on this suggestion hinges to some extent on how one views the clinical significance of an intraclass medication error, which may be made more likely by the use of color-coding, versus an interclass error, which presumably will be made less likely. However, some examples are quite nuanced: A common syringe swap error involves giving more neuromuscular blocking agent (red label) when a reversal agent was intended (red label with white slashes). An extreme example of the line of thinking that opposes the use of color in this way suggests that all medications should be made to look alike, to force practitioners to read the labels (108). This idea seems to us to be completely out of kilter with any of the objectives and principles of the science of human factors.

Overall, the evidence on the value of color-coding in the context of safe medication administration is not conclusive. In a recent letter (110), Webster and Merry pointed out that the use of any single approach, on its own, cannot be expected to eliminate syringe swaps. The essence of building cognitive science into the processes of medication management is the use of a multifaceted approach. In this view, it makes sense to include color-coding of labels by class of medication, not as an alternative to other checks and measures (including that of always reading labels carefully), but as a supplement to them.

In many parts of the world, anesthesia personnel are now familiar and comfortable with the use of colored labels in the operating room. A single standard for the color-coding of user-applied syringe labels has been adopted in Canada (100), the United States (111), New Zealand and Australia (99), and the United Kingdom (101). As noted in the technology section, it is increasingly common for these to come pre-applied to prefilled syringes purchased from commercial suppliers or to be produced with printers in response to swiping the barcode on an ampule or vial, using software integrated with the anesthesia record.

9.4.2.3 Prefilled Syringes

Prefilled syringes may be prepared by a hospital pharmacy or commercially; in 2011 there were some 20 pharmaceutical companies providing over 50 different medications in prefilled syringes (112). Either way, good manufacturing practices (GMPs) should be used. This implies that multiple syringes containing the same medication are prepared at a time, with appropriate checks, a high standard of sterility, and in an environment that is free from distractions without any pressure of time. For all these reasons, one should be able to rely on the accuracy and sterility of the contents of a prefilled syringe to a much greater extent than one can on the contents of a medication drawn into a syringe from an ampule or vial in the operating room under the pressures and distractions of giving an anesthetic. In the latter context, each individual syringe contains just one agent, and that agent is selected from a draw or tray containing many ampules, and this process of drawing up a medication has to be repeated with many different medications for each patient. Although there is little literature on this point, one would assume that the prefilled syringes, which are held to a high standard of sterility, would also offer advantages regarding asepsis (see Box 11.3).

Some of the potential benefits of prefilled syringes include decreased needlesticks (because there is no need to draw up medications from vials and ampules) and a decrease in wastage, either via prepared but not used syringes that are discarded at the end of the case or the systematic 20%–30% "overfill" of vials and ampules (112). Although more expensive than the same dose in a vial, the savings in non-wasted doses make them cost-effective (113). Prefilled syringes have the potential to eliminate many of the inherent system "vulnerabilities" that lead to medication errors, particularly when used with barcode scanning (11,113). In fact, elimination of the multiple steps in selecting an intravenous medication, drawing it into the syringe aseptically, and then correctly labeling the syringe is one of the few genuine hard-engineering opportunities to improve the safety of medication administration during anesthesia. Furthermore, the majority of prefilled syringes come with a barcode that incorporates (at a minimum) medication name, concentration, expiration date, and often the generic and trade names. These barcodes make it both easy and effective to incorporate barcode scanning systems for the operating room and emergency areas.

In Chapter 6, we discussed the question of using prefilled syringes when suppliers of medications have to be changed because of medication shortages. Prefilled syringes make eminent sense for managing this problem, especially for anesthetizing locations, but this does require an understanding by the pharmacy that consistent and clear labeling of the syringes is required and that this should include color-coding by class of medication if that is the practice of the particular anesthesia department.

The 2018 revision of the Royal Pharmaceutical Society's "Professional Guidance on the Safe and Secure Handling of Medicines" (114) includes the following section:

C1 As outlined in the core guidance, manipulation of medicines in clinical areas is minimised and medicines are presented as prefilled syringes or other "ready-to-administer" preparations wherever possible, e.g. infusion bags.

It will be interesting to see how long it takes for this recommendation to be widely implemented.

9.4.2.4 The Storage, Preparation, and Concentrations of Medications

Multiple studies show that many healthcare workers struggle to perform accurate calculations for dilutions and dosing (115–118). For example, Wheeler et al. analyzed the discarded contents of infusion syringes prepared by staff in an English ICU. They found a substantial deviation from the intended concentration, including some examples that contained multiples of the intended concentration and some which contained no medication at all. These authors recommended the use of prefilled syringes for these infusions (119). We agree in general (not just for ICUs) that, when commercial prefilled syringes are not available, intravenous medications that require dilution to a standard concentration should be prepared by the hospital's pharmacy. However, in a global context, this is still not widely done.

If clinicians have to draw up and dilute medications themselves (as many do, around the world),

there are some important points that can improve the safety of the process. Various relevant guidelines have been promulgated on the basis of expert consensus, notably those of the Australian and New Zealand College of Anaesthetists (ANZCA, updated in 2017) (120). Among other things, the ANZCA guidelines emphasize the importance of an uncluttered work area, good lighting, and minimization of distractions. The guidelines suggest the following:

An agreed and consistent process should be in place to determine whether syringes are labeled prior to or after a drug is drawn up. Drugs should be drawn up using one syringe and one ampoule at one time. The label on the ampoule should be checked, and matched to that on the syringe.

The process of *matching* the name on the syringe label with that on the ampule label is different from simply reading the ampule label and does appear to be more reliable (although data to support this contention are absent). If the label is placed on the syringe before drawing up the medication, then this matching process can occur while the medication is being drawn up, which seems to offer an approach that is likely to be both reliable and efficient.

There should be standard concentrations, and ideally a single concentration, of medications that providers draw up to administer, especially for high-risk medications (e.g., insulin, heparin, epinephrine). The practice of double diluting a concentrated vasopressor – that is, drawing up 1 mL of a 1:1000 concentration and diluting into 9 mL, then drawing up 1 mL of the 1:10,000 dilution and further diluting it in another 9 mL of solution – should be avoided: virtually every anesthesiologist has experienced or knows of episodes of severe hypertension due to failure to perform the second dilution. There is a strong case to support the view that labeling should be based on mass concentration (e.g., 1 mg/mL), not on ratio (e.g., 1:1000) (119). Concentrated formulations of potent medications (e.g., 1 mg/mL epinephrine) should not be available as an immediate choice for clinicians in the clinical setting except in certain specific circumstances (e.g., as part of a crash/code cart or box, where the entire 1 mg may be an appropriate dose).

In locations where medications are not in automated dispensing cabinets, as is the case for many anesthesia locations, standardized tray or drawer systems should be used (17). They should be standardized across all locations within any institution. Each section should be clearly labeled with the medication that should be in that spot. It is suggested that the medications *not* be placed alphabetically but either by medication class or by where they are used in the anesthesia process (induction, maintenance, emergence) (76). Anesthesia drawers and trays should contain the minimum number of medications required to provide safe care (to reduce complexity). Unusual medications, if brought into the operating room, should be placed in a unique container and be removed at the end of the case. Local anesthetics should be segregated from other anesthetic agents, preferably in a separate cart for placing blocks. Only preservative-free solutions should be available on nerve block carts. Along those lines, unusual formulations should not be stored with standard formulations; for example, hypertonic saline should be segregated from normal saline solutions. Concentrated potassium chloride should not normally be kept in the operating room (except perhaps for use in cardiac anesthesia) (17).

These comments apply primarily to intravenous medications, whether given by bolus injection or by infusion. Given their high potential for serious harm from errors, intraspinal injections require redoubled attention to detail, and should always include meticulous double checking with a second person.

9.5 Pharmacy

9.5.1 Pharmacist Involvement in Care Delivery

Increased involvement of pharmacists has a significant impact on medication errors. In 2001, Bond and colleagues reviewed error rates and pharmacy characteristics of 1116 hospitals and found that the presence of decentralized pharmacists decreased overall error rate by 45% and decreased the rate of harmful errors by 94% (121). Follow-up studies in 2002 (122) and in 2006–7 (123,124) found that, as pharmacist staffing increased from approximately 1/100 beds to 5/100 beds, adverse medication reactions decreased by nearly 50%, and overall mortality rates reduced significantly (124). The reduction in adverse medication rates and mortality was associated with several pharmacy-related traits (123,124):

- Increased clinical pharmacist staffing
- Participation of pharmacist on the
  - Total parenteral nutrition team
  - Medicine service
  - CPR team
- Pharmacist-led
  - In-service education and preparation of educational materials
  - Medication protocol development
  - Provision of medication information
- Pharmacist conducted medication reconciliation at admission
- Pharmacist involvement in management of adverse medication reactions

Many other studies support these early findings and demonstrate improvement in medication safety with greater pharmacist participation. The involvement of a pharmacist improves medication reconciliation at admission (125–129) and at discharge (130–135). Pharmacist involvement at any transfer of care significantly reduces medication error (63,136,137). This improvement in reconciliation accuracy significantly decreases readmission rates (131,138) and decreases costs (138,139).

9.5.2 Decentralized Pharmacy Services

As previously noted, the presence of a pharmacist in the ICU decreases medication errors (122,124,140). With the advent of CPOE, pharmacists now review each medication order as written and make interventions, so future research is likely to focus on interception of errors (141,142). Studies have shown that nearly 16% of initial ICU medication orders are incorrect and may have resulted in patient harm without pharmacist intervention (143,144). Having a specialist critical care pharmacist (as opposed to centralized pharmacy review) significantly increased the number of pharmacist interventions (145). Unfortunately, as mentioned earlier, CPOE is not used during anesthesia, thus obviating any possibility of pharmacist review of the choice of medications. This reflects the dynamic nature of medication selection and administration in the operating room – it might be possible to include computerized support for the selection of medications. To a limited degree, some AIMS do provide this (e.g., SAFERsleep checks for allergies and other medication contraindications and provides a reminder to administer timely pro-phylactic antibiotics), but it is difficult to see how a pharmacist could be inserted into the process. Satellite operating room pharmacies, however, can significantly impact operating room medication safety by preparing all medication infusions as well as preparing the daily stock of diluted vasopressor (146). Ideally, a dedicated pharmacist should also be embedded into anesthesia departments. A sat-ellite pharmacist could liaise with the Department of Anesthesia over the purchase and presentation of medications. A genuine two-way engagement would likely reduce costs and improve the satis-faction of the clinicians who (as we observed in Chapter 6) are the people who actually have to use these medications. It could also reduce the element of surprise that currently characterizes changes in commonly used medications forced on hospitals by medication shortages. Multiple studies of operating room satellite pharmacies have demonstrated sig-nificant cost savings or revenue capture, increased use of pharmacy-prepared high-risk medications, and improvement in on-time case starts (146–149). It would be expected that the impact of pharmacist involvement will only increase, with the tremen-dous increase in new medications that continually are added to our formularies.

9.5.3 Medication Ordering, Supply, Distribution, and Inventory Control

There are virtually no randomized controlled tri-als or even case cohort studies of pharmacy-led versus non-pharmacy-led medication manage-ment. However, most medication safety guidance (e.g., from ISMP, TJC, American Society of Health-System Pharmacists) place the responsibility for the entire pharmaceutical supply chain with phar-macy. This includes (but is not limited to) decisions about which medications to have on formulary; choice of manufacturer, concentration, and prepa-ration for each medication with choices made to avoid look-alike products; stocking and inventory control, including management of dangerous med-ications and solutions such as hypertonic saline or local anesthetics; the number and location of satel-lite pharmacies; the choice of technologies to sup-port medication management; and management of medication shortages (148,150). Expert opinion suggests that pharmacists should be involved in a "clean sweep" of every operating room between

cases to remove all used and unusual medications prior to the next case (17).

9.6 Teamwork, Communication, and Other Nontechnical Skills

Although there are few data specifically concern-ing communication or teamwork and medication errors, communication failure is possibly the most significant contributor to medical error that results in patient harm (151). Several analyses of medical malpractice claims have supported this conten-tion (152,153). Medication reconciliation failures often include communication failures between patients and caregivers or between clinicians (e.g., on discharge to primary care). Poor com-munication between clinicians is more common than between patients and clinicians (153,154). Handoffs between clinicians rarely include a for-mal review of medication status, especially in the operating room. As patients move across the continuum of care, information degrades, which presents a real danger to patients (155,156). Other teamwork skills that may be lacking include situ-ational awareness (e.g., failing to recognize that a surgeon is injecting local anesthesia after a large volume has already been injected by the anesthe-siologist for an analgesic block) and team checking (e.g., by nursing or other colleagues of critical steps in the medication administration process).

9.6.1 Team Training

Implementation of a comprehensive team train-ing program in 74 hospitals in the Veterans Affairs Health System reduced surgical mortality by 18% compared to a 7% decrease in 34 hospitals that had not received this training; for every quarter of the training program, the surgical mortality decreased by 0.5 per 1000 procedures (157). Smaller studies have shown that team training or training in non-technical skills reduces surgeons' technical errors (158,159), improves safety climate (160), improves communication skills (161), and improves team performance (162). As noted, an important part of teamwork is team checking, where team members actively check one another and intervene when they see an error or unsafe act being committed. Although the impact of team training on medica-tion error in particular is unknown, it seems highly likely that the improvement in communication and other teamwork skills resulting from such training will translate into safer medication practices.

9.6.2 Structured Communication Protocols

9.6.2.1 Speak Back, Read Back, Phonetics

Closed-loop communication and specific phonetic techniques are uniformly used in aviation and the military but are inconsistently used in healthcare, even in high-stakes settings (163). Perfusionists have incorporated this into their profession (163), and the Association of periOperative Registered Nurses has made this a priority for operating room nurses' communication with surgeons, especially regarding verbal orders. In Australia and New Zealand, all anesthesiology trainees are required to undertake simulation-based training that includes these principles, and many senior anesthesiologists chose to do this as well (164). The Royal Australasian College of Surgeons has recently instituted its Operating with Respect program (see www.surgeons.org/education/skills-training-courses/operating-with-respect-owr-course, accessed January 20, 2020), which also includes some of these principles. It is unfortunate (and somewhat ironic) that these programs have tended to operate in professional silos. However, in New Zealand, following a successful feasibility study (165), the Accident Compensation Corporation (ACC; see www.acc.co.nz/, accessed January 20, 2020; and see Chapter 12) has funded a 5-year program, called NetworkZ, to roll out in situ simulation training for entire operating room teams across the whole country over 5 years.

In one study of medication errors in the emergency department, verbal orders accounted for 32% of all medication errors (166). Although closed-loop communication would eliminate many of these errors, many institutions have taken the approach of simply prohibiting verbal orders except in code situations (167). Speak back or read back of critical information also has the potential to prevent serious medication errors, but it needs to be clear and explicit (Box 9.1). Strict attention to communication is key to preventing patient harm, not just medication harm.

9.6.2.2 Briefings and Handoffs

In the operating room, briefings have been shown to significantly reduce delays (168), technical errors (169), and mortality (170,171). Briefings have also

> **Box 9.1 A local case**
>
> A patient known to be diabetic was admitted to the emergency department, disoriented. A nursing assistant was asked to do a point-of-care glucose reading, and verbally reported to the nurse a blood glucose result of 27. The nurse heard 527, but did not speak this back to the assistant and simply asked the assistant to repeat the test. The second point-of-care testing showed a glucose of 29, but when reporting this to the nurse, the assistant simply said, "It's the same." An insulin infusion was subsequently ordered. Fortunately, the nursing assistant checked on the patient a bit later, recognized the error, and disaster was averted. *Source*: Personal communication, JW.

been shown to significantly decrease the number of medication omissions, notably those involving preoperative antibiotics and venous thrombosis prophylaxis (172,173).

As outlined in Chapters 2 and 3, patients undergo many transfers of care in the surgical continuum; errors in medication reconciliation are common, and review of medication plans seldom happens during the handoffs at these transitions. It is clear that, in the absence of a structured protocol for handoffs, significant omissions are likely to occur (155), and (as previously noted) information about a patient degrades progressively across the continuum of care (156). Within the operating room, handoffs between anesthesia providers have been associated with increased mortality (174,175); whether this is due to medication errors or omissions is not known. Structured protocols for handoffs have repeatedly been shown to reduce errors of omission, whether from the operating room to the ICU (176,177), within the operating room between providers, or between providers on the ward (178). Structured handoffs should include a review of the current medication plan, what medications have been suspended, last doses of critical medications, and upcoming administrations of medications (e.g., redosing of antibiotics).

9.6.3 Multitasking, Fatigue, and "Hero" Mentality

Much of the medication process involves skill-based tasks and is dependent on System I thinking rather than System II thinking. This is true whether typing a medication order, drawing up a medication from a vial, or administering a medication. These predominantly automatic tasks are at high risk for errors during disruptions, interruptions, distractions, or haste (e.g., because of production pressure). Although most of us pride ourselves on being excellent multitaskers, studies show that unless the task is an entirely automatic one (e.g., walking, chewing gum), the brain actually performs task switching and focuses on a single task at a time (179). This continual task switching actually slows completion of either task (180) and opens the door to error (181). Each time a skill-based schema is interrupted to perform a different task, there is a risk that we will return to the schema in the wrong spot – either repeating an already completed task or omitting a step. For this reason, many hospitals have sought ways to limit or prohibit interruptions of nurses performing medication administration. They have gone so far as to have nurses on medication administration rounds wear neon or orange vests to prevent interruptions. Unfortunately, these interventions have not yet been found to reduce administration errors (182) and more studies are warranted.

It is clear that those in healthcare are incredibly dedicated to their patients and are willing to work incredible hours when needed. It is also clear that this "hero" mentality ignores the deleterious effects of fatigue on human performance. We discussed the complex effects of fatigue on human performance in detail in Chapter 8. Unfortunately, there are only a few studies that have investigated whether reductions in workload or increased staffing actually reduce medication error in particular or outcomes in general (183,184); none of these are systematic or prospective. However, data from other contexts strongly suggest that sensible management of fatigue, and of one's health more generally, is likely to improve medication safety.

9.7 Conclusions

There are a host of expert-identified and recommended interventions to improve medication safety. Although few individual elements of these interventions have been rigorously tested and proven to actually reduce error, let alone save lives, many make sense and have little downside. Adoption of electronic medication processes (notably computerized order entry, pharmacist checking and verification, automated medication cabinets, and barcode administration) clearly can and has reduced medication error, both on the wards and in the operating room. More recently, comprehensive patient safety programs (including rigorous investigation of critical incidents, team training in high-reliability behaviors, a focus on identifying and correcting system vulnerabilities, use of checklists, and other elements) have been shown to reduce errors and even mortality. The reduction of any form of human error in medicine, and specifically a reduction in medication-related error, is likely to require a comprehensive bundle of interventions rather than any single silver bullet. We have cited several examples in which even the partially successful implementation of such bundles of interventions has resulted in a reduction in the rate of medication error. The data reviewed in Chapters 2 and 3 show clearly that the status quo is not good enough. In this chapter we covered many things that most institutions and practitioners could do today. Each of these may make only a small difference, but the key to substantially improving medication safety undoubtedly lies in the aggregation of minimal gains (8,185).

Our patients have a right to expect greater investment into medication safety by healthcare institutions and greater engagement with medication safety by the clinicians whose responsibility it is to care for them safely. The APSF's "Consensus Recommendations for Improving Medication Safety in the Operating Room" (see Figure 9.1) is authoritative and consistent with other expert guidelines on medication safety in the operating room, such as that of ANZCA (120). Although their time in the operating room is only part of the surgical patient's perioperative journey, it is an important part. The implementation of these recommendations should be a minimum expectation for institutions and anesthesia departments today. Furthermore, doing so would provide an excellent foundation from which initiatives to improve medication safety can be extended to the rest of the surgical patient pathway.

References

1. Miller MR, Robinson KA, Lubomski LH, Rinke ML, Pronovost PJ. Medication errors in paediatric care: a systematic review of epidemiology and an evaluation of evidence supporting reduction strategy recommendations. *Qual Saf Health Care.* 2007;16(2):116–26.

2. Singer SJ, Gaba DM, Falwell A, et al. Patient safety climate in 92 US hospitals: differences by work area and discipline. *Med Care.* 2009;47(1):23–31.

3. Pronovost PJ, Holzmueller CG, Martinez E, et al. A practical tool to learn from defects in patient care. *Jt Comm J Qual Patient Saf.* 2006;32(2):102–8.

4. Gazarian M, Graudins LV. Long-term reduction in adverse drug events: an evidence-based improvement model. *Pediatrics.* 2012;129(5):e1334–42.

5. Breeding J, Welch S, Whittam S, et al. Medication Error Minimization Scheme (MEMS) in an adult tertiary intensive care unit (ICU) 2009–2011. *Aust Crit Care.* 2013;26(2):58–75.

6. Keiffer S, Marcum G, Harrison S, Teske DW, Simsic JM. Reduction of medication errors in a pediatric cardiothoracic intensive care unit. *J Nurs Care Qual.* 2015;30(3):212–9.

7. McClead RE Jr, Catt C, Davis JT, et al. An internal quality improvement collaborative significantly reduces hospital-wide medication error related adverse drug events. *J Pediatr.* 2014;165(6):1222–9.e1.

8. Durrand JW, Batterham AM, Danjoux GR. Pre-habilitation. I: aggregation of marginal gains. *Anaesthesia.* 2014;69(5):403–6.

9. Prakash V, Koczmara C, Savage P, et al. Mitigating errors caused by interruptions during medication verification and administration: interventions in a simulated ambulatory chemotherapy setting. *BMJ Qual Saf.* 2014;23(11):884–92.

10. Moreira ME, Hernandez C, Stevens AD, et al. Color-coded prefilled medication syringes decrease time to delivery and dosing error in simulated emergency department pediatric resuscitations. *Ann Emerg Med.* 2015;66(2):97–106.e3.

11. Merry AF, Hannam JA, Webster CS, et al. Retesting the hypothesis of a clinical randomized controlled trial in a simulation environment to Validate Anesthesia Simulation in Error Research (the VASER Study). *Anesthesiology.* 2017;126(3):472–81.

12. Estock JL, Murray AW, Mizah MT, et al. Label design affects medication safety in an operating room crisis: a controlled simulation study. *J Patient Saf.* 2018;14(2):101–6.

13. Siebert JN, Ehrler F, Combescure C, et al. A mobile device app to reduce time to drug delivery and medication errors during simulated pediatric cardiopulmonary resuscitation: a randomized controlled trial. *J Med Internet Res.* 2017;19(2):e31.

14. Nuckols TK, Smith-Spangler C, Morton SC, et al. The effectiveness of computerized order entry at reducing preventable adverse drug events and medication errors in hospital settings: a systematic review and meta-analysis. *Syst Rev.* 2014;3:56.

15. Jensen LS, Merry AF, Webster CS, Weller J, Larsson L. Evidence-based strategies for preventing drug administration errors during anaesthesia. *Anaesthesia.* 2004;59(5):493–504.

16. Sackett DL, Rosenberg WM, Gray JA, Haynes RB, Richardson WS. Evidence based medicine: what it is and what it isn't. *Br Med J.* 1996;312(7023):71–2.

17. Wahr JA, Abernathy JH 3rd, Lazarra EH, et al. Medication safety in the operating room: literature and expert-based recommendations. *Br J Anaesth.* 2017;118(1):32–43.

18. Eichhorn J. APSF hosts medication safety conference: consensus group defines challenges and opportunities for improved practice. *APSF Newsletter.* 2010;25(1):1–7. Accessed January 3, 2020. https://www.apsf.org/article/apsf-hosts-medication-safety-conference/

19. Weick KE, Sutcliffe KM. *Managing the Unexpected: Resilient Performance in an Age of Uncertainty.* 2nd ed. San Francisco, CA: Jossey-Bass; 2007.

20. Singer SJ, Falwell A, Gaba DM, et al. Identifying organizational cultures that promote patient safety. *Health Care Manage Rev.* 2009;34(4):300–11.

21. Valentin A, Schiffinger M, Steyrer J, Huber C, Strunk G. Safety climate reduces medication and dislodgement errors in routine intensive care practice. *Intensive Care Med.* 2013;39(3):391–8.

22. Singer SJ, Vogus TJ. Reducing hospital errors: interventions that build safety culture. *Annu Rev Public Health.* 2013;34:373–96.

23. Frankel AS, Leonard MW, Denham CR. Fair and just culture, team behavior, and leadership engagement: the tools to achieve high reliability. *Health Serv Res.* 2006;41(4 pt 2):1690–709.

24. Pronovost PJ, Weast B, Bishop K, et al. Senior executive adopt-a-work unit: a model for safety improvement. *Jt Comm J Qual Saf.* 2004;30(2):59–68.

25. Committee on Data Standards for Patient Safety Board on Healthcare Services Institute of Medicine. Executive summary. In: Aspden P, Corrigan JM, Wolcott J, Erikson S, eds. *Patient Safety: Achieving a New Standard for Care.* Washington, DC: National Academies Press;

2004. Accessed July 18, 2020. https://www.ncbi
.nlm.nih.gov/books/NBK216103

26. Brilli RJ, McClead RE Jr, Crandall WV, et al.
A comprehensive patient safety program
can significantly reduce preventable harm,
associated costs, and hospital mortality. *J Pediatr.*
2013;163(6):1638–45.

27. Elden NM, Ismail A. The importance of
medication errors reporting in improving the
quality of clinical care services. *Glob J Health Sci.*
2016;8(8):243–51.

28. Pronovost PJ, King J, Holzmueller CG, et al.
A web-based tool for the Comprehensive Unit-
based Safety Program (CUSP). *Jt Comm J Qual
Patient Saf.* 2006;32(3):119–29.

29. Berenholtz SM, Hartsell TL, Pronovost PJ.
Learning from defects to enhance morbidity
and mortality conferences. *Am J Med Qual.*
2009;24(3):192–5.

30. Pronovost P, Needham D, Berenholtz S, et al.
An intervention to decrease catheter-related
bloodstream infections in the ICU. *N Engl J Med.*
2006;355(26):2725–32.

31. Pronovost PJ, Goeschel CA, Colantuoni E,
et al. Sustaining reductions in catheter related
bloodstream infections in Michigan intensive care
units: observational study. *BMJ.* 2010;340:c309.

32. Sexton JB, Berenholtz SM, Goeschel CA, et al.
Assessing and improving safety climate in a large
cohort of intensive care units. *Crit Care Med.*
2011;39(5):934–9.

33. Deming WE. *The New Economics.* Cambridge,
MA: Massachusetts Institute of Technology,
Center for Advanced Engineering Study; 1994.

34. Ramsay AI, Turner S, Cavell G, et al. Governing
patient safety: lessons learned from a mixed
methods evaluation of implementing a ward-level
medication safety scorecard in two English NHS
hospitals. *BMJ Qual Saf.* 2014;23(2):136–46.

35. Bowdle TA, Jelacic S, Nair B, et al. Facilitated
self-reported anaesthetic medication errors before
and after implementation of a safety bundle
and barcode-based safety system. *Br J Anaesth.*
2018;121(6):1338–45.

36. Marx D. *Patient Safety and the "Just Culture": A
Primer for Health Care Executives.* New York, NY:
Columbia University; 2001.

37. Haller G, Myles PS, Stoelwinder J, et al.
Integrating incident reporting into an electronic
patient record system. *J Am Med Inform Assoc.*
2007;14(2):175–81.

38. Abstoss KM, Shaw BE, Owens TA, et al.
Increasing medication error reporting rates while
reducing harm through simultaneous cultural and

system-level interventions in an intensive care
unit. *BMJ Qual Saf.* 2011;20(11):914–22.

39. Frey B, Buettiker V, Hug MI, et al. Does critical
incident reporting contribute to medication error
prevention? *Eur J Pediatr.* 2002;161(11):594–9.

40. Vincent C, Taylor-Adams S, Chapman EJ,
et al. How to investigate and analyse clinical
incidents: clinical risk unit and association of
litigation and risk management protocol. *BMJ.*
2000;320(7237):777–81.

41. Wilbur K, Scarborough K. Medication safety
huddles: teaming up to improve patient safety.
Can J Hosp Pharm. 2005;58:151–5.

42. Morvay S, Lewe D, Stewart B, et al. Medication
event huddles: a tool for reducing adverse drug
events. *Jt Comm J Qual Patient Saf.* 2014;40(1):
39–45.

43. Hughes RG, Blegen MA. Medication
administration safety. In: Hughes RG, ed. *Patient
Safety and Quality: An Evidence-Based Handbook
for Nurses.* Rockville, MD: Agency for Healthcare
Research and Quality; 2008. Accessed July 18,
2020. https://www.ncbi.nlm.nih.gov/books/
NBK2656

44. *2010–2021 Targeted Medication Safety Best
Practices for Hospitals.* Horsham, PA: Institute for
Safe Medication Practices; 2018. Accessed July
18, 2020. https://www.ismp.org/sites/default/files/
attachments/2017-12/TMSBP-for-Hospitalsv2.pdf

45. Nisly S, Shiltz ED, Vanarsdale V, Laughlin J.
Implementation of an order set to adhere to
national patient safety goals for warfarin therapy.
Hosp Pharm. 2013;48(10):828–32.

46. Alper SJ, Holden RJ, Scanlon MC, et al.
Self-reported violations during medication
administration in two paediatric hospitals. A
systematic review of safety violations in industry.
BMJ Qual Saf. 2012;21:408–15.

47. Trimble AN, Bishop B, Rampe N. Medication
errors associated with transition from insulin
pens to insulin vials. *Am J Health Syst Pharm.*
2017;74(2):70–5.

48. Atherton J. Development of the electronic health
record. *Virtual Mentor.* 2011;13(3):186–9.

49. Gray B, Johansen I, Koch S, Bowden T. Electronic
health records: an international perspective
on "meaningful use." *Commonwealth Fund
Newsletter.* November 17, 2011:28. Accessed
January 7, 2020. https://www.commonwealthfund
.org/publications/issue-briefs/2011/nov/
electronic-health-records-international-
perspective-meaningful

50. Metzger JB, Welebob E, Turisco F, Classen
DC. The Leapfrog Group's CPOE standard

and evaluation tool. *Patient Safety and Quality Healthcare Newsletter.* July/August 2008. Accessed December 30, 2019. https://www.psqh.com/julaug08/cpoe.html

51. Guo Y, Chung P, Weiss C, Veltri K, Minamoto GY. Customized order-entry sets can prevent antiretroviral prescribing errors: a novel opportunity for antimicrobial stewardship. *P T.* 2015;40(5):353–60.

52. Bates DW, Leape LL, Cullen DJ, et al. Effect of computerized physician order entry and a team intervention on prevention of serious medication errors. *JAMA.* 1998;280(15):1311–6.

53. Carayon P, Du S, Brown R, et al. EHR-related medication errors in two ICUs. *J Healthc Risk Manag.* 2017;36(3):6–15.

54. Kadmon G, Bron-Harlev E, Nahum E, et al. Computerized order entry with limited decision support to prevent prescription errors in a PICU. *Pediatrics.* 2009;124(3):935–40.

55. Gouyon B, Iacobelli S, Saliba E, et al. A Computer Prescribing Order Entry-Clinical Decision Support system designed for neonatal care: results of the "preselected prescription" concept at the bedside. *J Clin Pharm Ther.* 2017;42(1):64–8.

56. Balasuriya L, Vyles D, Bakerman P, et al. Computerized dose range checking using hard and soft stop alerts reduces prescribing errors in a pediatric intensive care unit. *J Patient Saf.* 2017;13(3):144–8.

57. Li Q, Kirkendall ES, Hall ES, et al. Automated detection of medication administration errors in neonatal intensive care. *J Biomed Inform.* 2015;57:124–33.

58. Prgomet M, Li L, Niazkhani Z, Georgiou A, Westbrook JI. Impact of commercial computerized provider order entry (CPOE) and clinical decision support systems (CDSSs) on medication errors, length of stay, and mortality in intensive care units: a systematic review and meta-analysis. *J Am Med Inform Assoc.* 2017;24(2):413–22.

59. Senger C, Kaltschmidt J, Schmitt SP, Pruszydlo MG, Haefeli WE. Misspellings in drug information system queries: characteristics of drug name spelling errors and strategies for their prevention. *Int J Med Inform.* 2010;79(12):832–9.

60. Vermeulen KM, van Doormaal JE, Zaal RJ, et al. Cost-effectiveness of an electronic medication ordering system (CPOE/CDSS) in hospitalized patients. *Int J Med Inform.* 2014;83(8):572–80.

61. Nuckols TK, Asch SM, Patel V, et al. Implementing computerized provider order entry in acute care hospitals in the United States could generate substantial savings to society. *Jt Comm J Qual Patient Saf.* 2015;41(8):341–50.

62. Gimenez-Manzorro A, Romero-Jimenez RM, Calleja-Hernandez MA, et al. Effectiveness of an electronic tool for medication reconciliation in a general surgery department. *Int J Clin Pharm.* 2015;37(1):159–67.

63. Rizzato Lede DA, Benitez SE, Mayan JC 3rd, et al. Patient safety at transitions of care: use of a compulsory electronic reconciliation tool in an academic hospital. *Stud Health Technol.* 2015;216:232–6.

64. Pevnick JM, Palmer KA, Shane R, et al. Potential benefit of electronic pharmacy claims data to prevent medication history errors and resultant inpatient order errors. *J Am Med Inform Assoc.* 2016;23(5):942–50.

65. Health Quality and Safety Commission New Zealand. eMedRec brings number of benefits for Counties Manukau Health and Northland DHB. *Med Saf.* May 2, 2016. Accessed January 20, 2020. https://www.hqsc.govt.nz/our-programmes/medication-safety/news-and-events/news/2512/

66. Agrawal A, Wu WY. Reducing medication errors and improving systems reliability using an electronic medication reconciliation system. *Jt Comm J Qual Patient Saf.* 2009;35(2):106–14.

67. Grissinger M. Safeguards for using and designing automated dispensing cabinets. *P T.* 2012;37(9):490–530.

68. Chapuis C, Roustit M, Bal G, et al. Automated drug dispensing system reduces medication errors in an intensive care setting. *Crit Care Med.* 2010;38(12):2275–81.

69. Tsao NW, Lo C, Babich M, Shah K, Bansback NJ. Decentralized automated dispensing devices: systematic review of clinical and economic impacts in hospitals. *Can J Hosp Pharm.* 2014;67(2):138–48.

70. Cottney A. Improving the safety and efficiency of nurse medication rounds through the introduction of an automated dispensing cabinet. *BMJ Qual Improv Rep.* 2014;3(1):u204237.w1843. doi:10.1136/bmjquality.u204237.w1843.

71. Institute for Safe Medication Practice. *Guidance on the Interdisciplinary Safe Use of Automated Dispensing Cabinets.* Horsham, PA: ISMP; 2008. Accessed April 14, 2018. https://www.ismp.org/Tools/guidelines/ADC_Guidelines_final.pdf

72. Poon EG, Keohane CA, Yoon CS, et al. Effect of bar-code technology on the safety of medication administration. *N Engl J Med.* 2010;362(18):1698–707.

73. Leape LL, Bates DW, Cullen DJ, et al. Systems analysis of adverse drug events. ADE Prevention Study Group. *JAMA*. 1995;274(1):35–43.

74. Poon EG, Cina JL, Churchill W, et al. Medication dispensing errors and potential adverse drug events before and after implementing bar code technology in the pharmacy. *Ann Intern Med*. 2006;145(6):426–34.

75. Shah K, Lo C, Babich M, Tsao NW, Bansback NJ. Bar code medication administration technology: a systematic review of impact on patient safety when used with computerized prescriber order entry and automated dispensing devices. *Can J Hosp Pharm*. 2016;69(5):394–402.

76. Merry AF, Webster CS, Mathew DJ. A new, safety-oriented, integrated drug administration and automated anesthesia record system. *Anesth Analg*. 2001;93(2):385–90.

77. Merry AF, Webster CS, Hannam J, et al. Multimodal system designed to reduce errors in recording and administration of drugs in anaesthesia: prospective randomised clinical evaluation. *BMJ*. 2011;343:d5543.

78. Jelacic S, Bowdle A, Nair BG, et al. A system for anesthesia drug administration using barcode technology: the Codonics Safe Label System and Smart Anesthesia Manager. *Anesth Analg*. 2015;121(2):410–21.

79. Douglas JR Jr, Ritter MJ. Implementation of an Anesthesia Information Management System (AIMS). *Ochsner J*. 2011;11(2):102–14.

80. Cooper RL, Merry A. Medication management. In: Stonemetz J, Ruskin K, eds. *Anesthesia Informatics. Health Informatics Series*. London: Springer; 2008:209–26.

81. Ohashi K, Dalleur O, Dykes PC, Bates DW. Benefits and risks of using smart pumps to reduce medication error rates: a systematic review. *Drug Saf*. 2014;37(12):1011–20.

82. Nuckols TK, Bower AG, Paddock SM, et al. Programmable infusion pumps in ICUs: an analysis of corresponding adverse drug events. *J Gen Intern Med*. 2008;23(suppl 1):41–5.

83. Borthwick M, Woods J, Keeling S, Keeling P, Waldmann C. A survey to inform standardisation of intravenous medication concentrations in critical care. *J Intensive Care Soc*. 2007;8(1):92–6.

84. Hilmas E, Sowan A, Gaffoor M, Vaidya V. Implementation and evaluation of a comprehensive system to deliver pediatric continuous infusion medications with standardized concentrations. *Am J Health Syst Pharm*. 2010;67(1):58–69.

85. Larsen GY, Parker HB, Cash J, O'Connell M, Grant MC. Standard drug concentrations and smart-pump technology reduce continuous-medication-infusion errors in pediatric patients. *Pediatrics*. 2005;116(1):e21–5.

86. Tran M, Ciarkowski S, Wagner D, Stevenson JG. A case study on the safety impact of implementing smart patient-controlled analgesic pumps at a tertiary care academic medical center. *Jt Comm J Qual Patient Saf*. 2012;38(3):112–9.

87. Irwin D, Vaillancourt R, Dalgleish D, et al. Standard concentrations of high-alert drug infusions across paediatric acute care. *Paediatr Child Health*. 2008;13(5):371–6.

88. Merry AF, Webster CS, Connell H. A new infusion syringe label system designed to reduce task complexity during drug preparation. *Anaesthesia*. 2007;62(5):486–91.

89. Kastrup M, Balzer F, Volk T, Spies C. Analysis of event logs from syringe pumps: a retrospective pilot study to assess possible effects of syringe pumps on safety in a university hospital critical care unit in Germany. *Drug Saf*. 2012;35(7):563–74.

90. Cook TM, Payne S, Skryabina E, et al. A simulation-based evaluation of two proposed alternatives to Luer devices for use in neuraxial anaesthesia. *Anaesthesia*. 2010;65(11):1069–79.

91. Kinsella SM, Goswami A, Laxton C, et al. A clinical evaluation of four non-Luer spinal needle and syringe systems. *Anaesthesia*. 2012;67(11):1217–24.

92. Australian Commission on Safety and Quality in Health Care. *2015 National Standard for User-Applied Labelling of Injectable Medicines, Fluids and Lines*. Sydney: ACSQHC; 2015. Accessed January 11, 2020. https://www.safetyandquality.gov.au/our-work/medication-safety/safer-naming-labelling-and-packaging-medicines/national-standard-user-applied-labelling-injectable-medicines-fluids-and-lines

93. Hellier E, Edworthy J, Derbyshire N, Costello A. Considering the impact of medicine label design characteristics on patient safety. *Ergonomics*. 2006;49(5-6):617–30.

94. Zhong W, Feinstein JA, Patel NS, Dai D, Feudtner C. Tall Man lettering and potential prescription errors: a time series analysis of 42 children's hospitals in the USA over 9 years. *BMJ Qual Saf*. 2016;25(4):233–40.

95. Lambert BL, Schroeder SR, Galanter WL. Does Tall Man lettering prevent drug name confusion errors? Incomplete and conflicting evidence suggest need for definitive study. *BMJ Qual Saf*. 2016;25(4):213–7.

96. Emmerton L, Rizk MF, Bedford G, Lalor D. Systematic derivation of an Australian standard for Tall Man lettering to distinguish similar drug names. *J Eval Clin Pract*. 2015;21(1):85–90.

97. Webster CS, Anderson D, Murtagh S. Safety and peri-operative medical care. *Anaesthesia*. 2001;56:496–7.

98. Webster CS, Larsson L, Frampton CM, et al. Clinical assessment of a new anaesthetic drug administration system: a prospective, controlled, longitudinal incident monitoring study. *Anaesthesia*. 2010;65(5):490–9.

99. Standards New Zealand. *User-Applied Labels for Use on Syringes Containing Drugs Used during Anaesthesia*. Wellington: Standards New Zealand; 1996. *AS/NZS 4375:1996*. Accessed January 20, 2020. https://shop.standards.govt.nz/catalog/4375%3A1996%28AS%7CNZS%29/view

100. CSA Group. *Standard for User-Applied Drug Labels in Anaesthesia and Critical Care*. Etobicoke, Canada: Canadian Standards Association; 1998. CAN/CSA-Z264.3-98. Accessed January 20, 2020. https://store.csagroup.org/ccrz__ProductDetails?sku=2700729

101. International Organization for Standardization. *Anaesthetic and Respiratory Equipment – User-Applied Labels for Syringes Containing Drugs Used during Anaesthesia – Colours, Design and Performance*. Geneva: International Organization for Standardization; 2008. *ISO 26825:2008*. Accessed January 20, 2020. https://www.iso.org/standard/43811.html

102. Russell WJ. Getting into the red: a strategic step for safety. *Qual Saf Health Care*. 2002;11(1):107.

103. Rowe D. Red plunger syringes for neuromuscular blocking drugs. *Anaesthesia*. 2015;70(1):107.

104. Fasting S, Gisvold SE. Adverse drug errors in anesthesia, and the impact of coloured syringe labels. *Can J Anesth*. 2000;47(11):1060–7.

105. Orser BA. Medication safety in anesthetic practice: first do no harm. *Can J Anaesth*. 2000;47(11):1051–4.

106. Cheeseman JF, Webster CS, Pawley MD, et al. Use of a new task-relevant test to assess the effects of shift work and drug labelling formats on anesthesia trainees' drug recognition and confirmation. *Can J Anesth*. 2011;58(1):38–47.

107. Pandit JJ, Cook TM. *NAP5: Accidental Awareness during General Anaesthesia in the United Kingdom and Ireland: Report and Findings*. London: National Audit Projects; 2014. Accessed January 20, 2020. https://www.nationalauditprojects.org.uk/NAP5home#pt

108. Grissinger M. Color-coded syringes for anesthesia drugs-use with care. *P T*. 2012;37(4):199–201.

109. Rupp SM. Color-coding of syringes may not enhance safety. *Reg Anesth Pain Med*. 2005;30(6):589–90.

110. Webster CS, Merry AF. Colour coding, drug administration error and the systems approach to safety. *Eur J Anaesthesiol*. 2007;24(4):385–6.

111. American Society for Testing and Materials. *Standard Specification for User Applied Drug Labels in Anesthesiology*. Philadelphia: American Society for Testing and Materials; 1995. ASTM *D4774-94*. Accessed January 20, 2020. https://www.astm.org/DATABASE.CART/HISTORICAL/D4774-94.htm

112. Makwana S, Basu B, Makasana Y, Dharamsi A. Prefilled syringes: an innovation in parenteral packaging. *Int J Pharm Invest*. 2011;1(4):200–6.

113. Yang Y, Rivera AJ, Fortier CR, Abernathy JH 3rd. A human factors engineering study of the medication delivery process during an anesthetic: self-filled syringes versus prefilled syringes. *Anesthesiology*. 2016;124(4):795–803.

114. Royal Pharmaceutical Society. *Professional Guidance on the Safe and Secure Handling of Medicines*. London: Royal Pharmaceutical Society; 2018. Accessed November 16, 2019. https://www.rpharms.com/recognition/setting-professional-standards/safe-and-secure-handling-of-medicines/professional-guidance-on-the-safe-and-secure-handling-of-medicines

115. Stucki C, Sautter AM, Wolff A, Fleury-Souverain S, Bonnabry P. Accuracy of preparation of i.v. medication syringes for anesthesiology. *Am J Health Syst Pharm*. 2013;70(2):137–42.

116. Weeks KW, Hutton BM, Young S, et al. Safety in numbers 2: competency modelling and diagnostic error assessment in medication dosage calculation problem-solving. *Nurse Educ Pract*. 2013;13(2):e23–32.

117. Avidan A, Levin PD, Weissman C, Gozal Y. Anesthesiologists' ability in calculating weight-based concentrations for pediatric drug infusions: an observational study. *J Clin Anesth*. 2014;26(4):276–80.

118. Venkataraman A, Siu E, Sadasivam K. Paediatric electronic infusion calculator: an intervention to eliminate infusion errors in paediatric critical care. *JICS*. 2016;17(4):290–4.

119. Wheeler DW, Degnan BA, Sehmi JS, et al. Variability in the concentrations of intravenous drug infusions prepared in a critical care unit. *Intensive Care Med*. 2008;34(8):1441–7.

120. Australian and New Zealand College of Anaesthetists. *Guidelines for the Safe Administration of Injectable Drugs in Anaesthesia*. Melbourne: Australian and New Zealand College of Anaesthetists; 2017.

Policy document PS 51. Accessed January 20, 2020. https://www.anzca.edu.au/resources/professional-documents

121. Bond CA, Raehl CL, Franke T. Medication errors in United States hospitals. *Pharmacotherapy*. 2001;21(9):1023–36.

122. Bond CA, Raehl CL, Franke T. Clinical pharmacy services, hospital pharmacy staffing, and medication errors in United States hospitals. *Pharmacotherapy*. 2002;22(2):134–47.

123. Bond CA, Raehl CL. Clinical pharmacy services, pharmacy staffing, and adverse drug reactions in United States hospitals. *Pharmacotherapy*. 2006;26(6):735–47.

124. Bond CA, Raehl CL. Clinical pharmacy services, pharmacy staffing, and hospital mortality rates. *Pharmacotherapy*. 2007;27(4):481–93.

125. Leguelinel-Blache G, Arnaud F, Bouvet S, et al. Impact of admission medication reconciliation performed by clinical pharmacists on medication safety. *Eur J Intern Med*. 2014;25(9):808–14.

126. Smith L, Mosley J, Lott S, et al. Impact of pharmacy-led medication reconciliation on medication errors during transition in the hospital setting. *Pharm Pract*. 2015;13(4):634.

127. Contreras Rey MB, Arco Prados Y, Sanchez Gomez E. Analysis of the medication reconciliation process conducted at hospital admission. *Farm Hosp*. 2016;40(4):246–59.

128. Marinovic I, Marusic S, Mucalo I, Mesaric J, Bacic Vrca V. Clinical pharmacist-led program on medication reconciliation implementation at hospital admission: experience of a single university hospital in Croatia. *Croat Med J*. 2016;57(6):572–81.

129. Mendes AE, Lombardi NF, Andrzejevski VS, et al. Medication reconciliation at patient admission: a randomized controlled trial. *Pharm Pract*. 2016;14(1):656.

130. Allison GM, Weigel B, Holcroft C. Does electronic medication reconciliation at hospital discharge decrease prescription medication errors? *Int J Health Care Qual Assur*. 2015;28(6):564–73.

131. Eisenhower C. Impact of pharmacist-conducted medication reconciliation at discharge on readmissions of elderly patients with COPD. *Ann Pharmacother*. 2014;48(2):203–8.

132. Garcia-Molina Saez C, Urbieta Sanz E, Madrigal de Torres M, Vicente Vera T, Perez Carceles MD. Computerized pharmaceutical intervention to reduce reconciliation errors at hospital discharge in Spain: an interrupted time-series study. *J Clin Pharm Ther*. 2016;41(2):203–8.

133. Musgrave CR, Pilch NA, Taber DJ, et al. Improving transplant patient safety through pharmacist discharge medication reconciliation. *Am J Transplant*. 2013;13(3):796–801.

134. Pourrat X, Corneau H, Floch S, et al. Communication between community and hospital pharmacists: impact on medication reconciliation at admission. *Int J Clin Pharm*. 2013;35(4):656–63.

135. Bishop MA, Cohen BA, Billings LK, Thomas EV. Reducing errors through discharge medication reconciliation by pharmacy services. *Am J Health Syst Pharm*. 2015;72(17 suppl 2):S120–6.

136. Ensing HT, Stuijt CC, van den Bemt BJ, et al. Identifying the optimal role for pharmacists in care transitions: a systematic review. *J Manag Care Spec Pharm*. 2015;21(8):614–36.

137. Mekonnen AB, McLachlan AJ, Brien JA. Pharmacy-led medication reconciliation programmes at hospital transitions: a systematic review and meta-analysis. *J Clin Pharm Ther*. 2016;41(2):128–44.

138. Anderegg SV, Wilkinson ST, Couldry RJ, Grauer DW, Howser E. Effects of a hospitalwide pharmacy practice model change on readmission and return to emergency department rates. *Am J Health Syst Pharm*. 2014;71(17):1469–79.

139. Sebaaly J, Parsons LB, Pilch NA, et al. Clinical and financial impact of pharmacist involvement in discharge medication reconciliation at an academic medical center: a prospective pilot study. *Hosp Pharm*. 2015;50(6):505–13.

140. Leape LL, Cullen DJ, Clapp MD, et al. Pharmacist participation on physician rounds and adverse drug events in the intensive care unit. *JAMA*. 1999;282(3):267–70.

141. Samaranayake NR, Cheung ST, Chui WC, Cheung BM. The pattern of the discovery of medication errors in a tertiary hospital in Hong Kong. *Int J Clin Pharm*. 2013;35(3):432–8.

142. Galanter W, Falck S, Burns M, Laragh M, Lambert BL. Indication-based prescribing prevents wrong-patient medication errors in computerized provider order entry (CPOE). *J Am Med Inform Assoc*. 2013;20(3):477–81.

143. Rudall N, McKenzie C, Landa J, et al. PROTECTED-UK – Clinical pharmacist interventions in the UK critical care unit: exploration of relationship between intervention, service characteristics and experience level. *Int J Pharm Pract*. 2017;25(4):311–9.

144. Shulman R, McKenzie CA, Landa J, et al. Pharmacist's review and outcomes: treatment-enhancing contributions tallied, evaluated, and documented (PROTECTED-UK). *J Crit Care*. 2015;30(4):808–13.

145. Richter A, Bates I, Thacker M, et al. Impact of the introduction of a specialist critical care pharmacist on the level of pharmaceutical care provided to the critical care unit. *Int J Pharm Pract*. 2016;24(4):253–61.

146. Shaw RE, Litman RS. Medication safety in the operating room: a survey of preparation methods and drug concentration consistencies in children's hospitals in the United States. *Jt Comm J Qual Patient Saf*. 2014;40(10):471–5.

147. Fiala D, Grady KP, Smigla R. Continued cost justification of an operating room satellite pharmacy. *Am J Hosp Pharm*. 1993;50(3):467–9.

148. Thomas JA, Martin V, Frank S. Improving pharmacy supply-chain management in the operating room. *Healthc Financ Manage*. 2000;54(12):58–61.

149. Ziter CA, Dennis BW, Shoup LK. Justification of an operating-room satellite pharmacy. *Am J Hosp Pharm*. 1989;46(7):1353–61.

150. Wahr JA, Merry AF. Medication errors in the perioperative setting. *Curr Anesthesiol Rep*. 2017;7(3):320–29.

151. Leonard M, Graham S, Bonacum D. The human factor: the critical importance of effective teamwork and communication in providing safe care. *Qual Saf Health Care*. 2004;13(suppl 1):i85–90.

152. Greenberg CC, Regenbogen SE, Studdert DM, et al. Patterns of communication breakdowns resulting in injury to surgical patients. *J Am Coll Surg*. 2007;204(4):533–40.

153. Gawande AA, Thomas EJ, Zinner MJ, Brennan TA. The incidence and nature of surgical adverse events in Colorado and Utah in 1992. *Surgery*. 1999;126(1):66–75.

154. ElBardissi AW, Regenbogen SE, Greenberg CC, et al. Communication practices on 4 Harvard surgical services: a surgical safety collaborative. *Ann Surg*. 2009;250(6):861–5.

155. Nagpal K, Vats A, Lamb B, et al. Information transfer and communication in surgery: a systematic review. *Ann Surg*. 2010;252(2):225–39.

156. Nagpal K, Vats A, Ahmed K, et al. A systematic quantitative assessment of risks associated with poor communication in surgical care. *Arch Surg*. 2010;145(6):582–8.

157. Neily J, Mills PD, Young-Xu Y, et al. Association between implementation of a medical team training program and surgical mortality. *JAMA*. 2010;304(15):1693–700.

158. Hull L, Arora S, Aggarwal R, et al. The impact of nontechnical skills on technical performance in surgery: a systematic review. *J Am Coll Surg*. 2012;214(2):214–30.

159. Mishra A, Catchpole K, Dale T, McCulloch P. The influence of non-technical performance on technical outcome in laparoscopic cholecystectomy. *Surg Endosc*. 2008;22(1):68–73.

160. Carney BT, West P, Neily J, Mills PD, Bagian JP. Changing perceptions of safety climate in the operating room with the Veterans Health Administration medical team training program. *Am J Med Qual*. 2011;26(3):181–4.

161. Awad SS, Fagan SP, Bellows C, et al. Bridging the communication gap in the operating room with medical team training. *Am J Surg*. 2005;190(5):770–4.

162. Armour Forse R, Bramble JD, McQuillan R. Team training can improve operating room performance. *Surgery*. 2011;150(4):771–8.

163. Santos R, Bakero L, Franco P, et al. Characterization of non-technical skills in paediatric cardiac surgery: communication patterns. *Eur J Cardiothorac Surg*. 2012;41(5):1005–12.

164. Weller J, Morris R, Watterson L, et al. Effective management of anaesthetic crises: development and evaluation of a college-accredited simulation-based course for anaesthesia education in Australia and New Zealand. *Simul Healthc*. 2006;1(4):209–14.

165. Weller J, Cumin D, Torrie J, et al. Multidisciplinary operating room simulation-based team training to reduce treatment errors: a feasibility study in New Zealand hospitals. *N Z Med J*. 2015;128(1418):40–51.

166. Patanwala AE, Sanders AB, Thomas MC, et al. A prospective, multicenter study of pharmacist activities resulting in medication error interception in the emergency department. *Ann Emerg Med*. 2012;59(5):369–73.

167. Rask K, Culler S, Scott T, et al. Adopting National Quality Forum medication safe practices: progress and barriers to hospital implementation. *J Hosp Med*. 2007;2(4):212–8.

168. Nundy S, Mukherjee A, Sexton JB, et al. Impact of preoperative briefings on operating room delays: a preliminary report. *Arch Surg*. 2008;143(11):1068–72.

169. Einav Y, Gopher D, Kara I, et al. Preoperative briefing in the operating room: shared cognition, teamwork, and patient safety. *Chest*. 2010;137(2):443–9.

170. Haynes AB, Weiser TG, Berry WR, et al. A surgical safety checklist to reduce morbidity and mortality in a global population. *N Engl J Med*. 2009;360(5):491–9.

171. de Vries EN, Prins HA, Crolla RMPH, et al. Effect of a comprehensive surgical safety system on patient outcomes. *N Engl J Med.* 2010;363(20):1928–37.

172. Paull DE, Mazzia LM, Wood SD, et al. Briefing guide study: preoperative briefing and postoperative debriefing checklists in the Veterans Health Administration medical team training program. *Am J Surg.* 2010;200(5):620–3.

173. Lingard L, Regehr G, Cartmill C, et al. Evaluation of a preoperative team briefing: a new communication routine results in improved clinical practice. *BMJ Qual Saf.* 2011;20(6): 475–82.

174. Hudson CC, McDonald B, Hudson JK, Tran D, Boodhwani M. Impact of anesthetic handover on mortality and morbidity in cardiac surgery: a cohort study. *J Cardiothorac Vasc Anesth.* 2015;29(1):11–16.

175. Saager L, Hesler BD, You J, et al. Intraoperative transitions of anesthesia care and postoperative adverse outcomes. *Anesthesiology.* 2014;121(4):695–706.

176. Joy BF, Elliott E, Hardy C, et al. Standardized multidisciplinary protocol improves handover of cardiac surgery patients to the intensive care unit. *Pediatr Crit Care Med.* 2011;12(3):304–8.

177. Petrovic MA, Aboumatar H, Baumgartner WA, et al. Pilot implementation of a perioperative protocol to guide operating room-to-intensive care unit patient handoffs. *J Cardiothorac Vasc Anesth.* 2012;26(1):11–16.

178. Wayne JD, Tyagi R, Reinhardt G, et al. Simple standardized patient handoff system that increases accuracy and completeness. *J Surg Educ.* 2008;65(6):476–85.

179. Skaugset LM, Farrell S, Carney M, et al. Can you multitask? Evidence and limitations of task switching and multitasking in emergency medicine. *Ann Emerg Med.* 2016;68(2):189–95.

180. Dreher JC, Koechlin E, Ali SO, Grafman J. The roles of timing and task order during task switching. *Neuroimage.* 2002;17(1):95–109.

181. Reason J. *Human Error.* New York, NY: Cambridge University Press; 1990.

182. Wimpenny P, Kirkpatrick P. Roles and systems for routine medication administration to prevent medication errors in hospital-based, acute care settings: a systematic review. *JBI Libr Syst Rev.* 2010;8(10):405–46.

183. Whitman GR, Kim Y, Davidson LJ, Wolf GA, Wang SL. The impact of staffing on patient outcomes across specialty units. *J Nurs Adm.* 2002;32(12):633–9.

184. Picone DM, Titler MG, Dochterman J, et al. Predictors of medication errors among elderly hospitalized patients. *Am J Med Qual.* 2008;23(2): 115–27.

185. Jones S, Blake S, Hamblin R, et al. Reducing harm from falls. *N Z Med J.* 2016;129(1446):89–103.

10 Medication Safety in Special Contexts

10.1 Introduction

In previous chapters, we have discussed medication safety in perioperative settings: for the most part, we have used literature and data from high-income countries (HICs) and have focused primarily on broad categories of the medication process (transitions of care, intraoperative, postoperative, etc.) to differentiate risks in each location. In this chapter, we turn our attention to some special contexts where medication safety has unique aspects. First, we review data from low- and middle-income countries (LMIC), as their special circumstances open them to different medication risks and significantly limit which of the recommendations we have made can be implemented. Both of the authors have traveled to a variety of LMIC, and we have been deeply impressed with the expertise, dedication, and resourcefulness of healthcare workers who often have to work under very difficult conditions with very limited resources. Information is usually accessible, in large part due to the penetration of the Internet into nearly all countries, which provides online access to current literature, books, and web-based guidelines that is not limited by borders, although it may be by economic considerations. However, in many countries, particularly in Sub-Saharan Africa, there is a dearth of trained physicians in general, and trained anesthesiologists in particular (1). Many anesthetics are administered by nurses or technicians with variable levels of training in anesthesia. Often these anesthesia providers earn poor salaries, have poor working conditions, and are not in a strong position to exercise influence on behalf of themselves or their patients. There may also be shortages of nursing staff trained to care for postoperative patients, and in some places, the burden of this care may fall heavily on families, who, of course, seldom have any relevant training.

Without the foundational blocks of a sound medical or nursing education, the ability to interpret the literature or even basic textbooks is limited. In particular, as we indicated in Chapters 2 and 3, the pharmacology of anesthesia and perioperative medicine is difficult and continuously developing, and a sound current knowledge of this subject is the foundation of medication safety. There is an enormous need for anesthesia training in most LMIC (2). But even when knowledge is up to date, LMIC anesthetists often lack the costly technologies and equipment that we in HICs believe are foundational for medication safety. More importantly, their access to the full range of medications required for the safe perioperative care of patients is often very restricted – in some countries patients are not only required to pay for the necessary medications but may also be expected to purchase them and bring them to the hospital for the clinicians to use.

A comprehensive discussion of the challenges of providing safe surgery, obstetrics, and anesthesia to the 5 billion people among the world's population of 7 billion who currently lack essential health services (3) is beyond the scope of this book. In this chapter, we touch on some of the unique challenges our LMIC colleagues face and consider some potential opportunities for improvement. We also discuss the dangers presented by substandard and falsified medications, which have a particular impact in LMIC, and briefly touch on the particular challenges of medication pricing, which can put life-saving medications out of the reach of many patients, regardless of whether they live in a high-income or low-income country. Indeed, some of our LMIC patients may paradoxically have better access to third-generation medicines (antivirals) than uninsured and financially constrained patients in HICs without universal healthcare, such as the United States.

We then turn to the particular issue of medication shortages, which has come to be a continual source of frustration in all countries and has considerable potential to undermine medication safety: directly by forcing the use of alternatives to the best available medications, and indirectly by promoting medication errors. We next expand on the topic of wrong-route administrations, which we have touched on previously, and then conclude with a brief look at the unique challenges in mental health medicines and the intersection with anesthesia.

10.2 Medication Safety in Low- and Middle-Income Countries

Medication safety in any country is dependent, in large part, on the safety and quality of the healthcare that is present. The overall topic of health policy in LMIC is vast (4–7). Therefore, in this chapter, we focus primarily on the significant barriers to medication safety in LMIC. We must, nevertheless, note that a primary failure in the healthcare policies of many LMIC lies in the inequitable distribution of the available resources within countries (8). Substantial inequities can also be found between countries (Box 10.1) (9). It is common for certain hospitals in wealthy areas of major cities to be of a similar appearance and standard to those in HICs with access to all the medications that one would expect to find in the United States or Europe. At the same time, hospitals in rural or poor regions can look like those in Westernized countries a century ago, and the levels of staffing, equipment, and medications may be totally inadequate. As we previously noted, inequity in the distribution of resources for healthcare is not confined to low-income countries (LICs) but can be found to varying degrees in many HICs as well.

10.2.1 Access to Healthcare in Low- and Middle-Income Countries

Most patients in LMIC struggle to gain access to any level of healthcare, and when they do, the costs are disproportionately borne by the patient, often leading to impoverishment (Box 10.1). This has a huge cost in terms of human suffering, compounded by the consequent financial impact of inadequate or absent healthcare on the productivity and economies of these countries (3).

> **Box 10.1 Universal health coverage**
>
> Universal health coverage is a critical health agenda around the world given the significant disparities between and within many countries (2,3,10–13).
> - At least half the world's population lacks access to essential health services.
> - Approximately 60% of surgical procedures are performed in countries with high expenditure on healthcare, representing 15.6% of the global population, while 3.2% are performed in countries with low expenditure on healthcare, representing 60% of the global population.
> - Five billion people lack access to safe and affordable surgery and anesthesia care when they need it, including 9 out of 10 people in low and middle-income countries (LMIC).
> - Each year, 143 million additional surgical procedures are needed in LMIC to save lives and prevent disability.
> - In 2015, it was estimated that the worldwide shortage of surgical, obstetric, and anesthesia providers was over 1 million in 136 LMIC.
> - It is estimated that 1.27 to 2.28 million additional surgical, obstetric, and anesthesia providers will be required by 2030 to achieve universal health coverage (the estimates depend on the workforce density considered to be adequate).
> - Some 800 million people spend more than 10% of their household budget on healthcare.
> - Nearly 100 million people each year are pushed into extreme poverty because of out-of-pocket health expenses; 33 million individuals face catastrophic expenditure for the direct costs of surgery and anesthesia and a further 48 million for the nonmedical costs of accessing such care.
> - On average, out-of-pocket payments represent about 32% of national health expenditure.

These issues exist in large part due to the dearth of funding pools, which, when present, effectively "level" the costs of healthcare across populations. Only 38% of healthcare financing in LICs comes from such pools, versus 60% in middle-income countries (MICs) and 80% in HICs (4). As a result, more than 50% of healthcare is typically paid for out-of-pocket in low-income locations, in contrast to only 30% in MICs and only 14% in HICs (4). The high cost of healthcare relative to incomes can easily push a family below the poverty line (Box 10.1) and often leads to patients not seeking healthcare (4). Clinics and healthcare staff are few and far between, especially in rural communities, and patients often walk days to reach one (Figure 10.1). In the 75 countries with the highest maternal and infant mortality rates, only 64% of births are attended by trained personnel (4). The constraints to accessing adequate healthcare are numerous (Table 10.1 and Figure 10.1), including shortage and uneven distribution of healthcare providers coupled with low staff pay, lack of infrastructure (facilities, equipment, even roads and bridges to access remote villages), poor funding, corruption, weak programs with lack of oversight and supervision, poor governance and policy frameworks, corruption, political instability, weak laws, little or no public accountability, and on and on (4).The difficulty in accessing healthcare in many countries led to unanimous adoption by the United Nations General Assembly, on December 12, 2012, of Resolution 72/138 (see www.un.org/en/ga/73/resolutions. shtml, accessed December 26, 2019), urging all countries to accelerate progress toward universal health coverage (UHC). December 12 has become International Universal Health Coverage Day, with assemblies, demonstrations, and parades in many countries across the world (see www.un.org/en/observances/universal-health-coverage-day, accessed January 8, 2020). The World Federation of Societies of Anaesthesiologists (WFSA) has also issued a "Position Statement on Anaesthesiology and Universal Health Coverage" (2). The United Nations, of course, only has a bully pulpit and cannot force any particular action or in any way

censure nations who make no progress toward UHC. In many countries, even some who have ratified this UN Resolution, not only is there little or no movement toward UHC, there is, to the contrary, misappropriation of healthcare resources by governmental individuals and bodies for personal enrichment. Indeed, infant mortality and the Corruption Perception Index are highly correlated: the countries perceived to be the most corrupt have the highest infant mortality (14). Clearly this is not just misappropriation of direct healthcare dollars or supplies but also of elements critical to good health, namely, clean water, sanitation, and food (14). Corruption can also be expected to increase the cost and potentially lower the quality of medications (see the discussion of substandard and falsified medications, later in this chapter).

Perhaps even more problematically, across the world, healthcare workers experience personal attacks, primarily verbal abuse but on occasion physical attacks (15,16). In LMIC, particularly in areas of armed conflict, healthcare workers may be targeted and killed, often as collateral damage in armed conflict (17). At the worst, healthcare workers, even as they risk their lives to treat patients with highly infectious diseases such as the Ebola virus, are attacked and killed. Sometimes, this is in the mistaken belief that the foreign workers are the source of the disease or that outside agencies are spreading the virus as a form of genocide (18).

A discussion of possible responses to the constraints in access to healthcare in LMIC is far beyond the scope of this book, but one notable example, based on cooperation between community, private funding, and governmental support, is summarized in Box 10.2.

Referral system

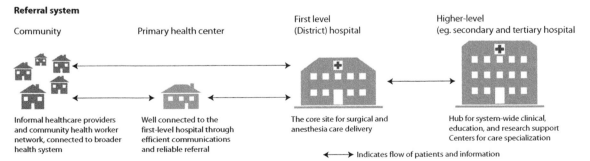

| Community | Primary health center | First level (District) hospital | Higher-level (eg. secondary and tertiary hospital |

Informal healthcare providers and community health worker network, connected to broader health system

Well connected to the first-level hospital through efficient communications and reliable referral

The core site for surgical and anesthesia care delivery

Hub for system-wide clinical, education, and research support Centers for care specialization

◄──────► Indicates flow of patients and information

Figure 10.1 The ideal surgical system as an interdependent network of individuals and institutions that reside within the wider health system and are supported by facilities in the community (such as those providing transportation). In reality, delays in accessing the parts of the system that a patient needs may occur in seeking care, reaching care, and receiving care. Reproduced with permission from Meara et al. 2015 (3).

Box 10.2 Mano a Mano

Over the past two decades, Mano a Mano has built 170 clinics in remote Bolivia (see https://manoama-no.org/about-us/our-model/, accessed January 21, 2020). Although it receives significant financial support from United States donors, the organization and operations in Bolivia are Bolivian. Remote communities are encouraged to request medical support from the organization in Cochabamba; the parent organization does not solicit requests. The requesting community is expected to provide unskilled labor to build the clinic (which takes 4000 hours, on average) and to provide 2%–3% of the costs. Standardizing the clinic floor plan minimizes costs: building supplies are the same for each clinic, down to the number of bricks. Furniture (e.g., examination tables, desks, cabinets) is typically built by Mano a Mano in Cochabamba; windows and doors are made by hand as well. For each clinic built, the local and national health ministries typically pledge to provide a nurse and a physician; lodging for these workers is built into the clinic plan. The Health Ministry provides essential medicines and reimbursement for vaccinations and basic services; the United States chapter often provides other supplies such as wheelchairs, canes, and stethoscopes, which are often donated by United States donors or US hospitals. The unique local, national, and private cooperation is highly effective, and this grassroots community partnership model has provided basic medical care to 700,000 Bolivians living in impoverished and rural communities.

10.2.2 Access to Medications in Low- and Middle-Income Countries

Recognizing that, worldwide, medication errors cost US$42 billion a year, which represents 0.7% of the total global health expenditure, the World Health Organization (WHO) in 2017 issued its Third Global Patient Safety Challenge: *Medication Without Harm* (Table 10.2; www.who.int/patient-safety/medication-safety/en/, accessed December 26, 2019) (19–21).Countries who can least afford to treat disease (i.e., the poorest ones), not surprisingly, also carry the greatest burden of disease in terms of sheer numbers and mortality. This applies to both communicable and noncommunicable diseases. This burden of disease occurs in the face of significantly restricted or nonexistent access to healthcare providers, facilities, and medicines. The

WHO estimates that one-third of people world-wide face significant challenges with access even to essential medicines (22). The WHO defines "essential medicines" as medicines that "satisfy the priority health care needs of the population," that should "be available within the context of functioning health systems at all times in adequate amounts, in the appropriate dosage forms, with assured quality and at a price the individual and the community can afford" (see www.who.int/medicines/publications/essentialmeds_committeereports/en, accessed July 19, 2019). The first list of essential medicines for adults was published in 1977; the first list for children was published in 2007. The most recent publication of "Selection and Use of Essential Medicines" was published in 2019 and includes lists for adults and children. Although the merit of some of the included medications is debatable (e.g., halothane given its potential hepatotoxicity), for the most part, the list incorporates all critical classes of medication and typically includes at least two options in each class. This recognizes that any given country may be able to get and afford one of the alternatives (e.g., thiopental, halothane) and not the other (e.g., propofol, isoflurane). Although the majority of medicines on the "essential" list are available in generic form and thus should be relatively more affordable, the fact that a medication is on the WHO "essential" list does not assure access at an affordable price or access to a pure product (see the discussion of pharmacovigilance, later).

As noted earlier, one-third of the world's population either has no access to, or cannot afford, even the most essential medicines. This problem is most marked in LICs, but it is increasingly becoming an issue even in MICs, and even some HICs. Unconscionably, with the drastic increase in some medication prices in the United States, even middle-class individuals may find it difficult to access essential medications. In a well-publicized case, Alex Smith, a patient with type I diabetes, died in 2018, a few months after he turned 26 years old and was no longer covered by his parent's insurance (23). Without insurance, he could not afford the $1300 monthly cost of insulin, which had increased 300% since 2002 (24); attempting to ration his insulin, Alex fell into a diabetic coma and died.

Many HICs and some LMIC negotiate for and purchase medications on a national basis, typically

Table 10.1 Healthcare system constraints and responses

Healthcare system level	Constraints	Responses
Community	Lack of local demand for effective intervention	Mobilize communities, provide incentives to healthcare provider to encourage use of services
	Physical, financial, social, and infrastructural barriers to use of interventions	Expand services within community, decrease financial constraints
Service delivery	Limited numbers and poor distribution of healthcare workers	Increase training programs, task shifting (train community members to manage simple diseases)
		Increase incentives to work in remote areas
	Low pay, poor conditions of employment, low motivation	Increase pay, support, and supervision; improve employment conditions
	Inadequate program management	Strengthen training, supervision; contract program management, utilize WHO, NGO programs
	Inadequate medicines, supplies, equipment, clinics/hospitals; poor physical access	Improve existing, build new clinics / Improve supply chain, efficiencies
		Public/private partnerships (e.g., Mano a Mano in Bolivia: see Box 10.2)
Government policy and strategic management in healthcare	Weak and overly centralized systems of planning, management	Decentralize, increase local responsibility for management
	Weak medicine policies, regulation; inadequate pharmaceutical regulation, support	Increase government oversight of medicine regulation / Provide inexpensive tools for detection of substandard medicines
	Lack of coordination between government and NGO and community organizations	Solicit (require) community involvement in planning and management
	Governmental bureaucracy, potential corruption	More efficient governmental structures with explicit monitoring capacity to ensure transparency and detect corruption
	Corruption and excess emphasis on profit by private companies	Greater use of private sector funding and management opportunities within governmental frameworks and structures (as mentioned earlier)
		Greater use of public-private partnerships, with caveats as mentioned earlier
		Greater community oversight and management of local HC services
Global	Brain drain: flight of doctors and nurses to high-income countries[a]	Voluntary agreements on migration of trained HC workers
		Improve pay, working conditions for HC workers

Source: Modified from Mills et al. 2014 (4).
Abbreviations: HC, healthcare; NGO, nongovernmental organization; WHO, World Health Organization.
[a] A major cause of the problem of brain drain lies in political instability (particularly, but not only, war) and associated risks to personal security (including the security of healthcare workers' families) and security of property.

as part of universal healthcare; these countries typically have much lower pharmaceutical costs than countries without universal healthcare. Patents allow manufacturers to set their own price, at least during the period of protection. Generic products,

which may be sold once the patent period is over, are typically much cheaper, but efforts to bring generics forward may be hampered by tactics of the brand-name manufacturer, including actually paying a generic manufacturer to delay introduction

Table 10.2 World Health Organization Third Global Patient Safety Challenge: *Medication Without Harm* – high-level actions with explanatory or more detailed comments on these

Actions	Comments
Focus on three priority areas:	• High-risk situations • Polypharmacy • Transitions of care
Design programs of action for improving medication safety in four domains:	• Healthcare professionals' behavior • Systems and practice of medication • Medicines • Patients and the public
Use convening and advocacy role to:	• Improve quality of monitoring for medication harm • Provide guidance and help develop strategies, plans, and tools • Produce a strategy for research priorities • Monitor and evaluate impact of this challenge • Engage with regulatory agencies to improve medication packaging and labeling • Design tools to help patients manage their own medications

Source: Sheikh et al. 2017 (19), Donaldson et al. 2017 (20), World Health Organization (21).

of the generic equivalent (25). Prices for anesthetic medications vary widely by country and may, consequently, drive the choice of anesthetic. An ampule of propofol, for example, in 2010 cost less than $1 in South Africa but $1.90 in Senegal and $10 in Guatemala; ketamine, however, cost $4 in South Africa but just $0.46 in Senegal and $2.32 in Guatemala (all prices in USD) (26). These price differences were in effect in 2010 and may not reflect today's costs, but they do demonstrate how price differences, which do not appear to be related to cost of manufacturing, may limit the choices an anesthesia provider has for a given patient. True life-saving biologics, such as sofosbuvir (a treatment for hepatitis C), are often priced in the tens to hundreds of thousands of dollars (USD); even though they may be cost effective compared to conventional treatments, these prices clearly

affect the overall cost of healthcare and the number of patients who have access to them. The price charged for a new medication by the manufacturer is, in general, determined by the willingness of the market to pay for it and often has no relationship to the costs of development and production (Box 10.3) (27). Some companies will charge differentially between high- and low-income settings, but others may worry that to do this would undermine the perception of the medication's value in HICs.

The solutions to this problem of access and affordability vary between settings. In our opinion, wealthy countries should recognize that healthcare is an "inalienable right" and allocate the necessary resources to it while effectively negotiating for equitable pricing. LMIC solutions are much more complex and require innovative approaches with participation by the pharmaceutical industry, international entities (e.g., United Nations, WHO, European Federation of Pharmaceutical Industries and Associations), philanthropic organizations (e.g., the Bill and Melinda Gates Foundation), and local governments (28). Such innovative approaches may take the form of public-private partnerships or product-development partnerships that use new models of knowledge and technology transfer that can effectively be codified in trade and investments agreements, such as the Transatlantic Trade and Investment Partnership (29).

In 2018, the WHO Executive Board proposed a draft road map with two strategic objectives: ensuring the quality and safety of health products and improving equitable access to medicines, vaccines, and health products (30). This road map specifically identifies weak government as a significant barrier to achieving these goals, by "fueling inefficiencies, distorting competition and leaving the system vulnerable to undue influence, corruption, waste, fraud and abuse" (31).

10.2.3 The Influence of Recreational Use of Medications

Access to some anesthesia-related medicines is further complicated by the overlap between them and the growing appetite for and supply of recreational drugs with narcotic or psychotropic ingredients, termed "novel (or new) psychotropic substances" (NPSs) (32). NPSs are often called "bath salts" in

---

Box 10.3 The price of a life-saving medication

- It is too simplistic to compare the cost of one medication's development and production expenses with the return on that medication. It is necessary to amortize the costs of all the medications that fail, which are the majority, into the ones that succeed.

- However, the price of a medication is, in the end, determined by market dynamics, not by the cost of production, however calculated. These dynamics reflect the benefit the medication brings, the amount governments and other funders are willing to pay, and how the medication compares with competing products. A medication that can save lives can be expected to command a higher price than one that provides a less impactful benefit.

- The willingness of pharmaceutical companies to develop and produce a new medication depends on the potential return from that medication (if it proves successful). This can be seen when comparing the much greater investment

into developing therapies for cancer than into new anesthetic agents in recent years. A new anesthetic agent would have to have a high enough price to justify its development, and that would likely make it too expensive to compete with current agents that are already very good and, increasingly, quite inexpensive in most countries.

- Pharmaceutical development is extremely risky – the odds of producing a highly profitable medication are small. Although governments fund basic research, they have seldom entered seriously into developing medications because they are (rightly) cautious about putting the public purse at risk. Thus, this is left to private enterprise.

- The question of reasonableness in relation to the overall return on investment of private funders is clearly moot. That of social responsibility for ensuring access to new and effective agents in economically challenged parts of the world is even more complex, but it is an important one.

---

news reports. Although the majority of these "legal high" drugs are focused on the synthetic cathinones, with pathological patterns comparable with amphetamines (32), many contain ketamine and other psychotropic drugs. While these drugs have been designed to reproduce the effects of common legal and street drugs such as ecstasy, ketamine ("vitamin K, Super K"), and cocaine, the NPSs are likely to contain far more "ingredients" than traditional street drugs, and thus pose a greater risk (33). A wide variety of dangerous effects, including many deaths, have been associated with their use (34). The majority of the NPS supply is from South East Asia, with a significant proportion from China (35). Mind-altering drugs have been sought by humans since the dawn of civilization, but the Internet has provided a substantial increase in access through the Dark Web (which provides anonymity through encryption) (34,36) and through smartphone apps such as Twitter, Facebook, and Instagram (Figure 10.2) (34).

10.2.3.1 The Story of Ketamine

Ketamine is a dissociative anesthetic agent that provides both analgesia and amnesia like other anesthetic agents but which preserves airway reflexes, does not result in respiratory depression, and typically preserves hemodynamic stability (in

particular, it does not produce hypotension). These characteristics make it an ideal anesthetic agent for many LICs, enabling nonanesthesia clinicians to provide anesthesia for essential surgical procedures, particularly cesarean sections, with a wide margin of safety. Given its perceived low risk and major benefits, ketamine was approved without being assigned to any of the controlled substance schedules in the United States between 1970 and 1999 (Table 10.3 [37]); most other countries during that same time period also did not place ketamine on any sort of controlled substance list. Although ketamine rapidly found favor as a recreational drug (news accounts surfaced within a year of its approval by the United States Food and Drug Administration [FDA]), the illegal manufacture and trafficking of this drug only became a global issue in the mid to late 1990s; many UN nations began reporting ketamine use disorder as a significant concern in the early 2000s and began more tightly regulating its production and importation. At the present time, the control and regulation of ketamine has significantly increased but still varies widely among nations. The United States, for example, now lists ketamine as a Schedule III drug, one with the potential for abuse but with moderate or high therapeutic benefit. By contrast, China, a major manufacturer of the drug,

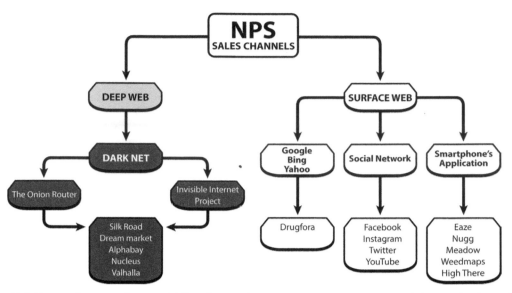

Figure 10.2 New psychotropic substances (NPS) marketing, advertising, and communication network. Reprinted with permission from Miliano et al. 2018 (34).

places ketamine in Schedule I, together with heroin, cocaine, and methamphetamine, as drugs with high risk of abuse with little to no therapeutic value. To date, the United Nations has declined to place ketamine into any of the Schedule Classes of the 1971 convention (see Table 10.3), despite repeated efforts by China to place it into Schedule I (2014), and more recently into Schedule IV (35). The decision to keep ketamine unscheduled was based on the WHO's Expert Committee on Drug Dependence assertion that "ketamine abuse does not pose a global public health threat, while controlling it could limit access to the only anesthetic and pain killer available in large areas of the developing world" (see www.who.int/medicines/access/controlled-substances/recommends_against_ick/en/, accessed December 26, 2019). This decision was supported by many health agencies providing care in LMIC (including the WFSA).

10.3 Falsified and Substandard Medicines

The presence of medicines that are, in some way, falsified or substandard has become widespread (Box 10.4). Increasingly, this problem is emerging

Table 10.3 The United Nations 1971 Convention on Psychotropic Substances: Schedules

Schedule	Potential for harm	Degree of control	Examples
I	Substances presenting a high risk of abuse, posing a particularly serious threat to public health with very little or no therapeutic value	Very strict: use is prohibited except for scientific or limited medical purposes	LSD, MDMA, mescaline, psilocine, THC
II	Substances presenting a risk of abuse, posing a serious threat to public health with low or moderate therapeutic value	Less strict	Amphetamines, and amphetamine-type stimulants, dronabinol
III	Substances presenting a risk of abuse, posing a serious risk to public health with moderate or high therapeutic value	These substances are available for medical purposes	Barbiturates, including amobarbital, buprenorphine
IV	Substances presenting a risk of abuse, posing a minor threat to public health with a high therapeutic value	The substances are available for medical purposes	Tranquilizers, analgesics, narcotics; including allobarbital, diazepam, lorazepam, phenobarbital

Source: From United Nations 1971 (37).
Abbreviations: LSD, lysergic acid diethylamide; MDMA, 3,4-methylenedioxymethamphetamine ("ecstacy"); THC, tetrahydrocannabinol.

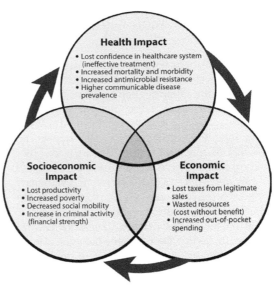

Figure 10.3 Individual, local, and global impact of substandard and falsified products.

> **Box 10.4 Some key facts about substandard medicines**
>
> - They affect every region of the world.
> - They have occurred in all main therapeutic categories.
> - Antimalarials and antibiotics are among the most commonly reported.
> - They can be found in illegal street markets, via unregulated websites, and through pharmacies, clinics, and hospitals.
> - They contribute to antimicrobial resistance.
> - An estimated 10%–30% of all medicines in LMIC are substandard or falsified.
>
> *Source*: See www.who.int/news-room/fact-sheets/detail/substandard-and-falsified-medical-products, accessed December 26, 2019.

in HICs as well as well as LMIC, particularly since the advent of medication shortages globally. However, it is particularly problematic in LMIC and has added to the extent and complexity of the issue of access, affordability and safety of medicines in these countries.

10.3.1 Nature and Scope of the Problem

Over the years, many terms have been used to refer to these products, including "counterfeit," "substandard," "falsified," and "degraded." More recently, the WHO has moved to only using the terms "substandard" and "falsified" to describe these illegitimate medicines. Use of the term "counterfeit" has been largely discarded, because of the legal connotation of the term, which implies infringement of a registered trademark. Substandard medicines are those that do not meet national or pharmacopeia specifications for the ingredients, whether due to original improper manufacturing (e.g., wrong ingredients including possibly toxic substitutions) or through improper storage or handling (e.g., nonrefrigeration). Some substandard medicines may have originated as legitimate medicines and subsequently been adulterated or degraded during storage or transport (38,39). Falsified medicines are those that carry a false representation of the identity or ingredients. Falsified medicines are substandard by definition. Therefore, we assume the term "substandard" refers to all of these medicines, and reserve the term "falsified" for specific reference to this group (i.e., not all substandard medicines are falsified).

Although these medical products can be found throughout the world, they are particularly prevalent in LMIC, through poor or absent controls on the pharmaceutical industry, on medication manufacturing or compounding, or within the marketplace. The WHO estimates that up to 30% of medicines sold in MICs are substandard, and the percentage is even higher in LICs – some 64% of antimalarial medicines in Nigeria in 2011 were found to be falsified (40). There are various ways in which medications can be substandard: all pose a substantial risk to patients, in LMIC and worldwide as shown in Figure 10.3, especially in treatment of communicable diseases (38,41,42).

Some of the most striking cases have resulted in deaths by poisoning from falsified medicines, but by far the greatest impact of these medicines arises from the fact that many of them simply do not work (Figure 10.3). All too often, neither the patient nor the physician consider the possibility that the resulting disease progression is due to ineffective, substandard medicine, and they may therefore continue an ineffective medicine, or even increase its dose. Although much attention has been brought to substandard antimalarial agents, a recent case of substandard propofol demonstrates that anesthetic agents are also at risk (Box 10.5) (43). The failure to treat communicable diseases appropriately through the use of substandard medicines has serious consequences for patients (including death)

Box 10.5 The case of substandard propofol in Zambia

In 2015, the occurrence of an unusual number of adverse events was noticed in Zambia in association with the administration of a particular brand of propofol (Unimed Propofol Injection British Pharmacopoeia, 1% w/v), manufactured in Amritsar, India (43). The adverse events experienced with this medication included urticaria, bronchospasm, and hypotension. A number of suspect vials were sent to Canada for analysis with mass spectroscopy and were found to contain between 45% and 57% of the stated quantity of propofol. Fortunately, in this instance, there were no additional toxic ingredients, but the provision of inadequate anesthesia with a standard dose could have led to awareness, serious harm, or even fatal outcomes. In one case, chest compressions were needed to resuscitate a patient who received this medication.

and the world (notably the development of resistant organisms). It has been estimated that, in 2013, in 39 countries in sub-Saharan Africa, 122,350 deaths of children younger than 5 years of age were directly due to substandard antimalarial medicines, accounting for 3.75% of all "under-5" deaths in those countries that year (44). Perhaps the greatest global risk is that substandard medicines promote antimicrobial resistance by exposing pathogens to what is termed the "mutation selection window," where the antimicrobial serum concentration of the active agent is too low to kill but high enough to exert selection pressure (38). Substandard antimalarials are believed to have contributed substantially to the rise of resistant forms of *Plasmodium falciparum* (38). Thus, the overall effect of substandard medicines goes far beyond being ineffective in disease management and even beyond direct poisoning of patients, with substantial socioeconomic, economic, and health impacts on individual patients, on local and national economies, and on the entire world, including HICs (see Figure 10.3).

Although the problem of substandard medicines has typically been thought of as a LMIC problem, the growth of ever more sophisticated organized crime networks has led to greater penetration of these medications, particularly falsified ones, even into HICs and into well-organized agencies such as

Medicines Sans Frontiers. In a recent case, a falsified version of the cancer medication bevacizumab (Avastin), was found in the United States; it contained salt and starch but not the active ingredient (45). More seriously, in 2008, a substandard heparin is believed to have been responsible for 81 deaths in the United States (46). It contained a contaminant (oversulfated chondroitin sulfate), structurally similar to heparin but about 100 times cheaper; the deaths were primarily due to hypotension caused by the contaminant (47). Detection of these counterfeit medicines can be extremely difficult, as many legitimate medications used in the United States and other HICs are made overseas. Furthermore, of the medicines manufactured in the United States, nearly 80% of the active ingredients are imported (40). Whether in LMIC or in wealthy countries without universal healthcare, patients prescribed a critically important but unaffordable medication will seek, and will often find, a cheaper, but potentially substandard, version on the Internet. Perhaps more worrisome, in the era of medication shortages, even some hospital pharmacies have unwittingly purchased substandard medications when forced to go outside of traditional supply chains. In the United States, online pharmacy sales were an estimated US$11 billion in 2009, but 97% of the online pharmacies investigated by the United States National Association of Boards of Pharmacy were found to be noncompliant with federal, state, or industry laws/standards. In the United States, many online pharmacies, purporting to be located in Canada, give the impression that the purchaser will be obtaining Canadian medications. The implication is that these will be as good as those in the United States but cost a lower price, but there is no way to verify their quality. One 2005 study found that only 214 of 11,000 so-called "Canadian" Internet pharmacies were actually registered in Canada (40).

The FDA, increasingly with international cooperation, has made considerable efforts to counter the sales of these medications. For example, Pangea VI shut down 1677 illegal websites and seized US$41 million of falsified medicines. The increasing complexity of supply chains, whether for ingredients or finished products, has provided multiple points where substandard medications can enter the market. A number of countries have responded to this challenge by adopting a mandatory track and trace system, which permits a specific medication to be followed from a legitimate manufacturer to a purchasing pharmacy (40). This will certainly decrease the number of substandard medications reaching pharmacies but will do little to alter the risk of falsified raw materials from reaching a legitimate manufacturer and will not protect online purchasers. In addition to substandard medicines being extraordinarily lucrative, the penalties when caught are woefully inadequate to act as a deterrent. Experts estimate that selling counterfeit medications can yield a profit margin 10 times that of heroin or 2000% more profitable than cocaine, but in the United Kingdom, selling a counterfeit designer handbag carries a heavier penalty than selling falsified medicines (40). These incredible profit margins and weak penalties make this trade irresistible for organized criminal and terrorist groups internationally.

10.3.2 Interventions to Protect Against Falsified and Substandard Medicines

A comprehensive review of the efforts that will be required to defend against this growing wave of substandard medicines is beyond the scope of this book, and the interested reader is referred to the systematic review by Hamilton et al. on this subject (38). It is clear that there will need to be concerted and coordinated international, national, and local efforts. International pharmacovigilance and global reporting systems include those maintained by WHO, the Medical Product Alert service, the Pharmaceutical Security Institute Counterfeit Incident System, and VigiBase. These reporting systems typically rely on national medicine regulatory agencies (NMRAs) that are responsible for medicine regulation in their own countries; unfortunately, 30% of sub-Saharan countries have no NMRA, and only 7% have NMRAs with moderately developed capacity to actually regulate medicines (38). Similar limitations exist in Arabic-speaking countries, leaving a vast number of patients exposed to the dangers of substandard medicines.

Simple pharmacovigilance, even if it were far more developed than it currently is, will not suffice. Supranational policing and law enforcement are needed. Pharmacovigilance relies heavily on activities within pharmaceutical and health organizations; international agencies such as the UN's Office of Drugs and Crime or the International Criminal Police Organization (INTERPOL) will

need to develop international regulations and attendant penalties to deter widespread proliferation of these falsified medicines. Unfortunately, to date, law enforcement seems sometimes to have focused more on protection of intellectual property for pharmaceutical companies than on safeguarding the health of individuals or nations. Individual penalties for trafficking in these substandard medicines vary widely among countries: France imposes a 3-year incarceration, while Norway and the Netherlands impose a sentence of only 4 or 6 months (48).

10.3.3 Preventing Substandard Medicines from Entering the Supply Chain

As noted previously, the increasing complexity and globalization of the pharmaceutical supply chain provide many points of entry for substandard medicines or ingredients. Even nations with highly developed NMRAs are at risk; LMIC, in addition to financial and human capital constraints that limit the scope of NMRAs, are more susceptible than highly regulated countries to corruption, notably in medication registration and inspection at ports of entry (38). There are pockets of hope: for example, Rwanda has had significant success in controlling falsified medicines, with centralized purchasing (limited to purchases of medicines to those with WHO certificates), pharmacovigilance at all health centers, centralized reporting, quality control testing of imports, routine systematic sampling for thorough testing, and effective collaboration between government agencies, including the Ministry of Health and the Customs services (49).

10.3.4 Detection of Falsified and Substandard Medicines

As detailed earlier, detection of a substandard medicine often begins with a suspicion that all is not well. Unfortunately, despite the substantial size of the problem, a high degree of suspicion is often absent, and substandard medicines go undetected. One successful detection example is that of the substandard propofol found in use in Zambia in 2015 (see Box 10.5) (43).

The Zambian case highlights some of the difficulties in detecting substandard medicines. Zambia is a country with a national NMRA, medicine purchasing is typically centralized, and medicines purchased by the Ministry of Health are identified with a logo that ostensibly verifies the medicine. For many countries, the only protection against substandard medicines is inspection of every batch of medicine entering the country or perhaps entering a local pharmacy. Technologies for detecting substandard medications are improving and are increasingly being applied, even when there is no reason to be suspicious that the medicine is substandard.

Technologies to detect substandard medications run the gamut from the very simple and inexpensive, such as the WHO or *United States Pharmacopoeia* checklist for visual appearance of packaging,

to the highly sophisticated and expensive, such as atomic force microscopy to verify validity of increasingly elaborate watermarks. Some of the technologies (although not all) are shown in Table 10.4; fortunately, some are designed specifically to be used in LMIC. These are portable, do not require electricity or trained lab personnel, can be used with minimal training, and are inexpensive.

The workflow for detection (see Table 10.4) begins with simple observation of the medication's packaging, the trademark, the information sheet, and the appearance of the tablets. The WHO and the International Pharmaceutical Federation checklists for detecting these counterfeits are inexpensive, straightforward, and can be used with

Table 10.4 Techniques and technologies for detecting falsified and substandard medications

Technique	What detected	Technology	Requirements	Performance; price
Inspection of packaging, materials; comparison to known authentic packaging	Misspelling of manufacturer or medicine; country of origin; container, sealing; illegible and indelible printing; tablet broken, not smooth; incorrect strength and dosage units, manufacturer's address, logo, or hologram, expiry and manufacture dates	WHO, USP checklist for visual examination FDA CD#3 (handheld scanner using range of light wavelengths) inspection of packaging and tablets	None; CD#3 is battery powered	Moderate; checklist is free; FDA CD#3 is low cost
	Label or tablets (these differ from real products under various wavelengths)			
	High-quality watermark (counterfeiters are increasingly sophisticated regarding watermarks)	Atomic force microscopy	Electricity, trained chemist, basic lab	High; high
Detection, classification, quantification of API	Presence of correct API	Colorimetry	Regents, UV light, lab tech, portable	High; low
	Classification of API	Paper chromatography cards	Water, lab tech, portable	High; low
	Identification, quantification of amount of API	Capillary electrophoresis	Regents, electricity, lab tech, physical lab	Moderate; medium
	Identification, quantification of API	HPLC	HPLC columns, pump, reagents, electricity, highly trained tech, research lab	High (gold standard); medium cost
	Chemical profiling for API, visual inspection	Counterfeit Device #3 (CD#3)	None, no electricity, minimal training, portable	High sensitivity, moderate specificity; low cost

Abbreviations: API, active pharmaceutical ingredient; FDA, Food and Drug Administration; HPLC, high-performance liquid chromatography; USP, *United States Pharmacopoeia*; WHO, World Health Organization.

minimal training (see www.who.int/news-room/fact-sheets/detail/substandard-and-falsified-medical-products; and www.fip.org/files/fip/counterfeit/VisualInspection/A%20tool%20for%20visual%20inspection%20of%20medicines%20EN.pdf, accessed December 26, 2019).

Medicines that are suspicious at this point can be sent to a more sophisticated laboratory for check of the watermark. Atomic force microscopy is a technology at the other end of the affordability spectrum and is capable of reading the molecular watermarks imprinted by manufacturers of genuine medications (50). These highly sophisticated instruments cost $100,000 or more, require well-equipped laboratories and skilled personnel, and thus are beyond the capabilities of a local clinic or pharmacy, especially in LMIC. These instruments are used at the national and international levels to verify suspected falsity detected with simpler tools and have an important role in criminal investigations of suppliers of falsified medicines (50). Alternatively, medicines that fail visual inspection, and those that pass this simple testing but are suspect for any other reason (e.g., adverse events, expected effect absent), can be checked for presence or absence of the correct active pharmaceutical ingredient (API) using simple and inexpensive technologies such as colorimetry or paper chromatography cards. If the medicine does contain the API, further testing can determine the concentration of the API (such as with the substandard Zambian propofol), although instruments capable of quantification typically require trained laboratory technicians, electricity, and various reagents. If no API is present, the falsified product can be sent for forensic examination, including mass spectrometry, to identify what agents actually are present, and nuclear magnetic resonance can be used to identify the geographic sources of the false ingredients (50).

One of the most LMIC-friendly detection instruments, the Counterfeit Detection Device #3, was designed by the FDA specifically for low resource settings (51). It is portable and does not require temperature controls, electricity (it is battery powered), elaborate laboratory settings, or reagents; it can be used with minimal training; and it is low cost. The current version has been significantly improved from the first versions and has an impressive array of LEDs covering a wide range of frequencies from the ultraviolet (UV) and visible wavelengths into the infrared (IR) region. The CD#3 includes a short-wave UV source, an anti-Stokes source, an electromagnetic field frequency detector, a digital handheld optical microscope, oscillating LED light sources (for hologram imaging), and tungsten as a source of rich IR (for document examination) (52). Although reliable and low cost, it does require an authentic sample of the medicine in question for comparison. It can be used both for inspecting packaging and for inspecting the contained tablets or capsules, although we found no literature on its use with liquid medications. When used to examine antimalarial tablets, it was found to have a very high sensitivity but only moderate specificity, meaning that it will identify virtually every sample that is falsified but will also wrongly identify some legitimate medicines (51). In addition, it will not detect legitimately produced medicines that have been rendered substandard due to improper handling or storage through the supply chain. Given its low cost, portability, and ease of use with minimal training, these false-positive identifications are perhaps not an issue, as medications flagged in the field or at port of entry as potentially falsified can then be sent to a more sophisticated laboratory for confirmation. This tool is not often used by anesthesiologists, because external packaging (rather than vial label) is often the most easily identified as false, and vials and ampules are often unpacked by supply chain staff or technicians prior to being placed in medication carts. In locations where the trust in these processes is low or where patients bring their own medications for their anesthetic, there could be a place for anesthesiologists to adopt such a tool.

10.4 Interventions for Improving Medication Safety in Low- and Middle-Income Countries

In Chapter 9, we referenced the framework of the Anesthesia Patient Safety Foundation (APSF) for improving medication safety. This framework focuses on four major areas: technology, standardization, pharmacy (including prefilled, premixed formulations and syringes), and culture. It can be applied with good effect in LMIC, but it needs some revision for this purpose.

10.4.1 Standardization

Despite financial challenges, anesthesia personnel working in LMIC can still implement many of the standardization techniques discussed in Chapter 9. Maintaining a consistent layout of medications in every anesthesia cart and on the top of the anesthesia cart does not cost much money; similarly, having a single concentration of any infusion or high-risk medication across all anesthetizing locations should be feasible. All personnel can agree to standardized and uniform labeling of syringes and infusion bags. Local anesthetics can be segregated from other anesthetic medications. Elimination of concentrated forms of high-risk medicines (e.g., insulin, epinephrine, heparin) may be more of a challenge, as providers may need to prepare all dilutions in their own operating room, because of lack of pharmacy support. Nevertheless, concentrated medications can then be kept strictly segregated from usual medications and clearly marked with "must be diluted." Route-specific connectors are highly unlikely to be available in LMIC, seeing that they are only now penetrating HICs, but it is inexpensive to label every line with the route (e.g., arterial, venous, epidural, or neuraxial). The APSF recommendations include a "uniform curriculum for medication administration safety": this should be feasible even in LMIC. The WHO has a medication safety curriculum available online (see https://www.who.int/patientsafety/education/curriculum/Curriculum_Tools/en/, accessed September 13, 2020) that although not specific to anesthesia providers, covers the key concepts for each step in the medication process.

10.4.2 Pharmacy and the Use of Prefilled and Premixed Syringes

Our LMIC colleagues will face significant challenges implementing the APSF suggestions for pharmacy and prefilled syringes. It is highly unlikely that enough pharmacists will be available in LMIC to provide specific support to operating room settings; this is not surprising, as many hospitals do not have satellite pharmacies in the operating room suite even in HICs. In addition, in the authors' experience, anesthesia personnel in LMIC almost always prepare all of their own medications (as they do in many HIC settings). As always, LMIC anesthesia providers will need to

be especially vigilant to check every label prior to drawing up or administering intravenous medications and, where possible, employ second-person checks for high-risk medications and routes of administration and when preparing dilutions of concentrated medications.

Easy access to medication information may be harder to obtain in the absence of 24/7 pharmacy support; the increasing prevalence of smartphones, medication libraries on apps, and Internet access may reduce this difficulty. One significant part of medication safety that HIC anesthesiologists rarely think of is appropriate storage; in areas with inconsistent electricity, maintenance of refrigeration can put the potency of some medications at risk. Also, given the difficulty in obtaining some medications, providers in LICs may feel obliged to resort to using recently expired medications or sharing the contents of multidose vials between several patients.

10.4.3 Technology and Equipment

As discussed in Chapter 6, providers in HICs are generally able to depend on the quality and reliability of the equipment used to deliver anesthesia and medications; anesthesia equipment available to HIC providers, particularly anesthesia machines and infusion pumps, have become progressively safer, with the total redesign of many components. Technological advances include pin-indexing for gas canisters and vaporizers for inhaled agents, coupling mechanisms to prevent hypoxic mixtures of nitrous oxide and oxygen, automated checks for leaks, oxygen pressure failure alarms, and many others. Similarly, the advent of computerized provider order entry systems and the networked surveillance between computerized provider order entry systems, pharmacy, automated dispensing cabinets, and the bedside (often incorporating barcoding) have increased patient safety; smart pumps with computerized dosing limits, often termed "guard rails," are widely used. With the possible exception of pin-indexing, these technologies are rare in LMIC, where practitioners may sometimes resort to third- and fourth-hand anesthesia machines, infusion pumps, and other discards from wealthy countries to administer anesthesia. In fact, donations of this type can be difficult to maintain and frequently end up doing nothing more than consuming storage space. Electronic medical records and CPOE systems rarely exist in low-income regions, so handwritten prescriptions are the norm, and thus electronic decision support and alerts for allergies or drug-drug interactions are missing. The issues with handwritten prescriptions have already been addressed in Chapter 3. In many LICs, hospitals struggle simply to provide reliable supplies of disposable needles and syringes.

Thus, LICs and many MICs face substantial, if not insurmountable, barriers to accessing most of the technology-based medication safety interventions proposed in Chapter 9. To put things in context, this lack of technology for medication safety may not be quite as antiquated as it appears. Many of these technologies have only become widely available relatively recently. Both authors of this book trained at a time (one in Harare, Zimbabwe, and then Auckland, New Zealand, the other in San Francisco, California, and Ann Arbor, Michigan) when anesthesia providers (and ward nurses) diluted their own medications, compounded infusions, and even delivered infusions, including vasoactive agents such as nitroglycerin and norepinephrine, using minibags with minidrip chambers controlled with simple wheel clamps. Infusion rates were determined literally by counting the number of drops per minute, and by titrating to effect. Monitoring under anesthesia was at times limited to a finger on the pulse and an esophageal or precordial stethoscope. Even today, in many HICs (including New Zealand), anesthesiologists and nurses in intensive care units or on the ward often dilute most of their own medications and may have only some of the available technology. Like providers in LMIC, they still need to rely on interventions known to be flawed, such as carefully reading the label and double-checking as much as possible when diluting or compounding high-risk medications, as some technological interventions are seen as cost prohibitive.

In the debate about exactly how much investment should be made into technology to improve medication safety, it is important to acknowledge the tension faced by any government in trying to improve the overall health of its population affordably. A high level of medication safety is possible with a restrained but well-directed level of investment that provides essential equipment with adequate numbers of well-trained staff working within a functional overall healthcare system. Decisions have to be made on the optimal allocation of resources. As indicated earlier, it is far better to invest in ensuring all the hospitals in a country are adequately staffed and equipped than in putting excessive resources into one or two flagship hospitals while underfunding others that serve large portions of the population. The key is to include the active pursuit of medication safety within a balanced overall national strategy for high-quality healthcare founded on principles of equity and continuous quality improvement (53).

10.4.4 Injection Practices

In addition to not having access to the innovative interventions proposed in Chapter 9, some low-resource and rural areas may not even be capable of basic safe injection practices. For example, they may not have single-use needles and syringes, and even where these are uniformly available, many safe practices, such as the use of autodisable needles or the imperative to never recap needles, may not be well embedded into practice. In a study of safe injection practices in a secondary hospital in Iran, most providers were aware of safe practices, but only 58% actually adhered to them when observed (54). The WHO made Safe Injection Practice a goal in 2010: a manual as well as a toolkit for assessment of local safety are available online (55).

10.5 Medication Shortages

Medication shortages began to appear around the world in the early 2000s and rapidly grew to become a significant risk to patient safety, as well as adding substantially to the costs of obtaining medications. As with substandard medications, these shortages have been felt across the globe. Virtually all medication classes have been affected as well as all disciplines; cancer treatment in some cases has been delayed by such shortages (56). Surveys done by the Institute for Safe Medication Practices in 2010–2012 uncovered at least 17 deaths attributable to medication shortages, whether due to physician unfamiliarity with substituted medications, errors following the need to purchase look-alike medications, or confusion around potency or formulation (57).

As with medication errors, there is more than one definition of medication shortage, with resulting differences in the numbers presented in different studies. The FDA definition refers to "a product used to prevent or treat a serious or life-threatening disease or medical condition for which there is no other available source with sufficient supply of that product or alternative drug available" (58), while the American Society of Health-System Pharmacists (ASHP) definition is broader, namely, "a supply issue that affects how the pharmacy prepares or dispenses a drug product or influences patient care when prescribers must use an alternative agent" (59). The FDA considers no shortage "when supply is available from at least one manufacturer to cover total market demand" (see www.accessdata.fda.gov/scripts/drugshortages/, accessed December 26, 2019). Thus, they do not count cases where pharmacists must change how medications are supplied. For example, the recent shortage of atropine formulated as 0.4 mg/mL in 1 mL vials has required pharmacists to change suppliers or to prepare dilutions for anesthesia use (for current shortages, see www.ashp.org/Drug-Shortages/Current-Shortages/Drug-Shortages-List?page=CurrentShortages, accessed December 26, 2019). ASHP includes atropine 0.4 mg/mL as a medication shortage; the FDA does not. Figure 10.4 presents the annual new medication shortages experienced in the United States from 2005 to 2017, with both FDA and ASHP data. We tend to prefer the ASHP definition, as substitutions may not always be equivalent to the preferred medication. A recent hydromorphone shortage would not have been counted by the FDA, but we think most anesthesiologists would take the view that the substitute opioids such as morphine or meperidine are not equivalent in relation to side effects or addictive potential. There is some evidence that substitutions resulting from medication shortages may increase mortality. Reviewing data from 27,835 patients admitted with septic shock to one of 26 hospitals, the rate of in-hospital mortality was greater for patients admitted during periods of norepinephrine shortages (39.6%) than during times of normal supply (35.9%) (60). Chemotherapeutic agents pose a particular concern, especially among the pediatric population (61), so much so that a "Working Group on Drug Shortages in Pediatric Oncology" has published a consensus statement on how shortages should be addressed (56). Anesthesiologists have continuously been impacted by medication shortages of one type or another, including the discontinuation of thiopental and shortages of succinylcholine, neostigmine, propofol, and most recently (in 2018 and 2019), local anesthetics. The propofol shortage had a significant impact, given the importance of this medication for induction and maintenance of a balanced anes-

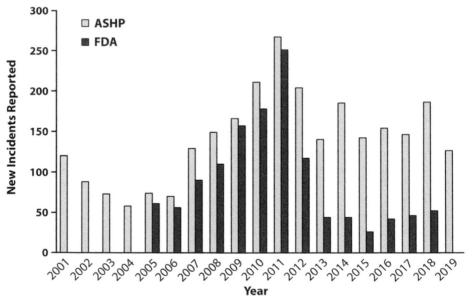

Figure 10.4 Number of new medication shortages reported to the United States Food and Drug Administration (FDA) and the American Society of Health-System Pharmacists (ASHP) 2001–2018 (note that this does not account for the total number of medication shortages at any given time, as this represents only new shortages. The number of active shortages at any given time has been between 174 for Q4 2016 and 282 for Q2 2019). Created with data from the FDA (www.accessdata.fda.gov/scripts/drugshortages/default.cfm, accessed December 26, 2019) and ASHP (www.ashp.org/Drug-Shortages/Shortage-Resources/Drug-Shortages-Statistics, accessed December 26, 2019).

thetic, provision of total intravenous anesthesia and sedation (62). At the time of the neostigmine shortage, sugammadex had not been approved by the FDA, and reversal of neuromuscular blockade became a significant problem. A national survey reported that most patients (72%) wanted to know of a medication shortage that would impact their anesthetic and that many would consider delaying surgery for this reason (62).

Even when an adequate substitute can be found, there are perils. Many hospital pharmacies will ration or aliquot existing supply during times of shortage (e.g., by dividing a 5 mg neostigmine vial into two doses of 2.5 mg each). This actually provides an opportunity to increase safety by the provision of medications in clearly and distinctively labeled prefilled syringes. Unfortunately, hospital pharmacists do not typically use color-coded labels, so anesthesia providers may be met by many look-alike syringes, all 5 mL in size, with plain white labels. Pharmacists may have to replace one manufacturer with another, thus changing the look of a given vial or ampule. Again, the use of prefilled syringes provides an opportunity to maintain consistent presentation of the generic agent to users but, unfortunately, this opportunity is often missed. Instead the result may be to create a look-alike issue when none existed with medications from the old supplier. Furthermore, the assumption that two versions of the same generic medication from different suppliers are equivalent may not be true. For example, various suppliers of heparin may specify equivalent units in a vial, but the potencies of formulations may vary widely (63). This may require cardiac surgery teams to determine heparin concentrations to monitor anticoagulation rather than using the more familiar and long-established activated clotting time (ACT).

As alluded to in the section on substandard and falsified medicines, severe shortages may cause even highly resourced pharmacy departments to search outside traditional supply chains to fill critical needs, potentially allowing substandard medicines to reach patients. Anesthesia providers in LMIC are likely much more aware of the risk of substandard medicines than are providers in HICs; providers in HICs thus may be less likely to be suspicious when a dose of anesthetic fails to achieve the expected outcome.

The extent to which medication shortages actually imperil health is not clearly known, but there is wide agreement that there is an impact and even stronger agreement that they are costly (64). This is due both to the need to use more expensive alternatives as substitutes and to the significant impact on pharmacists' time, to continually track shortages, search out alternatives, and educate staff members in potential shortages (59). Hernandez and colleagues analyzed price changes among medications prior to and after a shortage and concluded that medication prices clearly increase in the wake of a shortage (Box 10.6) (65).

Iacobucci estimated that medication shortages in the National Health Service cost the United Kingdom healthcare system £38M in a single month (66). It is highly unlikely that medication shortages will cease to exist in the foreseeable future. Increasingly, a medication may be offered by a single manufacturer, and if that one supplier runs into difficulties over quality or the supply of raw materials, or even faces a natural disaster (Hurricane Maria devastated manufacturing of intravenous solutions in Puerto Rico in 2017), there often is no easy solution. In the United States, Congress went so far as to pass a law directing the FDA to develop and implement a strategic plan to mitigate future shortages (codified in the Food and Drug Administration Safety and Innovation Act, 2012, Public Law

---

Box 10.6 Economic impact of medication shortages

Among medicines experiencing a shortage in the calendar year 2016 (617 dosages and 90 medications), prices increased an average of 16% in the 11 months after the shortage began, compared with 7.3% in the 11 months before the shortage (65).

Medications with three or fewer manufacturers increased by an average of 27.4% in the 11 months after a shortage; those with more than three suppliers saw price increases of only 4.8% in the same time period (65).

In addition to the direct increase in the costs of medications, there is a substantial increase in the time taken by pharmacists (and other staff) to access substitutes and costs associated with the reduced level of medication safety that results from these substitutions.

112–144, Title X). The strategic plan emphasizes the importance of early identification of problems and requires manufacturers to notify the FDA of any anticipated shortages as soon as possible. This triggers an assessment of the extent and impact of the problem, followed by working collaboratively to avoid or mitigate its impact. Unfortunately, these efforts do not appear to have mitigated the impact of medication shortages.

10.6 Wrong-Route Medication Errors

Wrong-route errors deserve a dedicated discussion in this chapter because they are important in anesthesia and perioperative medicine and can also occur in virtually any other hospital setting. Furthermore, although relatively rare compared to syringe swaps or omitted doses, they can have particularly devastating consequences.

One of the most notable cases of a wrong-route error, and one that received widespread attention, involved a young parturient admitted for induction of labor to St. Mary's Hospital in Madison, Wisconsin (67). The nurse attending to the parturient had completed two consecutive 8-hour shifts, slept at the hospital for approximately 6 hours, and then reported back to work at 8 a.m. Perhaps due to fatigue, she failed to place a barcoded ID band on a patient at admission. The nurse withdrew Pitocin, lactated Ringer fluid, and a bag of bupivacaine for epidural infusion from the automated dispensing cabinet in a single trip. On her way back into the room, another nurse handed her the bag of penicillin that had just been delivered from pharmacy. The nurse proceeded to hang what she thought was penicillin and administered it at a rapid rate. Within minutes the patient had seizure activity and cardiovascular collapse, which was initially attributed to penicillin anaphylaxis. Only after emergency delivery of the (healthy) baby and death of the parturient was it discovered that bupivacaine had been infused intravenously.

Many wrong-route errors, including the one previously noted, are made more likely by the ubiquitous presence of the Luer connector, which, until recently, has been used for virtually every infusion system in healthcare, including (until recently) pressure devices such as automated blood pressure cuffs. This uniformity of connections has allowed enteral feeds (68,69), epidural infusions (70), and bladder irrigation solutions (71) to be connected to a peripheral or central catheter. We discussed the *affordances* of things in Chapter 6. These connectors afford themselves to the administration of any medication in a standard syringe and thereby almost attract errors. In effect, injecting into a Luer connector *feels* right, even when it is catastrophically wrong. Other forms of misconnection are equally possible. One notable case involved attaching an automated blood pressure system to an intravenous catheter, resulting in a large air embolus and death (72).

One of the most troubling and stubbornly recurrent wrong-route errors involves the administration of a planned *intravenous* dose of vincristine into the subarachnoid space, which nearly always results in a slow, progressive encephalopathy and death (73–75). Although the reported numbers vary, there have been an estimated 135 deaths due to erroneous injection of vincristine into the intrathecal space between 1968 and 2011, with near 100% mortality. There are only a few reports of survivors, all with severe neurologic injury (76). Despite highly publicized recognition of this risk, prosecutions of some the doctors involved with them for manslaughter (77), and widespread educational efforts, these events have continued to occur regularly and with devastating results. Many of the publications about this problem have focused more on rescue after an erroneous intrathecal administration (78,79) than on finding a fail-safe solution. Despite many suggestions for safer procedures and policies (in particular, that vincristine should *only* be administered as an infusion, never as a syringe bolus), case reports continue to be published involving episodes when both intravenous and intrathecal medications were delivered to a patient's bedside in similar syringes (76). A survey of pharmacists in 2015 found that 30% of vincristine doses were still being prepared in a syringe rather than in an infusion bag (78). In 2014, the Institute for Safe Medication Practices (finally) made this process (vincristine as an infusion from a minibag, not in a syringe) a targeted medication best practice and, in 2019, it called upon the FDA "to lead the way internationally by requiring the removal of administration by syringe from the prescribing information for all vinca alkaloids" (see www.ismp.org/resources/ismp-calls-fda-no-more-syringes-vinca-alkaloids, accessed December 26, 2019). Again, the idea of affordances explains why this approach is safer: There are no medications that are routinely infused from a minibag into the intrathecal space, but we give many medications this way intravenously, making it feel right to give the syringe of methotrexate intrathecally and the minibag of vincristine intravenously.

Wrong-route errors are particularly dangerous and very difficult to prevent. Catheters can be placed in nearly every body cavity. Errors are inevitable, and the ubiquity of the Luer connection not only fails to provide protection against their occurrence but increases the likelihood of these errors occurring. As discussed in Chapter 9, the adoption in 2011 of the ISO standard 80369 that requires unique connector devices for each access mode (gastrointestinal, intrathecal, intravenously, arterial) will significantly reduce these errors but will likely not eliminate them, given the propensity for healthcare workers to jerry-rig devices when they do not fit or to find other workarounds for safety systems. Indeed, the tragic cases of injection of chlorhexidine into the epidural space, discussed in Chapter 4, would not have been prevented, as the presence of chlorhexidine in an open bowl could as easily been drawn up into a NRFit syringe as a Luer syringe, if mistaken for saline. These were certainly wrong-route errors (epidural instead of topical) and illustrate perfectly how dangerous the management of apparently innocent substances can be and how difficult it can be to design completely reliable systems to prevent them.

10.7 Psychiatry and Behavioral Health Units

Although medication errors among inpatients with psychiatric conditions are mostly consistent with errors described in other patients, there are some important differences. Patients with psychiatric conditions do present for surgery or for electroconvulsive therapy from time to time, so clinicians involved with the perioperative care of patients should be aware of these differences.

The Japan Adverse Drug Events (JADE) study from Japan found 398 medication errors among 448 inpatients with 27,733 patient days (17.5 errors per 1000 patient days) (80). Antipsychotics were associated with 50% of the ADEs; 34% were prescribing errors, while 39% were errors associated with monitoring, an error that has received much attention among the psychiatric community. It has been well documented that patients with mental illness in general and those with schizophrenia in particular are at increased risk for metabolic and cardiovascular diseases (81). To add to this risk, second-generation antipsychotic medications are associated specifically with increasing the risk for metabolic syndrome (82). Guidelines for management and monitoring of metabolic syndrome in this at-risk population have been available since 2004, but a recent systematic review and meta-analysis found that the rate of metabolic monitoring "is concerning low" (81). Prior to guideline implementation, fewer than 25% of patients had baseline lipid and glycosylated hemoglobin (HbA1c) monitoring. In nine studies of monitoring postguideline implementation, weight monitoring improved on average to 75%, but monitoring of glucose and lipid levels remained low (at an average of 56% and 29%, respectively). In one large academic medical center, even after implementation of a pop-up alert regarding the need for monitoring, the rate of metabolic monitoring did not significantly change (83).

In the JADE study, nonpsychiatric medications were three times as likely to cause an adverse event through an error, indicating that psychiatrists were especially prone to error when prescribing for nonpsychiatric conditions (80). In this study from Japan, few errors were associated with the administration phase, which is distinctly different from a study from Denmark, where administration errors accounted for 75%, prescribing for 8%, and dispensing for 10% of the 189 errors in 1082 opportunities for error (17% error rate) (84). Admission errors (100 discrepancies in 50 patients) (85), and errors at discharge (20.8% error rate) (86) appear to be similar to those seen in nonpsychiatric populations.

Given the dominant role of medication in the treatment of most psychiatric conditions, polypharmacy and medication interactions both pose potential hazard in this group of patients. A particular medication safety risk for patients with psychiatric conditions coming for anesthesia is the high likelihood of both psychiatric and anesthetic agents prolonging the QT interval. In the past, all anesthesia trainees were also educated on the dangers of monoamine oxidase (MAO) inhibitors, but

Box 10.7 Common medicines that prolong the QT interval; italics indicate medications common in anesthesia practice. This list is not comprehensive: to search for the QT effect of a medication, see www.credible-meds.org/index.php/drugsearch, accessed December 26, 2019

Antidepressants:	Mirtazapine, citalopram, venlafaxine, paroxetine, sertraline, trazodone, escitalopram, amitriptyline, nortriptyline
Antipsychotics:	Clozapine, ziprasidone, thioridazine, mesoridazine, risperidone, haloperidol, quetiapine, Lithium
Anti-arrhythmics:	Sotalol, amiodarone, procainamide, flecainide
Antimicrobials	Moxifloxacin, ciprofloxacin, trimethoprim-sulfa, azithromycin
Antihypertensive	Nicardipine, isradipine
Antinausea	Granisetron, *ondansetron, droperidol*
H₂ antagonist	*Famotidine*
Bronchodilators	*Albuterol, salmeterol, terbutaline, metaproterenol, levalbuterol, ephedrine, pseudoephedrine*
Anesthesia agents	*Sevoflurane* (propofol has been on this list, but recently risk has been downgraded), *cocaine*

Source: See Fazio et al. 2013 (87).

the frequency of these medications has diminished substantially, especially compared to the number of QT-prolonging medicines. Box 10.7 provides a list of some of the most common medicines recognized to prolong the QT interval: many antidepressant and antipsychotic medications are on this list. Because many of the patients on these medicines are otherwise healthy, they may not meet the guidelines for obtaining an ECG prior to anesthesia, and QT alterations can go unrecognized. Droperidol carries an FDA black box warning, and there are data to suggest that it carries a significantly higher risk than ones that do not carry such a warning, such as ondansetron (87). In our current state of opioid epidemic, many patients come to us on methadone, another medication recognized for its propensity to prolong the QT interval.

10.8 Conclusions

There are many more challenges to medication safety in LMIC than in HICs. Despite significant efforts by private, governmental, and international agencies, economic realities make achieving even basic aspects of medication safety in LICs particularly difficult. New recreational drugs, falsified and substandard medications, and medication shortages all add to the challenges of medication safety everywhere but perhaps more particularly in LMIC. Wrong-route errors occur in all countries within and beyond the boundaries of perioperative medicine. Although they are infrequent, their consequences can be severe. In patients with psychiatric conditions, the risks of prolonged QT interval and polypharmacy may be increased.

References

1. Kempthorne P, Morriss WW, Mellin-Olsen J, Gore-Booth J. The WFSA Global Anesthesia Workforce Survey. *Anesth Analg.* 2017;125(3):981–90.

2. WFSA Board and Council. WFSA Position Statement on Anaesthesiology and Universal Health Coverage. *Update in Anaesthesia.* 2017;32:6.

3. Meara JG, Leather AJM, Hagander L, et al. Global Surgery 2030: evidence and solutions for achieving health, welfare, and economic development. *Lancet.* 2015;386(9993):569–624.

4. Mills A. Health care systems in low- and middle-income countries. *N Engl J Med.* 2014;370(6):552–7.

5. Bennett S, Agyepong IA, Sheikh K, et al. Building the field of health policy and systems research: an agenda for action. *PLoS Med.* 2011;8(8):e1001081.

6. Gilson L, Hanson K, Sheikh K, et al. Building the field of health policy and systems research: social science matters. *PLoS Med.* 2011;8(8):e1001079.

7. Sheikh K, Gilson L, Agyepong IA, et al. Building the field of health policy and systems research: framing the questions. *PLoS Med.* 2011;8(8):e1001073.

8. Khan FA, Merry AF. Improving anesthesia safety in low-resource settings. *Anesth Analg.* 2018;126(4):1312–20.

9. Weiser TG, Haynes AB, Molina G, et al. Estimate of the global volume of surgery in 2012: an assessment supporting improved health outcomes. *Lancet.* 2015;385(suppl 2):S11.

10. Director-General. *Universal Health Coverage: Preparation for the High-Level Meeting of the United Nations General Assembly on Universal Health Coverage. A Report by the Director-General.* Geneva: World Health Organization; 2018. Accessed January 3, 2020. https://apps.who.int/gb/ebwha/pdf_files/EB144/B144_14-en.pdf

11. Meara JG, Greenberg SL. The Lancet Commission on Global Surgery Global surgery 2030: evidence and solutions for achieving health, welfare and economic development. *Surgery*. 2015;157(5):834–5.

12. Weiser TG, Regenbogen SE, Thompson KD, et al. An estimation of the global volume of surgery: a modelling strategy based on available data. *Lancet*. 2008;372(9633):139–44.

13. Daniels KM, Riesel JN, Meara JG. The scale-up of the surgical workforce. *Lancet*. 2015;385(suppl 2):S41.

14. Hanf M, Van-Melle A, Fraisse F, et al. Corruption kills: estimating the global impact of corruption on children deaths. *PLoS One*. 2011;6(11):e26990.

15. Franz S, Zeh A, Schablon A, Kuhnert S, Nienhaus A. Aggression and violence against health care workers in Germany – a cross sectional retrospective survey. *BMC Health Serv Res*. 2010;10:51.

16. Kowalczuk K, Krajewska-Kulak E. Patient aggression towards different professional groups of healthcare workers. *Ann Agric Environ Med*. 2017;24(1):113–16.

17. Ri S, Blair AH, Kim CJ, Haar RJ. Attacks on healthcare facilities as an indicator of violence against civilians in Syria: an exploratory analysis of open-source data. *PLoS One*. 2019;14(6):e0217905.

18. Schinirring L. WHO Ebola responder killed in hospital attack. *CIDRAP News*. April 19, 2019. Accessed January 3, 2020. https://www.cidrap.umn.edu/news-perspective/2019/04/who-ebola-responder-killed-hospital-attack

19. Sheikh A, Dhingra-Kumar N, Kelley E, Kieny MP, Donaldson LJ. The third global patient safety challenge: tackling medication-related harm. *Bull World Health Organ*. 2017;95(8):546-A.

20. Donaldson LJ, Kelley ET, Dhingra-Kumar N, Kieny MP, Sheikh A. Medication without harm: WHO's third global patient safety challenge. *Lancet*. 2017;389(10080):1680–1.

21. World Health Organization. *WHO Global Patient Safety Challenge: Medication Without Harm*. Geneva: World Health Organization; 2017. Accessed January 3, 2020. https://www.who.int/patientsafety/medication-safety/medication-without-harm-brochure/en/

22. World Health Organization, Regional Office for South-East Asia. *Equitable Access to Medicines for Universal Health Coverage by 2030*. Geneva: World Health Organization, Regional Office for South-East Asia; 2017. Accessed January 17, 2020. https://www.who.int/iris/handle/10665/258914

23. Anonymous. Woman says her son couldn't afford his insulin – now he's dead. CBS This Morning. January 4, 2019. Accessed December 26, 2019. https://www.cbsnews.com/news/mother-fights-for-lower-insulin-prices-after-sons-tragic-death/

24. Anonymous. What drove the 300% rise in insulin prices (and how to reverse it). Advisory Board. *The Daily Briefing*. November 7, 2018. Accessed December 26, 2019. https://www.advisory.com/daily-briefing/2018/11/07/insulin-prices

25. Federal Trade Commission Staff. *Pay-For-Delay: How Drug Company Pay-Offs Cost Consumers Billions: A Federal Trade Commission Staff Study*. Washington, DC: Federal Trade Commission; 2010. Accessed January 3, 2020. https://www.ftc.gov/reports/pay-delay-how-drug-company-pay-offs-cost-consumers-billions-federal-trade-commission-staff

26. Frye JE. *International Drug Price Indicator Guide*. Cambridge, MA: Management Sciences for Health; 2010.

27. Kesselheim AS, Avorn J, Sarpatwari A. The high cost of prescription drugs in the United States: origins and prospects for reform. *JAMA*. 2016;316(8):858–71.

28. Leisinger KM, Garabedian LF, Wagner AK. Improving access to medicines in low and middle income countries: corporate responsibilities in context. *South Med Rev*. 2012;5(2):3–8.

29. Stevens H, Huys I. Innovative approaches to increase access to medicines in developing countries. *Front Med*. 2017;4:Article 218.

30. World Health Organization. *Development of the Roadmap on Access to Medicines and Vaccines 2019–2023*. Geneva: World Health Organization; 2019. Accessed January 20, 2020. https://www.who.int/medicines/access_use/road-map-medicines-vaccines/en/

31. Director-General. *Medicines, Vaccines and Health Products: Access to Medicines and Vaccines*. Geneva: World Health Organization; 2018. Accessed January 3, 2020. https://apps.who.int/gb/ebwha/pdf_files/EB144/B144_18-en.pdf

32. Araujo AM, Valente MJ, Carvalho M, et al. Raising awareness of new psychoactive substances: chemical analysis and in vitro toxicity screening of "legal high" packages containing synthetic cathinones. *Arch Toxicol*. 2015;89(5):757–71.

33. Akhgari M, Moradi FMS, Ziarati P. The texture of psychoactive illicit drugs in Iran: adulteration with lead and other active pharmaceutical ingredients. *J Psychoactive Drugs*. 2018;50(5):451–9.

34. Miliano C, Margiani G, Fattore L, De Luca MA. Sales and advertising channels of New Psychoactive Substances (NPS): internet, social networks, and smartphone apps. *Brain Sci.* 2018;8(7):29.

35. Liao Y, Tang YL, Hao W. Ketamine and international regulations. *Am J Drug Alcohol Abuse.* 2017;43(5):495–504.

36. Wadsworth E, Drummond C, Deluca P. The dynamic environment of crypto markets: the lifespan of new psychoactive substances (NPS) and vendors selling NPS. *Brain Sci.* 2018;8(3):46. Accessed July 18, 2020. https://www.mdpi.com/2076-3425/8/3/46

37. United Nations. *Convention on Psychotropic Substances.* New York, NY: United Nations; 1971. Accessed January 20, 2020. https://www.incb.org/documents/Psychotropics/conventions/convention_1971_en.pdf

38. Hamilton WL, Doyle C, Halliwell-Ewen M, Lambert G. Public health interventions to protect against falsified medicines: a systematic review of international, national and local policies. *Health Policy Plan.* 2016;31(10):1448–66.

39. Institute of Medicine. *Countering the Problem of Falsified and Substandard Drugs.* Washington, DC: National Academies Press; 2013.

40. Blackstone EA, Fuhr JP Jr, Pociask S. The health and economic effects of counterfeit drugs. *Am Health Drug Benefits.* 2014;7(4):216–24.

41. World Health Organization. *A Study on the Public Health and Socioeconomic Impact of Substandard and Falsified Medical Products.* Geneva: World Health Organization; 2017. Accessed January 18, 2020. https://www.who.int/medicines/regulation/ssffc/publications/se-study-sf/en/

42. Ozawa S, Evans DR, Bessias S, et al. Prevalence and estimated economic burden of substandard and falsified medicines in low- and middle-income countries: a systematic review and meta-analysis. *JAMA Netw Open.* 2018;1(4):e181662.

43. Mumphansha H, Nickerson JW, Attaran A, et al. An analysis of substandard propofol detected in use in Zambian anesthesia. *Anesth Analg.* 2017;125(2):616–19.

44. Renschler JP, Walters KM, Newton PN, Laxminarayan R. Estimated under-five deaths associated with poor-quality antimalarials in sub-Saharan Africa. *Am J Trop Med Hyg.* 2015;92(6 suppl):119–26.

45. Mackey TK, Cuomo R, Guerra C, Liang BA. After counterfeit Avastin – what have we learned and what can be done? *Nat Rev Clin Oncol.* 2015;12(5):302–8.

46. Anonymous. Combating counterfeit drugs. *Lancet.* 2008;371(9624):1551.

47. Chess EK, Bairstow S, Donovan S, et al. Case study: contamination of heparin with oversulfated chondroitin sulfate. *Handb Exp Pharmacol.* 2012(207):99–125.

48. Nayyar GML, Breman JG, Herrington JE. The global pandemic of falsified medicines: laboratory and field innovations and policy perspectives. *Am J Trop Med Hyg.* 2015;92(6 suppl):2–7.

49. Binagwaho A, Bate R, Gasana M, et al. Combatting substandard and falsified medicines: a view from Rwanda. *PLoS Med.* 2013;10(7):e1001476.

50. Kovacs S, Hawes SE, Maley SN, et al. Technologies for detecting falsified and substandard drugs in low and middle-income countries. *PLoS One.* 2014;9(3):e90601.

51. Batson JS, Bempong DK, Lukulay PH, et al. Assessment of the effectiveness of the CD3+ tool to detect counterfeit and substandard antimalarials. *Malar J.* 2016;15(1):119.

52. Platek SF, Ranieri N, Batson J. Applications of the FDA's Counterfeit Detection Device (CD3+) to the examination of suspect counterfeit pharmaceutical tablets and packaging. *Microsc Microanal.* 2016; 22(suppl 3). Accessed July 26, 2019. https://www.cambridge.org/core/services/aop-cambridge-core/content/view/B527A009E3E4D4C248E53C0BD49AEEAB/S1431927616006206a.pdf/div-class-title-applications-of-the-fda-s-counterfeit-detection-device-cd3-to-the-examination-of-suspect-counterfeit-pharmaceutical-tablets-and-p-ackaging-div.pdf

53. Shuker C, Bohm G, Bramley D, et al. The Health Quality and Safety Commission: making good health care better. *N Z Med J.* 2015;128(1408):97–109.

54. Yusefzadeh H, Didarloo A, Nabilou B. Provider knowledge and performance in medication injection safety in anesthesia: a mixed method prospective crosses sectional study. *PLoS One.* 2018;13(12):e0207572.

55. World Health Organization. *WHO Best Practices for Injections and Related Procedures Toolkit.* Geneva: World Health Organization; 2010. Accessed January 18, 2020. https://www.who.int/infection-prevention/publications/best-practices_toolkit/en/

56. Decamp M, Joffe S, Fernandez CV, Faden RR, Unguru Y. Chemotherapy drug shortages in pediatric oncology: a consensus statement. *Pediatrics.* 2014;133(3):e716–24.

57. Fox ER, Sweet BV, Jensen V. Drug shortages: a complex health care crisis. *Mayo Clin Proc.* 2014;89(3):361–73.

58. Jensen V, Kimzey LM, Goldberger MJ. FDA's role in responding to drug shortages. *Am J Health Syst Pharm.* 2002;59(15):1423–5.

59. ASHP Expert Panel on Drug Product Shortages; Fox ER, Birt A, James KB, et al. ASHP guidelines on managing drug product shortages in hospitals and health systems. *Am J Health Syst Pharm.* 2009;66(15):1399–406.

60. Vail E, Gershengorn HB, Hua M, et al. Association between US norepinephrine shortage and mortality among patients with septic shock. *JAMA.* 2017;317(14):1433–42.

61. Jagsi R, Spence R, Rathmell WK, et al. Ethical considerations for the clinical oncologist in an era of oncology drug shortages. *Oncologist.* 2014;19(2):186–92.

62. Romito B, Stone J, Ning N, et al. How drug shortages affect clinical care: the case of the surgical anesthetic propofol. *Hosp Pharm.* 2015;50(9):798–805.

63. Thompson K, Alred J, Deyo A, Sievert AN, Sistino JJ. Effect of new heparin potency on activated clotting time during pediatric cardiac surgery: a retrospective chart review. *J Extra Corpor Technol.* 2014;46(3):224–8.

64. Davies BJ, Hwang TJ, Kesselheim AS. Ensuring access to injectable generic drugs – the case of intravesical BCG for bladder cancer. *N Engl J Med.* 2017;376(15):1401–3.

65. Hernandez I, Sampathkumar S, Good CB, Kesselheim AS, Shrank WH. Changes in drug pricing after drug shortages in the United States. *Ann Intern Med.* 2019;170(1):74–6.

66. Iacobucci G. Drug shortages cost NHS £38m in November. *BMJ.* 2017;359:j5883.

67. Smetzer J, Baker C, Byrne FD, Cohen MR. Shaping systems for better behavioral choices: lessons learned from a fatal medication error. *Jt Comm J Qual Patient Saf.* 2010;36(4):152–63.

68. Doring M, Brenner B, Handgretinger R, Hofbeck M, Kerst G. Inadvertent intravenous administration of maternal breast milk in a six-week-old infant: a case report and review of the literature. *BMC Res Notes.* 2014;7:17.

69. Simmons D, Phillips MS, Grissinger M, Becker SC; USP Safe Medication Use Expert Committee. Error-avoidance recommendations for tubing misconnections when using Luer-tip connectors: a statement by the USP Safe Medication Use Expert Committee. *Jt Comm J Qual Patient Saf.* 2008;34(5):293–6, 245.

70. Khan EI, Khadijah I. Intravenous bupivacaine infusion: an error in adminstration – a case report. *Middle East J Anaesthesiol.* 2008;19(6):1397–400.

71. Hicks RW, Becker SC. An overview of intravenous-related medication administration errors as reported to MEDMARX, a national medication error-reporting program. *J Infus Nurs.* 2006;29(1):20–7.

72. The Joint Commission. Avoiding catheter and tubing mis-connections. *Patient Safety Solutions,* volume 1, solution 7. 2007. Accessed July 19, 2020. www.who.int/patientsafety/solutions/patientsafety/PS-Solution7.pdf?ua=1

73. Slyter H, Liwnicz B, Herrick MK, Mason R. Fatal myeloencephalopathy caused by intrathecal vincristine. *Neurology.* 1980;30(8):867–71.

74. Reason J. Beyond the organisational accident: the need for "error wisdom" on the frontline. *Qual Saf Health Care.* 2004;13(suppl 2):ii28–33.

75. Berwick DM. Not again! *BMJ.* 2001;322(7281):247–8.

76. Noble DJ, Donaldson LJ. The quest to eliminate intrathecal vincristine errors: a 40-year journey. *Qual Saf Health Care.* 2010;19(4):323–6.

77. Merry AF, Brookbanks W. *Merry and McCall Smith's Errors, Medicine and the Law.* 2nd Edition. Cambridge: Cambridge University Press; 2017.

78. Gilbar P, Chambers CR, Larizza M. Medication safety and the administration of intravenous vincristine: international survey of oncology pharmacists. *J Oncol Pharm Pract.* 2015;21(1):10–18.

79. Reddy GK, Brown B, Nanda A. Fatal consequences of a simple mistake: how can a patient be saved from inadvertent intrathecal vincristine? *Clin Neurol Neurosurg.* 2011;113(1):68–71.

80. Ayani N, Sakuma M, Morimoto T, et al. The epidemiology of adverse drug events and medication errors among psychiatric inpatients in Japan: the JADE study. *BMC Psychiatry.* 2016;16:303.

81. Mitchell AJ, Delaffon V, Vancampfort D, Correll CU, De Hert M. Guideline concordant monitoring of metabolic risk in people treated with antipsychotic medication: systematic review and meta-analysis of screening practices. *Psychol Med.* 2012;42(1):125–47.

82. Rummel-Kluge C, Komossa K, Schwarz S, et al. Head-to-head comparisons of metabolic side effects of second generation antipsychotics in the treatment of schizophrenia: a systematic review

and meta-analysis. *Schizophr Res.* 2010;123(2–3):225–33.

83. Lee J, Dalack GW, Casher MI, Eappen SA, Bostwick JR. Persistence of metabolic monitoring for psychiatry inpatients treated with second-generation antipsychotics utilizing a computer-based intervention. *J Clin Pharm Ther.* 2016;41(2):209–13.

84. Soerensen AL, Lisby M, Nielsen LP, Poulsen BK, Mainz J. The medication process in a psychiatric hospital: are errors a potential threat to patient safety? *Risk Manag Healthc Policy.* 2013;6: 23–31.

85. Prins MC, Drenth-van Maanen AC, Kok RM, Jansen PA. Use of a structured medication history to establish medication use at admission to an old age psychiatric clinic: a prospective observational study. *CNS Drugs.* 2013;27(11):963–9.

86. Keers RN, Williams SD, Vattakatuchery JJ, et al. Medication safety at the interface: evaluating risks associated with discharge prescriptions from mental health hospitals. *J Clin Pharm Ther.* 2015;40(6): 645–54.

87. Fazio G, Vernuccio F, Grutta G, Re GL. Drugs to be avoided in patients with long QT syndrome: focus on the anaesthesiological management. *World J Cardiol.* 2013;5(4):87–93.

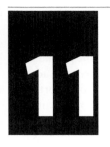

11 Legal and Regulatory Responses to Avoidable Adverse Medication Events, Part I: General Principles

11.1 Introduction

Thus far in this book, we have presented empirical data that show that too many patients suffer adverse medication events during anesthesia and the perioperative period. These adverse events include not only those attributable to undesired or unintended effects of medications but also those attributable to inappropriate omission or delay in the administration of indicated medications. A substantial proportion of these adverse events are avoidable, and many of these arise from errors, which by definition are unintentional. We think that an explicit intention to cause harm is very uncommon in the context of anesthesia and perioperative medicine, but we have argued that some of the decisions and actions that contribute to avoidable adverse medication events may involve violations rather than errors. These violations involve some element of disregard for patient safety. This disregard may manifest in the decisions and actions of individual practitioners. It may also manifest in the decisions and actions of the people responsible for leading, funding, and administering healthcare at institutional or national levels. Some institutions have made impressive and sustained efforts to improve the safety of their patients in this context (1), but there is considerable variation between institutions and between countries in their willingness to invest in initiatives to advance this cause, and between practitioners in their willingness to engage in such initiatives. The question arises, therefore, of how to hold all concerned accountable for the persistence of these avoidable adverse medication events and, in particular, accountable for doing everything reasonable to reduce their occurrence.

Therefore, in this chapter, we consider the role of regulation and the law in the promotion of safe medication practice in anesthesia and perioperative medicine, focusing on the underlying principles. In Chapter 12, we deal with the practical application of these principles in different parts of the world.

In Chapter 7, we outlined the story of an error in which an anesthetic registrar (i.e., resident) inadvertently administered 200 mg of dopamine as a bolus intravenous injection, instead of the intended medication, magnesium. The syringe had not been labeled, and a checking system based on barcodes that had been installed by that hospital at some cost was bypassed. These contributory actions were violations. Fortunately, rapid intervention by a consultant (i.e., attending) saved the day, and there were no long-term consequences for the patient. We also outlined a second story of an essentially similar, but fatal, error by another anesthesiologist some years earlier. We contrasted the low-level response that followed the first example with the prosecution and conviction for manslaughter of the doctor in the second.

It may be thought that the criminal prosecution of practitioners responsible for avoidable adverse medication events is so infrequent as to be hardly worth discussing. However, such prosecutions do occasionally follow fatal medication errors in various countries. For example in Nashville, Tennessee, a ward nurse, RaDonda Vaught, has recently been charged with the crime of reckless homicide after allegedly administering vecuronium instead of versed (midazolam) to a patient, with the intention of providing sedation during an imaging procedure (2). Two further examples from England, discussed in more detail elsewhere (3), involved tragic cases in which vincristine was inadvertently injected into patients' cerebrospinal fluid instead of methotrexate (4). A recent English case in which Jack Adcock (who was 6 years old) died some hours after being admitted acutely unwell to a pediatric service, involved a delay in the administration of antibiotics and has prompted extensive commentary and two major policy reviews (see Chapter 12) (5).

The extent of this variation in response to medication errors is remarkable: at one end of the spectrum we find very occasional criminal prosecutions of practitioners whose errors have proven fatal (often in response to understandable pressure from patients' families), and at the other is found little if any formal regulatory or legal response to the majority of failures in perioperative medication management. For the majority of medication errors, there seems to be nothing more than a nonmandatory expectation that an incident report will be submitted, and that some of these reports will be discussed at departmental mortality and morbidity meetings. Even at this low level of response, a comparison of the frequency of medication errors calculated from incident reports (6) with that identified through observational research (7,8) makes it clear that only a minority of such failures are reported, with an even smaller number followed up. In short, there seems to be a widespread acceptance by practitioners of avoidable adverse medication events as simply an inevitable part of providing patient care. However, this view is not matched by a parallel acceptance by patients and the courts when one of these events actually does cause serious harm.

In Chapter 8, we explained that the widespread toleration of minor violations of safe practices is called "normalized deviance." We suggest that an excessive willingness to tolerate errors and minor violations on the part of both practitioners and hospital management is a major barrier to safe medication practice. Equally, it is our opinion that the alternative extreme of criminal prosecution has only a very small role in improving medication safety and is typically unhelpful. Notwithstanding evidence that many adverse medication events reflect less than ideal practice, they nearly always involve well-intended, hardworking, and well-trained practitioners who are expected to administer medications safely in systems that are, to varying extents, poorly designed for this. It is our view, therefore, that a more proactive, but proportionate, regulatory approach to the numerous failures in medication management that occur daily in any hospital is required. An approach that genuinely held both practitioners and managers accountable for the management of medications would go a long way to improving safety and thereby reducing the number of tragic events that lead to these highly punitive criminal prosecutions.

Throughout the discussion in this chapter (and in Chapter 12), we take as given that the needs of the injured patient must always be the primary and central consideration in any response to an adverse medication event. However, it is also important to consider the overall need to improve healthcare and thereby minimize the risk of similar events occurring to future patients. Furthermore, as discussed in Chapter 5 and illustrated in the tragic story of Jack Adcock's death (outlined in Chapter 12), the clinicians involved in such cases may sometimes become victims themselves. Thus, we are also concerned with justice and with the needs of those clinicians who end up inadvertently harming patients in the process of doing their best to help them.

We begin this chapter with the main elements that should be considered in the overall response to any incident in which a patient is accidentally harmed during healthcare, but with particular reference to adverse medication events. We then consider ways in which regulatory and disciplinary processes might promote the achievement of these elements, beginning with those internal to any institution and then moving to those that operate at an external level, usually nationally and often through governmental agencies. We conclude with a consideration of the ethical responsibilities in this context and of who shares in these. We argue that the "team for safe medication management" must be seen as very broadly based and suggest that achieving the required changes will depend as much or more on the engagement of individual practitioners as on any particular regulatory framework. In these two chapters, we take a broad view of regulation. We include both voluntary and mandatory approaches to the promotion of safer practices and argue that professional self-regulation is as important as externally imposed regulation.

11.2 The Objectives of a Legal or Regulatory Response to an Unintended Adverse Medication Event

Five important objectives (discussed in previous chapters) that should be promoted by any legal or regulatory response to an unintended adverse medication event are listed as column headings in Table 11.1. After any adverse medication event (preventable or not), the priority should be the immediate and ongoing care of the injured patient, to ameliorate the harm to the extent possible. There should also be early provision of information to patients and families about what happened and why. Where the event was avoidable, compensation, a commitment to improving the system to prevent future such events, and when appropriate, retribution may also be appropriate. In Table 11.1, we also attempted to illustrate some of the legal or regulatory processes by which these objectives may be pursued.

Patients are central to these processes and to achieving these objectives. Clearly it is the patients and those close to them who are harmed by adverse medication events. Also, it is usually patients or their families who lodge complaints or initiate lawsuits or ask for criminal charges to be laid after such events. These people then have to live through the consequent processes, alongside the practitioners who set out to help them but ended up inadvertently harming them. These processes are often prolonged, emotionally distressing, and expensive for everyone concerned including patients and their loved ones. It is ironic that, whatever else they achieve, the legal responses to iatrogenic harm in healthcare often increase the net emotional and financial suffering associated with that harm, even for the patients. Thus, a sixth objective should be to make legislative and regulatory processes easily accessible and as supportive and comfortable as possible for the people who need to use them. The aim should be to improve the situation, not to make a bad state of affairs even worse.

Table 11.1 The objectives of a legal or regulatory response to the unintentional injury of a patient during healthcare (including by avoidable adverse medication events), the processes by which these might normally be achieved, and the extent to which the latter typically achieve the former

| | Objectives | | | | |
	Amelioration	Information	Compensation	Retribution	Accountability and prevention
	Treatment of the injury and consequential medical problems	Informed consent and/or open disclosure	Loss adjustment	Punishment	Improved practice
Internal processes					
Individual professionalism	√	√	Not usually	Not usually	√
Institutional responses[a]	√	√	√	√	√
Complaints and notifications[b]	√	√	√	√	√
External processes					
Media	Not usually	Probably	Not usually	Often	Possibly
Inquiries	Not usually	√	Possibly	Possibly	√
Tort	√	√	√	In practice yes, but not a primary purpose	Uncertain –controversial
No fault compensation	√	Not necessarily	√	Possibly via referral to other agencies	Possibly via referral to other agencies
Professional regulation	√	√	Not usually	√	Possibly
Criminal prosecution	Not usually, or very late	To some extent	Not usually	√	Uncertain – controversial

[a] Institutional responses typically include incident reporting, investigations or inquiries, discipline, root-cause analysis, and other efforts to improve relevant aspects of the quality and safety of care, risk management, complaints, resolution processes, and litigation resolution processes.

[b] In some countries, there are also external (sometimes national) processes for handling complaints (e.g., through the office of the Health and Disability Commissioner in New Zealand).

11.2.1 Amelioration

Immediate and adequate attention to amelioration of harm to a patient who has suffered an adverse medication event is clearly the right thing to do (9). Many medication errors are without consequence or have only minor or temporary adverse effects, so amelioration, if required at all, is straightforward. For a serious adverse medication event, more substantive action is needed. As explained in Chapter 4 (see Table 4.1), harm includes physical and emotional harm and may be short term or longer lasting. It may require a considerable amount of clinicians' time and often the expense of further procedures or medications or time in hospital or intensive care. These are expenses that a patient harmed by an adverse medication event should not bear. Regulatory and legal provisions should seek to ensure that patients do not have to do so. It should not be forgotten that emotional harm following an adverse medication event may extend beyond the patient to loved ones and to staff involved in the event (as discussed in Chapter 5).

The appropriate management of the consequences of an unexpected adverse event must take precedent over planned routine work. This may well require delaying or canceling the next scheduled case, and it will often involve asking for help or advice from others (such as surgeons, intensivists or internists, or other anesthesiologists). It may be necessary for the surgeon to stop operating so that efforts can be concentrated on the more pressing need to treat a medication reaction (anaphylaxis, hypotension, or an arrhythmia, for example). It may be appropriate for the practitioner whose error has caused the harm to be relieved of other duties to allow the practitioner to concentrate on attending to the patient, and/or to avoid further events during a period of emotional upset. Obviously, communication with colleagues in such situations needs to be frank and explicit about the exact nature of the error that has been made. It is sometimes overlooked that open disclosure starts with open disclosure to one's colleagues – a proper understanding of the nature of the problem by all concerned will typically facilitate its treatment. It may also alert colleagues to a systems failure, as in the cases of poisoned gas discussed in Chapter 6. This openness should extend to careful documentation of relevant events, and such documentation is generally expected by the courts.

It is, therefore, highly desirable that both the internal regulatory framework of any institution and the external laws within which the institution has to function encourage all of these things, and discourage a culture in which continuing with the next case is seen as a priority, perhaps because of financial pressures. It is also desirable to minimize anxiety about the consequences of openly sharing information. Obviously, care of the patient and the affected clinicians should take precedence over any concerns about legal or disciplinary risks. In fact, properly attending to the needs of the patient will usually have the effect of mitigating legal and regulatory risk both to the clinicians involved in the patient's care and to the institution, but an effective regulatory and legal system should seek to make this requirement explicit and to maximize the incentives for everyone concerned to do the right things. In particular, this patient-centered approach should be a strong focus for the internal systems and culture of any healthcare institution.

11.2.2 Information and Open Disclosure

Patients and their families who have suffered an adverse medication event will almost always want to be given information, and usually a sincere and empathic apology, if only for the fact that harm has occurred. As discussed in Chapter 4, in many high-income countries, forward-thinking institutions are increasingly embracing the principle of early open disclosure, embedding the requirement for it into their policies, and offering their staff training and support in communication and dispute resolution. Interestingly, recent data from England have shown that efforts to increase openness in the hospital system are associated with better quality of healthcare, manifest as a reduction in hospital mortality rates (10). It follows that as with patients' more general needs, discussed in the previous section, legal and regulatory approaches should encourage openness and transparency in general and even more particularly in the context of the adverse event.

We presented some evidence in Chapter 4 that transparency with patients is likely to decrease the risk of litigation, especially if disclosure is integrated into an effective process for dispute resolution. Conversely, few things are more likely to frustrate, distress, and anger an injured patient than difficulty in finding out what happened, and a desire for information is often the driver for a complaint, a lawsuit, or a request to the police to institute criminal proceedings.

On the other hand, even if empathic open disclosure reduces the overall cost of litigation, knowledge of an event may provide exactly the information needed by the occasional injured patient or family who does decide to take any of these actions, and such a decision is probably most likely when the adverse event has been very serious (11,12). For example, in the second case involving dopamine mentioned earlier, it was the anesthesiologist's own openness about his error that led to his conviction for manslaughter. On that occasion, as with many medication errors, he was the only person who understood that an error had occurred, so if he had chosen to remain silent, it is more than possible that no legal consequences would have followed. Furthermore, the subsequent abuse of legislative provisions related to the confidentiality of his report to a statutory committee on deaths related to anesthesia was very instructive (Box 11.1). Not only does this case illustrate the hazards of providing information, even under privilege, it also provides an interesting example of how motivated practition-

ers often are to learn from adverse events and how this can be facilitated or inhibited by legislation and policy (in this case, the policy decision of the police to access information that had been given in good faith under the impression that it was protected). Perhaps the most telling point is that legal mandate may be less effective than personal motivation in promoting activities to improve the quality and safety of healthcare.

It is one thing to send a confidential report to a statutory committee and quite another to tell patients the very things that one might include in such a report. Unfortunately, until quite recently, patients in many countries have often found it difficult to obtain information about what has happened to them during their healthcare; there continues to be considerable variation in this (14). As one example, a survey of European intensive care doctors found that patients were more likely to get complete information in the Netherlands than in Greece, Spain, and Italy (15). In most settings, the greatest source of anxiety in relation to the provision of "too much" information to patients is probably related to the possibility of civil litigation or perhaps to the possibility of a formal complaint. It seems likely

---

Box 11.1 How legislation and policy can influence clinicians' motivation to learn from adverse medication events

At the time of the event, outlined in Chapter 7, in which the inadvertent administration of dopamine instead of doxapram led to a patient's death in New Zealand, there was a statutory requirement to report deaths associated with anesthesia to a committee known as *The Anaesthetic Mortality Assessment Committee*. This committee had been set up in 1979 at the behest of a group of anesthesiologists and was very well supported by this professional group. Its function was not to allocate blame but to understand and learn from these events. Anesthesiologists believed that information supplied to this committee was privileged, but it turned out that there were limited exceptions, including for the "purposes of the investigation of crime." The police used these provisions to obtain the report submitted by the anesthesiologist, and once this became known, even though it was argued that the information was not actually used during his prosecution for manslaughter, reporting to the committee declined dramatically, despite the fact that it was a requirement under the law. Thus, after being very

well supported by the anesthesia profession during its first decade, the committee became "effectively defunct because of civil disobedience by those who campaigned for its establishment, namely the anaesthetists of New Zealand" (13). The extent of this civil disobedience was such that there was very little that could be done about it in practice. In fact, it would have been possible to comply with the law by submitting very short reports that provided little in the way of useful information, but we believe the anesthetic community in New Zealand was outraged, and seeking to make a point. The committee was eventually disestablished.

In 2010, some years after changes to the criminal law in 1997 made similar prosecutions much less likely, a new, multidisciplinary Perioperative Mortality Review Committee (see www.hqsc.govt.nz/our-programmes/mrc/pomrc/, accessed January 21, 2020) was established, again in response to strong representation to government from practitioners, notably anesthesiologists. This new committee is very active and well supported today.

that the overall culture and laws of a country influence not only the likelihood of open disclosure (as just discussed) but also the type of response to be expected from most patients on receiving information about failures in the standard of their care. The national culture may be as important in this regard as the culture within individual institutions.

In New Zealand and the Nordic countries, no-fault compensation schemes reduce the likelihood that a patient will sue for negligence (3). In fact, in New Zealand, civil actions for compensation for harm arising from any accident, whether associated with healthcare or not, are not permitted under the law. On the other hand, it is particularly easy to lay a complaint and have it followed up, either within hospitals or through the office of a national Health and Disability Commissioner (see www.hdc.org.nz/, accessed January 21, 2020). Thus, disclosure could inform a complaint. On the other hand, in New Zealand, Right 6 of the Code of Health and Disability Services Consumers' Rights (16) gives all consumers the right to be fully informed (i.e., to receive the information that a reasonable consumer in this situation would expect to receive), so failing to provide such information could itself constitute a breach of this code. Similarly, in the United Kingdom, doctors now have a legislated duty of candor when patients have suffered at least moderate harm (17).

Qualified privilege laws protect information disclosed as part of an apology from discovery in legal proceedings in some countries and in some states in the United States, but there is no such protection in many other countries, including New Zealand. Legislation also changes over time. For example, in New Zealand, prosecutions for negligence manslaughter have become very infrequent since the above-mentioned change in the law in 1997 (13), so the risk of criminal charges arising from open disclosure now seems to be very low. In the United Kingdom, the introduction of the duty of candor followed calls arising from the events at the Mid Staffordshire NHS Trust (18). Thus, one should not lose sight of the possibility that further legislative changes may have a role in advancing (or impeding) the cause of perioperative medication safety. This alone is reason for practitioners to take an interest in the laws and regulations of their own country.

Resourcing may also make a difference – in some low-income countries, patients may be less likely to complain simply because the overall resources for healthcare are so inadequate that minor failures in the system are accepted as normal. In addition, there may be no institutional policies, procedures, or dedicated staff to facilitate the filing of a complaint. It is also worth noting that (in any country) patients who feel deprived of the opportunity to complain may find their own ways to express their frustration and attempt to hold practitioners accountable. In some countries, physical violence directed by aggrieved patients or their families against doctors or other health professionals is a major problem (19). The increasing role of social media in modern life has also opened up new possibilities in almost all countries for direct reprisal by patients ("crowd regulation" as it were), perhaps informed by disclosed information, in addition to the possibilities that have always been provided through conventional media.

In summary, then, it is not easy to predict the likely effect of empathically disclosing information about an adverse medication event to any individual patient on that patient's subsequent decision to pursue retribution, even though, on balance, doing so seems likely to reduce that risk, probably substantially. This may be true whether there are legislative protections for such information or not, and in many parts of the world there are not. Regardless, the fact remains that, ethically, being open and transparent with patients while also engaging proactively in addressing the harm they have suffered are the right things to do (20–23).

Even after having decided to do the right thing in this respect, the question of exactly what information should be disclosed in relation to precisely which medication errors and when is quite nuanced. We have seen that many medication errors cause no harm to patients. Thus, if one takes the phrasing quoted earlier from New Zealand's Code of Patient Rights (which is simply a codified statement of a principle accepted in many countries), it might well be thought that information about a medication error that was without consequence does not constitute something that "a reasonable consumer in his or her situation would expect to receive." On the contrary, it could be argued that the provision of such information may be detrimental in that it might cause unnecessary worry or information overload to a patient. One could support this view with reference to the United Kingdom duty of candor for which the threshold is "at least moderate harm." However, an alternative viewpoint would be that disclosure of such information would align with a strong commitment to eliminate such errors and with transparency more generally. Box 11.2 contains a discussion of these points in relation to a particular example.

Box 11.2 Disclosing a medication error made during an anesthetic: a matter for judgment

In Box 7.5, we describe a medication error in which suxamethonium was inadvertently administered to a patient instead of pancuronium.

What disclosure and documentation should have occurred?

The issues weighed up by the anesthesiologist were as follows:

- The systems failure (or latent factor [24]) that created a situation promoting this error and the importance of preventing a recurrence in the future.
- The potential risk rather than the actual consequences – the same error could have been serious in certain (somewhat rare) circumstances in which suxamethonium is contraindicated.
- The fact that the information would have no particular value to this patient and that trying to explain this event to him or his family might well have been a distraction from the wider matter of ongoing information about all the other aspects of his care.
- The possibility that someone else would tell the patient what had happened (it is a sensible assumption that this is always quite likely to happen with information one would prefer not to disclose, unless no one else knows it) and that it might be better for the patient to hear about it from the anesthesiologist.

We suspect that consensus on what should have been done might be difficult to achieve. The following approach seems reasonable to us (and we understand it to be broadly consistent with what actually happened).

- The surgeon was informed immediately because this served to assure him that his concern had been noted, the cause identified, and the problem dealt with.
- Obviously other people in the operating room (the nurses and perfusionist) also learned about the error through this communication.
- The error and its correction were documented in the notes.
- An incident report was completed, and the management of the hospital was also notified,

directly. This resulted in a subsequent meeting between the anesthesiologist and a senior manager, which was quite stressful for the anesthesiologist but in the end resulted in an acceptance by the manager that the right things had been done and that the focus now should be on steps to prevent a recurrence. The manager undertook to follow up on this.

- Since the patient had severe heart failure and required support with inotropes, an intra-aortic balloon pump, and ventilation of the lungs for some days postoperatively, it was decided that no useful purpose would be achieved in informing him or his family about this minor event. Some people might see this as controversial, but the anesthesiologist felt that the decision would be defensible, taking into account that this was not an attempt to hide his error (which had been disclosed and documented) but rather to act as he would wish others to do if he were in that patient's position. Instead of distracting himself and them with a minor and resolved issue, he devoted his efforts as part of the team caring for the patient postoperatively to the important aspects of managing the patient's care, including communication with the family about the patient's ongoing management, likely progress, and ultimate outcome.

If this event had occurred in the United Kingdom, we think the threshold for candor would not have been met, and no disclosure would have been expected. Anecdotally, we know that many low-impact medication errors are not even documented, let alone declared to anyone. Indeed, often the person making a medication error does not even know that an error has been made. However, in this case, the substitution was not completely benign, so if the operation had been of lesser magnitude, the balance might have swung more toward disclosure of the matter to the patient. For example, after a minor procedure, postoperative muscle pain attributable to the inadvertently administered suxamethonium would have been reasonably likely and might have been of material consequence to the patient, so under these circumstances, we think disclosure would have been appropriate.

11.2.3 Compensation

It would be widely accepted within contemporary Western societies that a patient who has been harmed by an avoidable adverse medication event has a reasonable claim for compensation. Whatever arguments one might make about the inevitability of human error, an avoidable adverse medication event that results in harm to a patient constitutes a material failure in the standard of care. It is this failure (or "fault" or "wrong" or "tort") that is seen as the justification for compensation. Therefore, in many countries the provision of compensation for negligently caused harm in healthcare is achieved by civil actions based on tort law (i.e., the law of civil "wrongs").

Obviously, money does not truly compensate for injury or for the loss of a loved one. However, the award of damages can at least shift some of the financial burden of an avoidable adverse medication event from the patient to the practitioner. In particular, costs of healthcare required in consequence of the harm clearly can be covered in this way and so can the costs of loss of income. Compensation for pain and suffering is a little harder to quantify in financial terms, but there is considerable symbolic value in recognizing such pain and suffering through a financial payment.

An argument can be made that the primary aim of a civil lawsuit is compensation, rather than punishment (3), although the motivations of a patient in bringing a lawsuit may well include a desire to punish. However, because fault is central to tort law, it is likely that a lawsuit against a practitioner will bring reputation into question. This, alongside the emotional stress associated with defending such a suit, means that punishment does usually occur. At the same time, the need to prove fault in a court of law may make it difficult for many civil actions for alleged negligence to succeed, even when they have a just foundation. Thus, in some cases, the effect may be to punish a practitioner through the stress and reputational damage associated with the proceedings, but without obtaining compensation. Even in those cases where fault may be found and compensation awarded, the legal process may take years to complete, years where the patient has to bear the financial burden of consequent injury without compensation. Because of these disadvantages, there is a strong case for providing timely compensation through a mechanism that is genuinely separate from those for punishing fault.

On the other hand, tort law is not without its advantages. In particular, there is a strong argument that this secondary effect of punishment and potential deterrence is actually a desirable feature, rather than a disadvantage of civil litigation. If a tort is a wrong, why should it not generate punishment? Furthermore, it may be argued that an obligation on the part of practitioners and institutions to provide compensation for iatrogenic harm (whether personally or through insurance) is an important incentive for safer practice – this idea is based on the simple economic argument that the overall cost of investing in safety, or embracing safe practices, will presumably be lower than that of paying damages. It may be further argued that fear of reputational damage is a powerful motivator for safe practice.

The requirement on the part of harmed patients to demonstrate fault is, however, a more nuanced matter. This requirement for fault (rather than necessarily having to prove fault) is important and reasonable – not all harm caused by adverse medication events warrants compensation. For example, there is clearly a need to differentiate the known side effects of medications from harm arising out of a failure in some aspect of their management. A patient who suffers nausea and vomiting after receiving an indicated dose of morphine would have no claim for compensation in any system, notwithstanding that the suffering associated with nausea and vomiting may be considerable. Similarly, a patient who suffered from an anaphylactic reaction to a medication would be unlikely to be eligible for compensation under any system, even if the patient sustained serious consequential harm, unless there had been some failure to recognize a previously established allergy to the medication in question (Table 11.2). Although the patient was not at fault, neither was anyone else, so in most legislation this would be seen as simply a matter of individual misfortune. Another advantage often argued for tort law includes the fact that anyone can sue. However, this is only true in theory. In practice, an individual's capacity to bring, and then to win, a lawsuit is substantially related to that individual's financial situation. From the perspective of social justice, this is an important disadvantage. It is true that in some countries (including the United States), lawyers will take cases on contingency (i.e., on the basis of only being paid if the case suc-

Table 11.2 Adverse medication events related to the levels of blame proposed by Merry and McCall Smith in 2001. In each case a duty of care applies, and the adverse event has been caused by the administration of a medication by a practitioner, creating at least causal responsibility. The examples and comments are illustrative and not intended to cover every possible variation of circumstances or national legislation.

Level of blameworthiness	Examples of adverse medication events	Compensation	Punishment
1 – Causal blame	Nausea and vomiting after the appropriate administration of intravenous morphine (with antiemetics) for analgesia to a patient postoperatively	No compensation is provided in any system because this is a common and known (i.e., "normal") consequence treatment – like a scar after a surgical incision.	No punishment should apply.
	Anaphylaxis to a medication in the absence of a history of allergy: the clinician has caused the anaphylaxis, but there is no basis for blame either to the clinician or to the patient	Under tort, no responsibility for compensation would usually be accepted; in a no-fault system, no-fault compensation would be unlikely but might be considered on the basis that this event is uncommon and not a "normal" consequence of treatment.	
2 – Unavoidable error	A stroke, attributable to a cardiac arrest during anesthesia caused by a syringe swap between look-alike, sound-alike medications (dopamine instead of doxapram) by a conscientious clinician trying to do the right thing under pressure of time in an emergency	Since the standard of care was objectively imperfect (i.e., there was an error), compensation should (arguably) be available under tort law. Since this is not a normal consequence of treatment, compensation should also be provided under a no-fault system.	Little if any punishment is appropriate – assessment of this should consider the context and the extent to which due care was being taken – predisposing violations such as failing to label the syringes would arguably increase the level of blameworthiness.
3 – Negligence, minor violation	A postoperative infection resulting from poor aseptic technique during the drawing up and administration of intravenous medications	This should be compensated: causation would usually be impossible to prove in a lawsuit, but compensation might be provided through a no-fault system (see text).	Some form of proportionate punishment is reasonable, as well as remediation, taking into account the circumstances and extent of disregard for patient safety that had been displayed.
	A failure to conscientiously elucidate a full history of allergy resulting in inappropriate administration of a contraindicated medication with consequent anaphylaxis	This represents negligence, and compensation should be available under tort law and under a no-fault system.	
4 – Recklessness	Not even trying to elucidate a full history of allergy resulting in inappropriate administration of a contraindicated medication with consequent anaphylaxis	Compensation should clearly be available under tort or a no-fault system.	Some form of proportionate punishment is appropriate, including a review of the right to practice, or of conditions under which future practice is permitted.
5 – Sabotage	Death caused by an overdose of opioid administered with the objective of killing the patient, other than under legalized provisions for assisted euthanasia	Ironically, because this is a criminal matter, it might not reach the civil courts; some no-fault systems may provide minimal or no compensation for death.	Criminal charges are appropriate, leading to punishment if a conviction ensues. Also appropriate is a review of the right to practice.

Source: See Merry and Brookbanks 2017 (3) and Leslie and Merry 2015 (65).

ceeds), but they tend to be highly selective in which cases they take in this way, and there is a risk that the whole process may shift to being more about business than about justice. It often seems that the purpose of a lawsuit and trial from an attorney's perspective is not to find the truth but simply to win by arguing one's case as persuasively as possible, typically with substantial sums of money at stake. The judgement in an individual case can sometimes set a precedent for a subsequent, highly lucrative, group action, but the level of settlement for an adverse medication event may not otherwise be sufficient to warrant the costs of such an action, yet it might be of great material and symbolic value to a patient. Thus, once again, it is the need to *prove* fault in a court of law that can be both difficult and expensive for a patient to achieve, with the result that access to compensation for harm arising from an avoidable adverse medication (or any other) event tends to be very uncertain. In Chapter 12, we discuss approaches to compensation that do not require the demonstration of fault.

11.2.4 Retribution and Punishment

Clearly punishment is warranted in relation to intentional harm and serious violations involving recklessness (and arguably, gross negligence). Even then, it has been argued that excessive focus on the remote possibility that someone new may be deliberately murdering patients with overdoses of morphine, after the pattern of Harold Shipman in the United Kingdom, has the potential to introduce measures that may be very costly with little purpose and thus potentially counterproductive to high-quality healthcare (25). The problem is that the detection of dedicated criminal behavior is very difficult. Criminals can be very skilled at all forms of deception and can find their way through checks, audits, and other efforts to ensure good practice while at the same time pursuing their criminality. There are statistical approaches that can be integrated into healthcare governance with a view to detecting outlier behavior, whether of an individual doctor or an institution (26), but they need to be used with care and with triangulation to other sources of information to avoid unjust accusations (27,28). It seems probable that far more is to be gained through quality improvement initiatives addressing common practice problems than on excessive efforts to unearth the rare lurking healthcare assassin – after

all, most practitioners are honest. Nevertheless, punishment of serious crime or harm that reflects what has been called an attitude of "couldn't care less" does serve an important declarative or expressive role: this has been explained by Yeung and Horder as follows: "A criminal conviction amounts to a public proclamation that the conduct in question is seriously wrongful and worthy of condemnation and punishment, whether or not it leads directly to a substantial improvement in healthcare quality" (29). These authors make clear, however, that such convictions are only appropriate in serious circumstances of willful harm, neglect, or ill-treatment of a patient (see Table 11.2).

An important example of such a "couldn't care less" attitude of particular importance to safe medication management in anesthesia and perioperative medicine is provided by the crime of fraud in research. Over the last decade, the anesthesia community has come to realize that some of the allegedly seminal research underpinning perioperative management or medications and intravenous fluids has been fraudulent to the extent that data have been made up and institutional review board (or ethics committee) approvals have been counterfeited. Fraud of this type totally undermines the veracity not only of the published studies themselves but also of secondary reviews, book chapters, and lectures that base their advice for therapeutic decision-making on these sources (30). One might say that a little fraud in research goes a long way. Thus, even if the total number of truly fraudulent researchers is small, it is worth investing considerable effort into their detection and punishment and into assuring the integrity and quality of the research more generally. Journal editors have an important regulatory role in monitoring publications for evidence of fraud and in acting on such evidence when reason to suspect fraud is identified (31,32). It is worth noting, however, that the detection of fraud may not be straightforward, and that care is needed not to incorrectly impugn the innocent (33,34). It is also worth noting that many lesser forms of research misconduct also undermine the integrity of evidence used to inform treatment (35). These lesser failures in the sound and ethical conduct of research are probably much more common than outright fraud and when deliberate, must surely warrant some form of sanction.

11.3 Accountability and the Prevention of Future Harm

We come now to the question posed at the beginning of this chapter, about the place of accountability for avoidable adverse medication events involving the lower end of culpable behavior. This is important because, as discussed in Chapters 7 and 8, minor violations are likely to be as important as errors in the generation of iatrogenic harm. In these chapters, we argued that errors should not be seen as blameworthy, but that there should be some level of accountability for violations.

The classic example of a minor violation is that of poor compliance with aseptic practices, which may affect many aspects of patient care including the preparation and administration of intravenous medications perioperatively (36–42). On any one occasion, a failure in required hand hygiene (as one example of an aseptic practice) may be an error, but surely a persistent lack of engagement in hand hygiene with regular, repeated failures should be viewed as violation (43). The aseptic management of propofol provides a relevant example (Box 11.3).

The question here is whether the failures in accepted best practice described in various studies referred to in Box 11.3 should be construed as errors or violations. They reflect conscious decisions on the part of practitioners, so they ought to be preventable in a way that unintentional errors, such as occasional slips or lapses for example, are not. It is, however, likely that they reflect a genuine lack of appreciation of the issues on the part of the various anesthesia providers involved. This may be particularly true for the failures reported by Cilli et al. The technicians discussed in this report apparently receive only 2 years of anesthesia education after college, so it is conceivable that they may have been completely unaware of the risks associated with contamination of propofol. However, even if that were accepted, would it not be reasonable for patients to expect that someone in the institution would have known about the risk? There have been several previous reports of sepsis from the contamination of propofol (47,48), so it seems reasonable to expect that any anesthesiologist could be expected to be aware of the relevant risks. In fact, it is not clear from the report how much (if any) oversight of these technicians was provided by a physician. That leads to the question of the responsibility of the management and directors of the institution

> **Box 11.3 Propofol and the aseptic practices of anesthesia providers in the management of intravenous medications more generally**
>
> Cilli et al. recently reported a series of three patients in Turkey who developed sepsis postoperatively, which was attributed to contamination of propofol through "disobeying aseptic injection rules, reusing single-use ampules for multiple patients, using a common needle/syringe, and/or using prepared propofol after 12 hours" (44). In their report, these authors discuss the potential contributory influences of a performance-based payment system and other economic pressures on the anesthesia technicians who actually draw up propofol in their institution.
>
> Poor aseptic practices in the management of propofol, and in aseptic management of intravenous medications more generally, seem to be quite widespread, even in high-income countries (36,38,39,42). In fact, a clinical audit of 300 patients in New Zealand demonstrated that microorganisms would have been injected into 6.3% of these patients had they not been trapped by a 0.2 micron filter (37). Anecdotal, survey, and simulation-based observational data provide reason to believe that contamination of injected medications with microorganisms occurs through failures in aseptic technique by at least some (probably not all) anesthesiologists, not just in New Zealand but also in the United States (and presumably elsewhere as well) (36,40,45,46). Thus, the failures described at this Turkish institution are simply one part of a much wider failure in this particular aspect of safe medication practice, at least during anesthesia but probably more generally.

for their high-level decisions on funding and staffing and to governments in relation to their strategy for the health workforce.

In their report, "To Err Is Human," the Institute of Medicine stated that most errors in healthcare do not reflect recklessness or carelessness on the part of individuals (49). Instead, they arise out of faulty processes or systems. This view of the situation has recently been very clearly restated by Wachter and Pronovost, who wrote:

Most errors are committed by good, hard-working people trying to do the right thing. Therefore, the traditional focus on identifying who was at fault is a distraction. It is far more productive to identify error prone situations

225

and settings and to implement systems that prevent caregivers from committing errors, catch errors before they cause harm, or mitigate harm from errors that do reach patients. (50)

However, even if one accepts that for everyone concerned these three cases of sepsis were the manifestation of genuine error, surely the most important point here is that these patients should reasonably be able to expect that something will now be done to ensure better practices in the future. Now that the issues have been brought into clear view, it would be hard to accept any line of argument that attributed a persistence of them to error. A failure to address this problem would have to be construed as evidence of a lack of concern by all concerned, including the leadership of the institution, for the well-being of patients. Gratifyingly, a first giant step toward improvement has already been taken in this institution. The response to these cases of sepsis by the microbiologists who have written the report was successful in identifying the origins of the problem through an impressive process of analysis. The capacity to identify causes when something goes wrong in a complex and overstretched system is central to resilience in healthcare (51).

Unfortunately, this case series from Turkey is not an isolated example of this particular problem: in fact, as outlined in Box 11.3, lesser degrees of imperfection in the aseptic management of intravenous medications during anesthesia seems to be widespread. A recent recommendation has been made in the *United States Pharmacopoeia* (USP) that medications drawn up for a case should be discarded after 60 minutes unless they will be used in an ongoing case. For many this means that no one should draw up medications for a subsequent case during a current case, but this practice is routinely violated in our experience, at least in the United States. Even when prohibited by a policy, many anesthesia providers, citing pressure to turnover cases more quickly, surreptitiously continue this practice. The question then, is how regulatory and legal mechanisms can ensure appropriate accountability for important safety practices of this type within all institutions within any given country.

It seems hard to escape the conclusion that some form of sanction or punishment for persistent violation of important safety practices may be required, whether this is applied to the institution

as a whole (perhaps through fines) or to individuals in particular (perhaps through discipline), or both. On the other hand, the challenges of addressing embedded systematic failures or weaknesses within healthcare should not be underestimated, and there is a strong discourse to the effect that punishment is potentially counterproductive to quality improvement.

In no small part, this is because the challenges of improving healthcare practice are not trivial, and there is increasing recognition that the key to quality improvement lies in winning the hearts and minds of practitioners and managers alike. However, there may well be a place for the carefully considered inclusion of some form of sanctions within a consultative approach to changing practice on the basis of building consensus and redesigning key processes and structures within the system.

The Keystone ICU project (Box 11.4) illustrates such an approach, and also illustrates the considerable lengths that one needs to go to achieve change and embed improved practices within institutions and countries. As is now well known, the project was highly successful in reducing central line–associated bloodstream infection (CLABSI) at Johns Hopkins Hospital and subsequently across the state of Michigan (52). It might be thought that the publication in a leading journal of data documenting a major quality improvement success would be sufficient to spur the rest of the world on to adopt the successful initiative. Interestingly, to extend successes of this sort beyond the institution in which they were born, it seems that the key steps have to be repeated locally, taking into account the differences in culture and circumstances that prevail in different parts of the world. For example, this was done in New Zealand (as in many countries and states), where the same type of improvement was observed once again (53). In fact, it may take several iterations of effort to really embed changes in practice. This was seen in respect of the use of the World Health Organization (WHO) Surgical Safety Checklist at Auckland City Hospital. This hospital was one of the original eight sites in which this checklist was first evaluated (54), but several further projects were required to achieve excellent levels of engagement and compliance with its use (55–59). Furthermore, when use of the Surgical Safety Checklist was mandated in all Danish hospitals, variable response was seen: decreases in

---

Box 11.4 The Keystone ICU project and the balance of accountability

The *Keystone ICU project* illustrates the way in which such a balance can be struck in a way that involves both individual practitioners and those responsible for the overall system at institutional and national levels.

Until quite recently, it was widely believed that a certain rate of CLABSI was an inevitable accompaniment of the use of central venous lines. Pronovost, an anesthesiologist and intensivist at Johns Hopkins Hospital, questioned this perception and initiated a project to reduce this rate. He identified four elements required to successfully change practice and thereby improve quality of care. These requirements were as follows:

- Education – about the problem and the solution
- Facilitation of compliance (in the case of CLABSI, making compliance with good practice easier involved creating a catheter insertion cart containing everything needed to insert a central line sterilely)
- Use of process tools (in the case of CLABSI, this involved creating a checklist that outlined the key steps for sterile insertion and management of the lines)
- Enforcement of compliance (in the case of CLABSI, hospital leadership across the project agreed

to personally intervene if a provider refused to comply)

These four elements required a detailed analysis of both the problem and the solution, so an analysis of this sort could be seen as a fifth element and indeed the starting point in seeking to improve the quality of any aspect of practice. In fact, Pronovost and his colleagues began by looking in a generic way at the literature on human factors and barriers to the uptake of guidelines (63). Restating the points in simple English, a request for a change in practice should be supported by convincing evidence and, with the support of this evidence, agreement should be obtained from the affected clinicians that the problem matters and the response is warranted. The elements of the CLABSI bundle did not include every possible way to reduce central line infection but focused on those elements where the evidence was strong and where all could agree that they were best practice. The requested changes should be made as easy as possible to do. And finally, and most controversially, compliance should not be negotiable: in the case of the CLABSI initiative, nurses at Hopkins were empowered to stop physicians if they did not comply with the checklist. The autonomy of the individual practitioner to indulge in unwarranted variation in practice was overridden.

---

patient mortality were strongly related to checklist compliance. In hospitals where only a portion of the Checklist was implemented, no change in mortality was seen, but when all aspects were implemented, the original results were replicated (60).

The Keystone ICU project (like implementation of the WHO Surgical Safety Checklist) represents a systems-oriented approach to normalized deviance in which idiosyncratic variation characterizes a particular practice and in which room for improved patient outcomes is clearly discernable. One important element of the Keystone ICU project in each of its implementation phases was a requirement that all concerned would comply with the elements of the bundle introduced for the management of central venous catheters (CVCs). Notably, nurses were empowered to stop the procedure if a doctor did not comply with the prescribed checklist during the insertion of a CVC. Wachter and Pronovost have extended this idea of insisting on compliance by suggesting that we need to

stop accepting idiosyncratic behavior manifesting as repeated violations of accepted safety practices. Like us, they suggest that there is in fact a role for punishment in this regard, as part of an approach for promoting accountability within institutions (50). In a paper entitled "Balancing 'No Blame' with Accountability in Patient Safety," they explain that even after substantial efforts to improve the systemic elements of hand hygiene in many United States hospitals, compliance continued to be poor. They comment: "In 2009, low hand-hygiene rates are generally not a systems problem anymore; they are largely an accountability problem." Similar opinions had been articulated by Goldman (then a senior vice president of the Institute for Healthcare Improvement) in 2006 (61), Marx in 2001 (62), and James Reason in 1997. As quoted in Chapter 8, Reason argued for a just culture based on "an atmosphere of trust in which people are encouraged, even rewarded, for providing essential safety related information – but in which they are also clear about where the line must be drawn between acceptable and unacceptable behaviour" (24).

We agree with Reason about the line between acceptable and unacceptable behavior, but we believe that it can be very difficult to know where such a line should be drawn. It is also all too possible to misjudge situations (64). In 2001 Merry and McCall Smith suggested that it is possible to classify blame into five levels, on the basis of an understanding of human error and violation within complex systems along the lines discussed in Chapters 6, 7, and 8 (3). In Table 11.2 we have listed these levels and provided examples of adverse medication events illustrative of each level (3). We have also commented on the role of punishment at each level and the extent to which compensation should or might be provided for each event, whether through tort law or through no-fault systems of compensation. It is straightforward that no blame should apply at Level 1, and that Level 5 is completely unacceptable. Level 4 is also easily dealt with – it is not controversial that recklessness is blameworthy and that punishment of recklessness is appropriate. Level 2, involving human error, is more controversial, and this is why we have gone to considerable lengths to explain the nature of human error in Chapter 7. The previously popular idea of a no-blame culture for patient safety was based on the notion that many of the things that go wrong in healthcare reflect genuine errors and that it is most constructive to focus on redesigning the system to make such errors less likely. Uncertainty and tension arise over Level 3. This is the level of minor violations, of the type typically construed as simple rather than gross negligence. There is clearly quite a wide range of such decisions, and their consequent actions and arguments about the boundaries of negligence and recklessness can be highly nuanced. However, the key point here is that, like the failures in aseptic management with propofol, adverse events associated with failures at Level 3 are substantially avoidable through the active decisions and engaged attention of practitioners, in a way that errors at Level 2 are not. At the same time, though, decisions taken at this level of blameworthiness are not generally associated with the "couldn't care less" attitude mentioned earlier in this chapter, which is characteristic of Level 4. Most failures at Level 3 probably reflect a lack of awareness or conviction on the part of the people concerned that they actually matter. Unfortunately,

they often do matter, and a just culture requires that people be accountable for them.

This view of accountability is not always accepted by physicians, who have long cherished their right to practice autonomously. This belief in autonomy goes hand in hand with considerable influence, and manifests in various ways. For example, Wachter and Pronovost contrast the position of most staff within hospitals (e.g., nurses and pharmacists) who accept as uncontroversial that they work for the organization under clear lines of authority, with that of physicians. They explain that in the United States (as in many other countries), physicians often work in hospitals as "individual entrepreneurs" and are therefore less responsive to the institution's authority. They draw an interesting distinction between a hospital's willingness to discipline senior physicians over matters of administrative compliance required by external agencies and necessary for billing, and a hospital's reluctance to discipline them over matters of safety. We would add that even when physicians are directly employed by a hospital, they often see themselves as working primarily for patients. Thus, they may tend to see the proper role of hospital management as one of supporting them, the physicians, in their efforts to care for patients. In most countries, considerable support for this view can be drawn from the fact that physicians are indeed held accountable for their care of patients by licensing or regulatory bodies external to the hospitals in which they work, such as the General Medical Council (GMC) in the United Kingdom, for example. These bodies can, and sometimes do, discipline physicians for failures in safe practice. Sanctions may be severe and include the possibility of permanent removal of a license to practice. Thus, the argument that physicians are highly trained professionals with their own system of professional regulation, that their priority is to ensure that patients gain the best possible care, and that they should therefore be supported in this by managers (who are often less well qualified and who may not have any parallel accountability to registration authorities) is not necessarily unreasonable.

On the other hand, there is an obvious irony in combining an argument of this type with the assertion that a failure to engage in safety initiatives (such as hand hygiene) is simply part of any physician's right to autonomous practice. Wachter and Pronovost therefore advocate the adoption by hospitals of a system of accountability within a just culture that should apply equally to all clinical staff, including physicians. There is a moral imperative for this egalitarian approach (in that it would be quite wrong for a nurse to be dismissed while a physician was required only to undertake some remedial training for the same violation), but we think there is also a practical reason for it. The provision of healthcare is a team endeavor (65,66), and buy-in from all members of the team (of whatever discipline) can be expected to shift culture in a positive direction. If all clinicians (physicians, nurses, pharmacists, etc.) feel that they are in the same boat in this respect, this will presumably be better for morale, and practitioners from different disciplines will be more likely to respect and support each other in promoting and achieving the required safe practices than if resentment emerges in some groups toward others who are seen as receiving unjustifiable privileges. As stated by Bosk and Pronovost in their editorial *Reality Check for Checklists*, "What happened in Michigan involved the creation of social networks with a shared sense of mission, whose members were each able to reinforce the efforts of the other to cooperate with the interventions" (67).

For such an approach to be accepted, certain other prerequisites must also be in place: these are essentially the prerequisites for quality improvement that underpinned the Keystone ICU project (see Box 11.4 and Chapter 8). In essence, people should not be taken by surprise: they should be clearly informed about the relevant expectations, and deficiencies in the system should have been addressed so that compliance with safe practice is at least possible and preferably easy. Initial warnings and counseling should precede punishment. Finally, and importantly, punishment when administered needs to be proportionate to the violation in question and should ideally serve a remedial purpose. Wachter and Pronovost illustrate this idea with some "straw man" examples, such as "education and loss of patient care privileges for one week" (see Table 11.2 and Box 11.5).

As we indicated earlier in this chapter, one of the objectives of punishment is its declarative and motivational purpose. This implies that, at some point, it should be visible to other staff that sanctions are being applied appropriately when called

---

Box 11.5 A possible framework for sanctions for persistent violations of safe practice

Graded reprimand
- "Cup of coffee" with coworker (e.g., as with the Vanderbilt model for disruptive behavior [68,69])
- Formal reprimand with supervisor
- Letter to personnel file
- Required educational activity
- Financial penalties
- Suspension of privileges for a period of time
- Dismissal from staff

---

for. There is, however, a difficulty in relation to this point.

As we already observed, we live in a world where transparency within an institution is likely to extend beyond its boundaries, very quickly through social media and a little more slowly through traditional forms of media. This creates some risk that a punishment that is in itself reasonable and proportionate ends up having unintended consequences for the individual practitioner that are far more severe than intended. It would not be beyond the bounds of possibility for a process initiated in relation to a relatively minor matter to lead to substantial loss of reputation and income for a practitioner. It may increase not only the individual practitioner's emotional responses, with potential consequences for his or her health, it may reverberate to their local colleagues as well, and raise fears for his or her ability to practice as well. One might counter that patient safety is not a minor matter even if the violations in question seemed relatively trivial at the time to the practitioner in question, as with the example of sepsis from contaminated propofol. Nevertheless, the objective of advancing patient safety depends (among other things) on a general acceptance by staff that the institution's approach is indeed just, so considerable care should be taken in the choice, framing, and general notification of any sanction to minimize this risk. Much can be done in this regard, and some thoughts on possible options are provided in Box 11.5. Ideally, clinicians within institutions should work together to develop consensus on sanctions, appropriate to their own context, relevant to their own practices, and acceptable from the perspective of potential reputational impact.

11.3.1 Some Thoughts on Possible Sanctions for Persistent Violation of Important Safety Practices in General

Sanctions for persistent minor violations in healthcare should ideally be sufficiently inconvenient and undesirable for the person concerned to act as a moderate deterrent. Most practitioners are motivated to practice safely, and for many a formal reprimand from one's superior will often go a long way toward achieving this. Such a reprimand could be confidential in the first instance, and thus serve as a first step in a graded series of sanctions, with subsequent steps escalating in severity if an individual continues to refuse to comply with the practices in question. Vanderbilt University established a Co-Worker Observation Reporting System in which it has been found that something as minimalist as a conversation over a cup of coffee is often effective as a response to reports of disrespectful or unsafe behavior; however, a database of such reports is maintained, and the response is escalated in the case of recidivism (68,69). One could envisage a similar approach in relation to medication safety.

Suspension of privileges for a short period of time (as suggested by Wachter and Pronovost) would certainly be visible to other staff (and for many people would be a cause of some shame and some financial loss), but this is not a sanction that can be applied equitably across disciplines or even across different specialties in medicine. Furthermore, it may serve to damage the institution's capacity to deliver services, which may resemble cutting off one's nose to spite one's face.

Financial penalties in the form of fines have some attraction. These work well for road traffic offenses, for example, and would be relatively straightforward to administer. Fines could be accompanied by some form of publication of information about who had been fined and why, which would likely be perceived as more punitive than the fine itself. A drawback of this approach is that of equity: A fine that might be quite onerous for one type of healthcare worker might be seen as trivial for another. On the other hand, if the amounts were quite low, the real element of punishment would lie in the fact that a fine had been levied and the effect of this might be more evenly felt.

We are, however, drawn more to a requirement for the individual to participate in some relevant educational activity, specifically directed toward the aspect of practice that has been violated. It is probably moot whether the person sees such participation as a punishment or an opportunity, provided it succeeds in improving his or her practice. Furthermore, the sort of clinician who would welcome such an opportunity is perhaps less likely to be required to participate in training of this type than one who demonstrated a lack of understanding of the importance of the practice in question.

Careful thought is needed over the matter of who should be told that a sanction has been imposed, and how. Publication of the lists of people attending such courses in institutional newsletters (without differentiating between those required to do so and those participating of their own volition) might be sufficient. Colleagues would notice who was participating and might well draw their own conclusions. Alternatively, some phrasing such as "attending at the request of the service director" would be more explicit and should perhaps be considered.

Whatever other steps are included between the early ones listed previously and dismissal or permanent withdrawal of privileges, the latter must be part of the graded series of progressively more severe sanctions. At these more serious stages, a formal process is required which must include a fair hearing in line with all relevant legal requirements, bearing in mind the possibility that the employee may respond by taking a lawsuit against the institution. Nevertheless, at some point, an individual who continues to refuse to engage with the safety practices explicitly identified as important to an institution should be confronted with the fact that doing so is incompatible with working in that institution. The need to resort to dismissing an otherwise valued member of staff in this way should be rare, and the declarative value of doing so would be considerable. An institution that dismissed one senior physician for violating safety practices, after all the other steps envisaged here had been taken, would be unlikely to have to do this very often again.

11.4 Ethics, Professionalism, and "the Team for Medication Safety"

We already alluded more than once to an important role for individuals to take responsibility themselves for the advancement of medication safety,

> **Box 11.6 Ethical principles articulated by the Tavistock Group for those who shape and give healthcare**
>
> - Healthcare is a human right
> - The care of individuals is at the center of healthcare delivery but must be viewed and practiced within the overall context of continuing work to generate the greatest possible health gains for groups and populations.
> - The responsibilities of the healthcare delivery system include the prevention of illness and the alleviation of disability.
> - Cooperation with each other and those served is imperative for those working within the healthcare delivery system
> - All individuals and groups involved in healthcare, whether providing access or services, have the continuing responsibility to help improve its quality.
>
> Source: Smith et al. 1999 (70).

regardless of the internal or external legal or regulatory frameworks under which they work. In 1999, the Tavistock Group articulated five ethical principles for those who shape and give healthcare (Box 11.6) (70). These principles were to be used by people who work in healthcare delivery systems, healthcare organizations, insurers, employers, and governments and the public. The importance of cooperation "throughout a healthcare system" to produce "better outcomes and greater value for individuals and for society" was emphasized. The fifth point is particularly relevant to the present chapter. The question arises as to who is encompassed by the reference to "All individuals and groups involved in health care." In the present context, who is actually "on the team" for ensuring safe medication practices during anesthesia and the perioperative period? Members of the legal profession, the judiciary, and other regulators were not explicitly mentioned by the Tavistock Group, although insurers, employers, governments, and the general public were. We think they should have been.

Without question, effective regulation of healthcare is necessary, and the courts have an essential role in this. The methods of funding the legal and regulatory processes of healthcare vary from country to country, but it seems entirely reasonable to consider their cost as part of the overall cost of delivering healthcare in any country. Money

spent on expensive litigation or criminal prosecutions (and on the defense of those sued or accused) is money that could have been spent directly on healthcare. We find it disconcerting, therefore, that legal responses to adverse medication events often seem to be primarily reactive, adversarial, and expensive rather than proactive, inquisitorial, and cost effective. It is debatable whether lawsuits and criminal prosecutions are effective in promoting medication safety, but, whether they are or not, the cost of these processes is unquestionably considerable. Furthermore, it seems that the willingness to spend money on the aftermath of a serious adverse medication event is often much greater than the willingness to spend it on improving medication safety to reduce the likelihood of such an event. Obviously, the protection of patients' rights is both reasonable and necessary, but it has been suggested that, in doing this, the law has a responsibility to be *restorative*, and perhaps even *therapeutic* as well as more proactive in relation to the harm caused by healthcare (3). The concept of *therapeutic jurisprudence* is gaining traction in the context of psychiatry, and similar ideas could be applied to the present context (these ideas have been discussed elsewhere in some detail [3]). Such a sea change in approach is unlikely to be forthcoming in any reasonable time frame, but many governments review their relevant legislation from time to time and occasionally make changes to restrain upper limits of awardable damages or seek to streamline the processes of litigation. It seems to us that moves of this type are at least steps in the right direction.

In the meantime, however, we suggest that a greater degree of individual social conscience is called for. The Tavistock Group suggests that both the public and governments have a responsibility in this regard – that they are, in effect, also part of the team. Certainly, there are notable examples of individual members of the public who have been the drivers for improved practices, notably Julie Bailey in relation to the Mid Staffordshire NHS Foundation Trust (71). More generally, patients can often contribute substantially to the safety of their own medication usage, but not always: a patient who is anesthetized could hardly be expected to play an active role in this regard. The general public can and should also engage in a more general way, through social debates about the systems of funding and regulating healthcare. This implies that those people of influence who represent the public have a responsibility to learn more about specialized and potentially hazardous aspects of healthcare including the management of medications during anesthesia and the perioperative period. For the legal profession, we think this role for an individual social conscience encompasses such things as viewing healthcare-related lawsuits more as matters of justice than as potential business opportunities. For physicians, it implies at least some concessions in respect to their long-cherished authority to practice autonomously and to the traditional authoritarian hierarchy in healthcare that has often impeded attempts by other staff (notably nurses) and patients to speak up about seriously bad practices – in the Mid Staffordshire (72) and Gosport War Memorial Hospitals (73,74), for example. To be clear, we believe that many lawyers are deeply committed to justice, and many physicians have embraced the cause of working as a team to provide high-quality patient-centered care, but we also believe that there is still considerable room for improvement on both these fronts. Most importantly, there is a strong parallel between the acceptance of failures in care that occurred at these hospitals and the widespread ongoing acceptance of avoidable adverse medication events in anesthesia and perioperative medicine, despite numerous calls to engage in addressing this problem (75–77). There is surely an overdue responsibility on the part of all concerned to put an end to this epidemic of normalized deviance.

11.4.1 Professionalism

As already intimated, many physicians have traditionally argued strongly for self-regulation, seeing this as a core element of professionalism. In recent years, public sentiment has become skeptical of this view. In many countries, there has been a move toward including legal and laypeople on medical licensing bodies, disciplinary tribunals, and so forth. We accept that this shift has been necessary but not that there is therefore any less responsibility on the part of physicians to self-regulate, through both formal and informal (peer-to-peer) processes. There would be much less need for regulation through external mechanisms if all health professionals involved with medication management during anesthesia and the perioperative period collectively embraced their ethical responsibility to ensure safe practices for their patients, and engaged fully with such practices. We recognize that neither

speaking up about poor practices and facilities nor insisting that management invest in medication safety initiatives supported by strong consensus are easy matters (72), but if anesthesiologists and other practitioners do not do this, it is hard to see who will. The most obvious fact about current legal and regulatory approaches to improving medication safety is that they are not working as well as they should be, because too many avoidable adverse medication events continue to happen. Improvements in these regulatory and legal frameworks should be sought, but they are likely to be slow in coming. In the meantime, we think that the only way to achieve the changes that are needed to substantially improve medication safety lies in an increased acceptance by individual practitioners of their professional responsibility to make these changes happen. Martin et al. have referred to professionalism as "the third logic" in a healthcare system currently dominated by market and managerial logics and called for its reshaping and reinvigoration (78). We echo this call.

11.5 Conclusions

Regulatory and legal processes relevant to avoidable adverse medication events have the potential to advance the cause of patient safety, but it is expecting too much to believe that these processes alone will achieve the changes that need to be made, urgently and affordably, to reduce the persistently high rate of avoidable adverse medication events. Achieving the required change will require engagement by all concerned, from politicians, through directors of hospital boards and managers, and clinical leaders of hospital services to frontline clinicians – and also, of necessity, regulators and the legal profession. It has been argued elsewhere that there is an ethical imperative for greater engagement in patient safety (9), and we agree.

References

1. Bowdle TA, Jelacic S, Nair B, et al. Facilitated self-reported anaesthetic medication errors before and after implementation of a safety bundle and barcode-based safety system. *Br J Anaesth.* 2018;121(6):1338–45.

2. Gordon M. When a nurse is prosecuted for a fatal medical mistake, does it make medicine safer? *Health Inc.* April 10, 2019. Accessed January 8, 2020. https://www.npr.org/sections/health-shots/2019/04/10/709971677/when-a-nurse-is-prosecuted-for-a-fatal-medical-mistake-does-it-make-medicine-saf

3. Merry AF, Brookbanks W. *Merry and McCall Smith's Errors, Medicine and the Law.* 2nd ed. Cambridge, UK: Cambridge University Press; 2017.

4. *R v Prentice, R v Sullman, R v Adomako, R v Holloway* [1994] QB 302.

5. Ameratunga R, Klonin H, Vaughan J, Merry A, Cusack J. Criminalisation of unintentional error in healthcare in the UK: a perspective from New Zealand. *BMJ.* 2019;364:l706.

6. Webster CS, Merry AF, Larsson L, McGrath KA, Weller J. The frequency and nature of drug administration error during anaesthesia. *Anaesth Intensive Care.* 2001;29(5):494–500.

7. Nanji KC, Patel A, Shaikh S, Seger DL, Bates DW. Evaluation of perioperative medication errors and adverse drug events. *Anesthesiology.* 2016;124(1):25–34.

8. Merry AF, Webster CS, Hannam J, et al. Multimodal system designed to reduce errors in recording and administration of drugs in anaesthesia: prospective randomised clinical evaluation. *BMJ.* 2011;343:d5543.

9. Runciman B, Merry A, Waltnon M. *Safety and Ethics in Healthcare: A Guide to Getting It Right.* Aldershot: Ashgate Publishing; 2007.

10. Toffolutti V, Stuckler D. A Culture of openness is associated with lower mortality rates among 137 English National Health Service acute trusts. *Health Aff (Millwood).* 2019;38(5):844–50.

11. Studdert DM, Mello MM, Gawande AA, et al. Claims, errors, and compensation payments in medical malpractice litigation. *N Engl J Med.* 2006;354(19):2024–33.

12. Kachalia A, Kaufman SR, Boothman R, et al. Liability claims and costs before and after implementation of a medical error disclosure program. [Summary for patients in *Ann Intern Med.* 2010;153(4):I-28]. *Ann Intern Med.* 2010;153(4):213–21.

13. Skegg PDG. Criminal prosecutions of negligent health professionals: the New Zealand experience. *Med Law Rev.* 1998;6:220–46.

14. O'Connor E, Coates HM, Yardley IE, Wu AW. Disclosure of patient safety incidents: a comprehensive review. *Int J Qual Health Care.* 2010;22(5):371–9.

15. Vincent JL. Information in the ICU: are we being honest with our patients? The results of a European questionnaire. *Intensive Care Med.* 1998;24(12):1251–6.

16. Health and Disability Commissioner. *Code of Health and Disability Services Consumers' Rights.* Auckland: New Zealand Government; 2004. Accessed January 3, 2020. https://www.hdc.org.nz

17. Quick O. *Regulating Patient Safety: The End of Professional Dominance?* Cambridge, UK: Cambridge University Press; 2017. Laurie G, Ashcroft R, eds. Cambridge Bioethics and Law.

18. Quick O. Regulating and legislating safety: the case for candour. *BMJ Qual Saf.* 2014;23(8):614–18.

19. Hesketh T, Wu D, Mao L, Ma N. Violence against doctors in China. *BMJ.* 2012;345:e5730.

20. Studdert DM, Mello MM, Gawande AA, Brennan TA, Wang YC. Disclosure of medical injury to patients: an improbable risk management strategy. *Health Aff (Millwood).* 2007;26(1):215–26.

21. Lamb R. Open disclosure: the only approach to medical error. *Qual Saf Health Care.* 2004;13(1):3–5.

22. Iedema R, Jorm C, Wakefield J, Ryan C, Dunn S. Practising open disclosure: clinical incident communication and systems improvement. *Sociol Health Illn.* 2009;31(2):262–77.

23. Finlay AJ, Stewart CL, Parker M. Open disclosure: ethical, professional and legal obligations, and the way forward for regulation. *Med J Aust.* 2013;198(8):445–8.

24. Reason J. *Managing the Risks of Organizational Accidents.* London: Routledge; 1997.

25. Haines D. The legacy of Dr. Harold Shipman. *Med Leg J.* 2015;83(3):115.

26. Mohammed MA, Cheng KK, Rouse A, Marshall T. Bristol, Shipman, and clinical governance: Shewhart's forgotten lessons. *Lancet.* 2001;357(9254):463–7.

27. Mohammed MA, Rathbone A, Myers P, et al. An investigation into general practitioners associated with high patient mortality flagged up through the Shipman inquiry: retrospective analysis of routine data. *BMJ.* 2004;328(7454):1474–7.

28. Hamblin R, Shuker C, Stolarek I, Wilson J, Merry AF. Public reporting of health care performance data: what we know and what we should do. *N Z Med J.* 2016;129(1431):7–17.

29. Yeung K, Horder J. How can the criminal law support the provision of quality in healthcare? *BMJ Qual Saf.* 2014;23(6):519–24.

30. Shafer SL. Tattered threads. *Anesth Analg.* 2009;108(5):1361–3.

31. Klein AA. What *Anaesthesia* is doing to combat scientific misconduct and investigate data fabrication and falsification. *Anaesthesia.* 2017;72(1):3–4.

32. Carlisle JB. Data fabrication and other reasons for non-random sampling in 5087 randomised, controlled trials in anaesthetic and general medical journals. *Anaesthesia.* 2017;72(8):944–52.

33. Kharasch ED, Houle TT. Seeking and reporting apparent research misconduct: errors and integrity. *Anaesthesia*. 2018;73(1):125–6.

34. Carlisle JB. Seeking and reporting apparent research misconduct: errors and integrity – a reply. *Anaesthesia*. 2018;73(1):126–8.

35. Merry AF, Merry D. Ethics in research: bend it like Beauchamp. *Extra Corpor Technol*. 2006;38(4):312–17.

36. Gargiulo DA, Sheridan J, Webster CS, et al. Anaesthetic drug administration as a potential contributor to healthcare-associated infections: a prospective simulation-based evaluation of aseptic techniques in the administration of anaesthetic drugs. *BMJ Qual Saf*. 2012;21(10):826–34.

37. Gargiulo DA, Mitchell SJ, Sheridan J, et al. Microbiological contamination of drugs during their administration for anesthesia in the operating room. *Anesthesiology*. 2016;124(4):785–94.

38. Loftus RW, Koff MD, Brown JR, et al. The dynamics of Enterococcus transmission from bacterial reservoirs commonly encountered by anesthesia providers. *Anesth Analg*. 2015;120(4):827–36.

39. Loftus RW, Koff MD, Brown JR, et al. The epidemiology of *Staphylococcus aureus* transmission in the anesthesia work area. *Anesth Analg*. 2015;120(4):807–18.

40. Loftus RW, Koff MD, Birnbach DJ. The dynamics and implications of bacterial transmission events arising from the anesthesia work area. *Anesth Analg*. 2015;120(4):853–60.

41. Loftus RW, Brown JR, Patel HM, et al. Transmission dynamics of Gram-negative bacterial pathogens in the anesthesia work area. *Anesth Analg*. 2015;120(4):819–26.

42. Fernandez PG, Loftus RW, Dodds TM, et al. Hand hygiene knowledge and perceptions among anesthesia providers. *Anesth Analg*. 2015;120(4):837–43.

43. Weller JM, Merry AF. I. Best practice and patient safety in anaesthesia. *Br J Anaesth*. 2013;110(5):671–3.

44. Cilli F, Nazli-Zeka A, Arda B, et al. *Serratia marcescens* sepsis outbreak caused by contaminated propofol. *Am J Infect Control*. 2019;47(5):582–4.

45. Ryan AJ, Webster CS, Merry AF, Grieve DJ. A national survey of infection control practice by New Zealand anaesthetists. *Anaesth Intensive Care*. 2006;34(1):68–74.

46. Munoz-Price LS, Bowdle A, Johnston BL, et al. Infection prevention in the operating room anesthesia work area. *Infect Control Hosp Epidemiol*. 2019;40(1):1–17.

47. Cole DC, Baslanti TO, Gravenstein NL, Gravenstein N. Leaving more than your fingerprint on the intravenous line: a prospective study on propofol anesthesia and implications of stopcock contamination. *Anesth Analg*. 2015;120(4):861–7.

48. Sakuragi T, Yanagisawa K, Shirai Y, Dan K. Growth of *Escherichia coli* in propofol, lidocaine, and mixtures of propofol and lidocaine. *Acta Anaesthesiol Scand*. 1999;43(4):476–9.

49. Kohn LT, Corrigan JM, Donaldson MS, eds. *To Err Is Human: Building a Safer Health System*. Washington, DC: National Academy Press, Institute of Medicine; 1999.

50. Wachter RM, Pronovost PJ. Balancing "no blame" with accountability in patient safety. *N Engl J Med*. 2009;361(14):1401–6.

51. Braithwaite J, Wears RL, Hollnagel E. Resilient health care: turning patient safety on its head. *Int J Qual Health Care*. 2015;27(5):418–20.

52. Pronovost P, Needham D, Berenholtz S, et al. An intervention to decrease catheter-related bloodstream infections in the ICU. *N Engl J Med*. 2006;355(26):2725–32.

53. Gray J, Proudfoot S, Power M, et al. Target CLAB Zero: a national improvement collaborative to reduce central line-associated bacteraemia in New Zealand intensive care units. *N Z Med J*. 2015;128(1421):13–21.

54. Haynes AB, Weiser TG, Berry WR, et al. A surgical safety checklist to reduce morbidity and mortality in a global population. *N Engl J Med*. 2009;360(5):491–9.

55. Vogts N, Hannam JA, Merry AF, Mitchell SJ. Compliance and quality in administration of a surgical safety checklist in a tertiary New Zealand hospital. *N Z Med J*. 2011;124(1342):48–58.

56. Hannam JA, Glass L, Kwon J, et al. A prospective, observational study of the effects of implementation strategy on compliance with a surgical safety checklist. *BMJ Qual Saf*. 2013;22(11):940–7.

57. Devcich DA, Weller J, Mitchell SJ, et al. A behaviourally anchored rating scale for evaluating the use of the WHO surgical safety checklist: development and initial evaluation of the WHOBARS. *BMJ Qual Saf*. 2016;25(10):778–86.

58. Martis WR, Hannam JA, Lee T, Merry AF, Mitchell SJ. Improved compliance with the World Health Organization Surgical Safety Checklist is associated with reduced surgical specimen labelling errors. *N Z Med J*. 2016;129(1441):63–7.

59. Ong APC, Devcich DA, Hannam J, et al. A "paperless" wall-mounted surgical safety checklist with migrated leadership can improve

compliance and team engagement. *BMJ Qual Saf.* 2016;25(12):971–6.

60. van Klei WA, Hoff RG, van Aarnhem EE, et al. Effects of the introduction of the WHO "Surgical Safety Checklist" on in-hospital mortality: a cohort study. *Ann Surg.* 2012;255(1):44–9.

61. Goldmann D. System failure versus personal accountability – the case for clean hands. *N Engl J Med.* 2006;355(2):121–3.

62. Marx D. *Patient Safety and the "Just Culture": A Primer for Health Care Executives.* New York, NY: Columbia University; 2001. Accessed January 21, 2020. https://www.psnet.ahrq.gov/issue/patient-safety-and-just-culture-primer-health-care-executives

63. Cabana MD, Rand CS, Powe NR, et al. Why don't physicians follow clinical practice guidelines? A framework for improvement. *JAMA.* 1999;282(15):1458–65.

64. Goodyear-Smith F. *Murder That Wasn't.* Dunedin: Otago University Press; 2015.

65. Leslie K, Merry AF. Cardiac surgery: all for one and one for all. *Anesth Analg.* 2015;120(3):504–6.

66. Weller J, Civil I, Torrie J, et al. Can team training make surgery safer? Lessons for national implementation of a simulation-based programme. *N Z Med J.* 2016;129(1443):9–17.

67. Bosk CL, Dixon-Woods M, Goeschel CA, Pronovost PJ. Reality check for checklists. *Lancet.* 2009;374(9688):444–5.

68. Webb LE, Dmochowski RR, Moore IN, et al. Using coworker observations to promote accountability for disrespectful and unsafe behaviors by physicians and advanced practice professionals. *Jt Comm J Qual Patient Saf.* 2016;42(4):149–64.

69. Cooper WO, Guillamondegui O, Hines OJ, et al. Use of unsolicited patient observations to identify surgeons with increased risk for postoperative complications. *JAMA Surg.* 2017;152(6):522–9.

70. Smith R, Hiatt H, Berwick D. Shared ethical principles for everybody in health care: a working draft from the Tavistock Group. *BMJ.* 1999;318(7178):248–51.

71. Francis R. *Report of the Mid Staffordshire NHS Foundation Trust Public Inquiry.* London: HMSO; 2013. Accessed January 18, 2020. https://www.midstaffspublicinquiry.com/report

72. Jones A, Kelly D. Deafening silence? Time to reconsider whether organisations are silent or deaf when things go wrong. *BMJ Qual Saf.* 2014;23(9):709–13.

73. Walshe K. Gosport deaths: lethal failures in care will happen again. *BMJ.* 2018;362:k2931.

74. Gosport War Memorial Hospital. *The Report of the Gosport Independent Panel (HC1084).* London: HMSO; 2018. Accessed January 3, 2020. https://www.gosportpanel.independent.gov.uk/media/documents/070618_CCS207_CCS03183220761_Gosport_Inquiry_Whole_Document.pdf

75. Llewellyn RL, Gordon PC, Reed AR. Drug administration errors – time for national action. *S Afr Med J.* 2011;101(5):319–20.

76. Merry AF, Webster CS. Medication error in New Zealand – time to act. *N Z Med J.* 2008;121(1272):6–9.

77. Orser BA. Medication safety in anesthetic practice: first do no harm. *Can J Anaesth.* 2000;47(11):1051–2.

78. Martin GP, Armstrong N, Aveling EL, Herbert G, Dixon-Woods M. Professionalism redundant, reshaped, or reinvigorated? Realizing the "third logic" in contemporary health care. *J Health Soc Behav.* 2015;56(3):378–97.

12 Legal and Regulatory Responses to Avoidable Adverse Medication Events, Part II: Practical Examples

12.1 Introduction

Internationally, many different regulatory models reflect a common desire to ensure compliance by healthcare provider organizations and individuals with accepted minimal standards (in effect *quality assurance* [QA]) and to encourage them to exceed these (in effect, *continuous quality improvement* [CQI]). In many countries, the responsibilities for QA and quality improvement (QI) reside in government departments, often within ministries of health. In some countries, nongovernmental organizations have been set up to advance quality improvement. In addition to these external processes, most institutions have their own internal regulatory frameworks. In part, internal mechanisms are needed to ensure compliance with relevant national legal and regulatory requirements, but increasingly, many institutions go beyond these with internal processes aimed at achieving the highest possible levels of quality and safety in the services they provide to patients. Despite all of this, avoidable adverse medication events continue to occur everywhere.

Given the considerable variation between and within countries, a comprehensive review of all the relevant regulatory and legal mechanisms currently in use around the world would not be possible within the limitations of a single chapter. Furthermore, this would not be particularly useful. Instead, we have approached this topic from the perspective of trying to illustrate some approaches that seem to be working reasonably well at present and some that do not, and also to highlight what changes might make an overall regulatory and legal framework more successful in assuring safe medication practice in anesthesia and perioperative medicine. We have been particularly interested in the potential value of a middle road between the extremes (described in Chapter 11) of (infrequent) criminal prosecution of a small number of practitioners on one hand, and on the other hand, the almost total disregard of the vast majority of failures in medication safety by both practitioners and those who fund and administer hospital services. For the practitioners, funders, and administrators who are strongly motivated to promote patient safety, heavy-handed regulation and policy decisions can be counterproductive (see Box 11.1). At the same time, it can be very challenging to ensure that those who seem to have other priorities actually do embrace the cause of patient safety. A further problem is that high-level rules or laws that deal with patient safety in general, or even medication safety in particular, may fail to ensure the attention to detail required for safe medication management in anesthesia and perioperative medicine. Thus, in thinking about each specific legal and regulatory approach considered in this chapter, it is worth asking if and how each might have prevented the various examples of serious adverse medication events discussed in this book.

12.2 Internal Institutional Regulation of Medication Safety

Whatever laws and regulations may exist in any particular jurisdiction, their effectiveness depends on how they are translated into practice in the workplace. Furthermore, institutions can often go beyond externally applied regulations and apply the theoretical considerations discussed in Chapter 11 to create their own frameworks for ensuring that their patients receive the highest quality and safety of care that they are capable of providing. Thus, we believe that it is within institutions that the best opportunity exists to improve the safety of healthcare, and that the establishment of a just culture within each institution is essential for achieving this.

12.2.1 Examples of Bottom-Up Efforts to Improve Medication Practices

The Keystone ICU project, discussed in Chapter 11, is an excellent example of an institutional initiative to improve a particular aspect of patient safety (i.e., the aseptic management of central venous catheters) (1). A recent publication from the University of Washington describes a sustained initiative to reduce medication administration errors in anesthesia (2). At the University of Iowa, Dr. Loftus's group is presently implementing a bundle of aseptic practices for anesthesiologists which includes a focus on the intravenous administration of medications (see ClinicalTrials. gov Identifier:NCT03638947, accessed January 21, 2020). In Auckland, in the Anaesthetists Be Cleaner (ABC) study, a multidisciplinary group is implementing a somewhat similar bundle of aseptic practices for anesthesia teams in three major hospitals (3).

It is reasonable to assume that although all four of these projects were the product of the enthusiasm of concerned clinicians, they must have been supported by their institutional leadership, at least to some extent. An element that contributed to the success of the Keystone ICU project was the insistence by leadership that physicians complied with certain specified requirements for safe practice. This instance was, in effect, a form of institutional regulation. Wachter and Pronovost have listed certain prerequisites for an institution to impose regulation of this type successfully (4). In Table 12.1, we have reproduced this list in relation to the example of hand hygiene, with their matching comments in the second column. In the third column, we have added our own commentary on how the leadership of an institution might translate these prerequisites to safe medication management in anesthesia and, in the last column, to the safe aseptic management of propofol with reference to the ABC study (which includes this aspect of practice as an important part of the overall aseptic management of intravenous medications). In contrast to the Keystone ICU study, compliance with the bundle of measures at the center of the ABC study is voluntary, not regulated. Nevertheless, the ABC study does have the explicit endorsement of the leadership of the three hospitals in which it is being conducted, so there is arguably at least some institutional authority supporting it.

An important problem becomes apparent in the third column, which deals with the overall safety of medication management in anesthesia: there is sufficient evidence to demonstrate that failures in medication management during anesthesia are an important problem (the first listed prerequisite), but there seems to be a lack of hard evidence to support any particular strategy or strategies to address this overall problem. This difficulty has been discussed in the report of the "extensive literature search to identify publications pertaining to medication error and medication safety in the operating room" undertaken by Wahr et al. (5). These authors identified only one "true" randomized controlled trial (RCT) in medication safety in anesthesiology (6), and the primary outcome measure used in this trial involved errors rather than patient outcomes. The reason for the limitation in this RCT's outcome measures was that, despite involving 89 consenting anesthesiologists, 1075 cases, and 10,764 medication administrations, it was massively underpowered to show any difference between groups in respect to harm. Furthermore, although it demonstrated a significant reduction in errors in the administration and recording of medications during anesthesia when a multimodal system that included checking by means of barcodes was compared with conventional methods of medication administration, it was not entirely clear which elements of the system were important and which were not (see Table 12.1 [2,3,7–10]).

Notwithstanding this lack of RCTs, by using a modified Delphi process, Wahr et al. were able to identify 35 specific recommendations (which included the key elements investigated in the two published RCTs [6,11]) that are strongly supported by expert consensus. In a somewhat similar way, in an earlier systematic review of the literature, Jensen et al. identified 12 recommendations that they considered were supported by expert consensus at least (12). There is considerable congruity between these two lists and also between them and the consensus statement for a "New Paradigm" arising from two summits of the Anesthesia Patient Safety Foundation (APSF) (13). Thus, Wahr et al. found that "the level of consensus among published expert opinions is high, with a strong consistency of view." They comment that "The dearth of evidence from randomized controlled trials, however, is not permission for us to do nothing."

Table 12.1 Prerequisites for expecting accountability from practitioners for adhering to a particular patient safety practice, with illustrative examples

Prerequisite	Example of hand hygiene	Example of safe medication management in anesthesia	Example of aseptic practices in relation to the aseptic management of propofol
The patient-safety problem that is being addressed is important.	Rates of healthcare–associated infections are unacceptably high, resulting in serious morbidity and mortality.	Numerous studies and case reports testify to substantial harm arising from failures in safe medication practice, often referred to as "medication errors." This evidence has been summarized in Chapters 2 and 3.	First principles and several case series leave no doubt that propofol is a potent culture medium, and sepsis and death may follow poor aseptic practices in its use (7,8).
The literature or expert consensus strongly supports adherence to the practice as an effective strategy to decrease the probability of harm.	Many studies and long-standing expert consensus support the value of hand hygiene, and healthcare–associated infections are now reported publicly and are subject to "no-pay" initiatives.	There are several reviews, guidelines, and consensus statements that provide consistent consensus-based recommendations and are supported by some evidence but very little evidence from randomized trials showing differences in patient outcomes (see Chapter 9).	There is some uncertainty about exact time limits for safely keeping syringes of propofol once drawn up, but substantial growth of injected *Escherichia coli* can be demonstrated by 4 hours (9), and the general principle that drawn-up propofol should be kept for the shortest period practicable is clear. The grounds for meticulous asepsis in drawing up and injecting propofol are also not controversial.
Clinicians have been educated about the importance of the practice and the evidence supporting it.	Lectures, reminder systems, academic detailing, dissemination of literature, and other steps to educate caregivers have been completed.	Many papers, editorials, and presentations have been written or given, but in most institutions targeted education is needed. The University of Washington Medical Center is one example of an institution in which a sustained initiative to implement a comprehensive medication safety bundle has been undertaken (2).	In Auckland, through the Anaesthetists Be Cleaner (ABC) study (3), systematic education of relevant staff on a bundle of aseptic practices in relation to the management of intravenous medications in general during anesthesia, with explicit emphasis on the management of propofol, is being introduced into successive clinical units.[a]
The system has been modified, if necessary, to make it as easy as possible to adhere to the practice without disrupting other crucial work or creating unanticipated negative consequences; concerns by providers regarding barriers to compliance have been addressed.	Hand-gel dispensers have been placed in convenient locations throughout the building; dispensers are never empty and work well (e.g., they do not squirt gel onto providers' clothes).	Substantial modifications to the system for intraoperative medication administration have been achieved in some institutions (2,10), but the willingness to invest in such modifications and to actively implement guidelines such as those of the APSF is variable.	In the ABC study, many modifications had already been made in Auckland hospitals to facilitate hand hygiene in the operating room; the bundle of the ABC study includes further modifications, notably in modifying the requirements for hand hygiene to more accurately reflect the context of the operating room and incorporating a 0.02 micron filter into the intravenous line for injection of all intravenous medications except propofol, thus reducing "the ask" for better aseptic practices to propofol alone.

Table 12.1 (cont.)

Prerequisite	Example of hand hygiene	Example of safe medication management in anesthesia	Example of aseptic practices in relation to the aseptic management of propofol
Physicians, other providers, and leaders have reached a consensus on the value of the practice and the process by which it will be measured; physicians understand the behaviors for which they will be held accountable.	Meetings have been held with relevant provider groups, including medical staff, to review the evidence behind hand hygiene, the rates of hospital-acquired infections, and the steps that have been taken to optimize the system.	As previously indicated, there is reasonable consensus in the literature on many aspects of safe medication practice in the perioperative period, but anecdotally there seems to be a substantial diversity of opinion among individual practitioners that is also sometimes reflected in correspondence sections of anesthesia journals. Thus, some departments may have difficulty in achieving consensus.	The bundle for the ABC study was developed by a modified Delphi process and reflects broad consensus of both anesthesiologists and other relevant clinicians. This included specifying 1 hour as a practicable limit within which propofol that has been drawn up into a syringe must be used or discarded.
A fair and transparent auditing system has been developed, and clinicians are aware of its existence.	Providers know that observers will periodically audit hand-hygiene practices; observers can determine whether providers adhere to the practices, even if hands are cleaned inside patients' rooms (including the use of video or systems that sound an alarm when providers approach patients' beds without using nearby hand-cleaning dispensers).	The University of Washington initiative has involved ongoing facilitated self-reporting of incidents to auditing the rate of errors but no observational collection of audit data in relation to safe medication practices. Few departments are resourced to undertake such observations.	The ABC study is a quality improvement initiative. It includes measurement of clinically relevant outcomes and the collection of sequential observational data on the aseptic practices of the anesthesiology teams. Participating clinicians are aware of these measurements (formal consent is part of the protocol), but data will be deidentified, and there is no element of compulsion.
Clinicians who do not adhere to the practice have been counseled about the importance of the practice, about the steps that have been taken to make it easy to adhere, and about the fact that further transgressions will result in punishment; the consequences of failure to adhere have been described.	A physician, for example, might receive a warning note or be counseled by a department chair after the first or second observed transgression.		
The penalties for infractions are understood and applied fairly.	Chronic failure to clean hands will result in a 1-week suspension from clinical practice, accompanied by completion of a 2-hour online educational module on infection prevention.		

Source: First two columns reproduced with permission Wachter and Pronovost 2009 (4), table 1.

Note: The first two columns are reproduced verbatim from table 1 in Wachter and Pronovost 2009 (4), except that references and notes about no-pay initiatives have been removed (these can be found in their publication). The examples in columns 3 and 4 extend these ideas to aspects of safe medication management.

[a] At the University of Iowa, Dr. Loftus's group is undertaking a similar implementation of a bundle of aseptic practices for anesthesiologists. See ClinicalTrials.gov Identifier:NCT03638947, accessed January 21, 2020.

It is hardly surprising that we, the present authors, agree with this view, since we are, in effect, the converted. The difficulty lies in persuading those practitioners and healthcare funders who are less convinced, for whatever reasons, about what in fact should be done (if anything). After all, Wahr et al. had to concede that their list of recommendations was "based nearly entirely on expert opinion." It is also interesting that very little emerged on the aseptic management of intravenous medications in general, or of propofol in particular, from any of the three of these consensus-building processes, despite their broad and systematic approach to the problem of medication safety. In addition, the vast majority of the recommended interventions to improve safety were weak, in that they require voluntary compliance by the anesthetist. Even a relatively advanced technological intervention, that of barcode scanning, allows administration without scanning or with scanning after administration. Most of the other recommendations are even weaker, such as "carefully read every label" or "use a two-person check when preparing high risk medications such as insulin or heparin." Thus, an institution could introduce all the recommendations listed by Wahr et al., Jensen et al., and the APSF and still be confronted with failures in their voluntary adoption or in the aseptic management of propofol as outlined in Box 11.3. What this illustrates is the complexity involved in ensuring medication safety as a generalized objective.

We have already emphasized that the Keystone ICU project was a major undertaking, but in some ways initiatives to reduce the rate of postprocedural infection are more straightforward than those to improve medication safety overall. Central line–associated bacterial infection is a more unified problem, although it is not without complexity. The evidence for what needs to be done is relatively clear. There is also substantial national and international momentum in relation to reducing hospital-acquired infections in general. Thus, it is not overwhelmingly difficult to obtain buy-in from senior hospital clinicians and administrators to support calls to mandate compliance with the required bundle of practices (14–16). Finally, the adverse outcome to be improved is relatively common, is readily measurable, and carries a heavy patient and economic cost (e.g., mortality associated with sternal wound infection is

significant [17], as is the cost to the hospital [18]). By contrast, relevant serious adverse medication events are varied in nature. The outcomes that need to be measured include death, sepsis, paraplegia, awareness, arrhythmias, cardiac arrest, and so forth. Each of these is individually infrequent and may also represent different mechanisms of failure: The safety considerations related to the oral administration of a medication on the ward or in a postoperative recovery unit by a nurse are different from those associated with giving sedation in the holding area before induction of anesthesia, giving a muscle relaxant as part of the anesthetic, or injecting bupivacaine into the cerebrospinal fluid. Of course, there are many aspects of medication management in anesthesia which are already regulated and for which compliance is not negotiable in most countries and institutions – the use of pulse oximetry and other key monitoring techniques, the requirement for providers of anesthesia to be qualified, and so forth. These regulatory requirements have dramatically reduced certain subsets of medication error, notably associated with the administration of oxygen. The problem is the long list of other potential sources of failure that needs to be considered, and it is more challenging to encapsulate many of these into a simple list of practice expectations that can reasonably be made mandatory.

Given this, perhaps an institution seeking to improve the safety of medication management in general should do this by taking individual aspects of medication management separately and sequentially, with a view to gradually extending its framework of internal regulation until the entire range of interrelated aspects of the problem has been covered.

Thus, the highly specific example of propofol has been chosen in Table 12.1 as a promising starting point. It is unequivocal that propofol is a culture medium for bacteria and that sepsis is a serious risk if propofol is not drawn up and administered with adequate asepsis (7,19). It is also clear that retaining propofol for too long after drawing it up into syringes magnifies that risk markedly. The only thing that is not completely certain is the lower boundary for a limit on how long (20), but microbiological growth of some bacteria can be shown by 3 or 4 hours (8,19), and endotoxins can be demonstrated by 24 hours (19). Package inserts vary in recommending that such syringes should be discarded between 6 and 12 hours, with the shorter times pertaining particularly to propofol that does not contain preservative (21). Thus, there is a basis for providing practicable guidance. In short, it is quite clear that something needs to be done and also clear what needs to be done.

In fact, these conclusions can reasonably be extended to the aseptic management of all intravenous medications during anesthesia. In 2015 Loftus et al. (22), having summarized the data demonstrating that there is a serious problem in this respect, proposed that "a multimodal approach targeting improvements in intraoperative hand hygiene, patient screening and decolonization, and environmental decontamination, as well as improvements in intravascular handling and design, may reduce the risk of postoperative infections." Again, we know there is a problem for which it would be reasonable to insist on compliance with a relatively contained list of practices, yet we know of only two places that have yet responded to the challenge of implementing these practices (the University of Iowa and the three hospitals in Auckland, as indicated).

Perhaps the most telling point is that all three of the initiatives discussed in this section have arisen, not because of external regulation, but spontaneously from the bottom up. They represent the efforts of concerned individuals to address this particular problem. The publication from the institute in Turkey (see Box 11.3) suggests (implicitly) that their response to their three cases of sepsis thus far has also been bottom-up from clinical staff, although hospital policies may possibly have played a role. Although it is gratifying to see clinical leadership, supported by institutional leadership, translating evidence into actions to improve the quality of perioperative medication management, the public would surely expect that hospitals would have governance mechanisms for assuring the quality and safety of relevant practices and also for identifying failures in that quality. In fact, many do: The importance of what is now often called *clinical governance* has been embraced within institutions over recent decades.

12.2.2 Clinical Governance

The concept of clinical governance was introduced in the United Kingdom in the 1990s in response to several substantial failures in healthcare delivery, to address the imbalance between the priorities of managers (often predominantly financial) and those of clinicians (often predominantly patient centered). Clinical governance has been defined as "a system through which healthcare organisations are accountable for continuously improving the quality of their services and safeguarding high standards of care, creating an environment in which excellence in clinical care will flourish" (23).

Clinical governance is not the same thing as clinical leadership (24). Indeed, governance sometimes serves to counter failures in clinical leadership, but even then it does (and must) include the meaningful incorporation of clinicians into the overall leadership of healthcare institutions. In the same way that managers need to have a reasonable understanding of healthcare, clinician leaders need to develop a reasonable understanding of the various aspects of governance and management on which the functioning of any substantial organization depends. This reciprocal knowledge can break down the divisions and ensure that healthcare organizations deliver the services for which they are accountable and that these services are safe and of an adequate quality.

The governance of many healthcare organizations is through boards of directors, or trustees, who set the strategy that is implemented by managers under the direction of a chief executive officer (although the precise terms used for various roles vary somewhat between countries). Much work has been done in the United States and many other countries to broaden the focus of these boards from a narrow perspective on the financial performance of the institution to also encompass the quality of the care provided – in effect to engage the directors in clinical governance. Notably, the Institute for Healthcare Improvement in the United States has emphasized the importance of "getting boards on board" (25).

12.2.2.1 Quality Accounts

In the United Kingdom, since 2010, under statutory regulations (26), the directors of National Health Service Trusts are required to prepare and publish annual *quality accounts*. The aim of this legislation was to make reporting on quality as important as financial reporting for boards of directors. As an example, the quality account of Imperial College outlines a quality improvement plan, current priorities for quality improvement, and progress in relation to these priorities (27). Other countries have followed suit. For example, in New Zealand, in 2012 the Health Quality and Safety Commission recommended similar reporting by health and disability service providers (28). To be effective, the expectation set by external regulators should be not so much the publication of an annual glossy report but rather the regular review of progress on the quality priorities at every meeting of the board of directors, much as the accounts are reviewed. This provides a nice illustration of the importance of each institution's implementation of external requirements and also of the point that institutions can choose to adopt quality accounts whether required to or not. Clearly an active process of reviewing the quality of care within an institution in this way could provide a basis for a problem in the aseptic management of propofol, of perioperative medications in general, or of any other aspect of medication safety to become an agreed priority for an institution. Agreeing on such a priority implies that resources will be invested in addressing the problem, and progress toward explicit goals will be monitored. This is, therefore, one way in which improving the overall safety of medication management in anesthesia and perioperative medicine could feasibly become an explicit responsibility for the directors of an institution, as well as for its clinicians. One example of such an approach is that undertaken by the leadership of nationwide Children's Hospital in Columbus, Ohio. Faced with an unacceptable rate (to the board) of preventable adverse events, the board authorized increasing the budget of the Quality Department from US$690,000 to $3.3 million and increasing the quality and safety staff from 8 to 33 (29). Every employee of the hospital was trained in quality and safety, and over an 18-month period, the rate of preventable harm fell to nearly zero. Adverse medication events were the focus of one of eight domains, and a substantial reduction was achieved (30). This provides a striking illustration of how a leader-led focus improves all aspects of quality, including medication safety.

On the other hand, it is not completely clear how directors should select priorities, or even how key information to inform such selection might reach them. Unsurprisingly, there is also variation between institutions in how well quality accounts are instituted and used (31). In part this is because of turnover and selection of directors, the need for director education, and the somewhat overwhelming problem of deciding which particular problem out of the huge number that confront any hospital at any one time should be selected as a priority. In Australia, Bismark et al. found that most health service boards had quality performance as a standing item on their agendas (32). Importantly, 77% reviewed data on medication errors and hospital-acquired infections at least quarterly. About half benchmarked their quality performance against external comparators, and about half offered formal training in quality to their directors. Worryingly, however, although 82% of directors identified quality as a top priority for board oversight, many thought that boards had only a minor influence on their institution's quality of care.

In the United States, a white paper from the Lucean Leape Institute gives a rather more depressing impression of the engagement of boards in quality improvement in the United States (33,34). A research scan involving expert interviews found that director (or trustee) education often fails to prepare participants for governance in relation to quality, and in particular in relation to elements of quality other than safety. A national survey by Jha and Epstein in 2010 found that fewer than half of the surveyed boards rated quality of care as one of their top two priorities, and only a minority of trustees had received training in clinical quality (35). Importantly, this study also showed an association between the engagement of boards in quality and the overall performance of organizations. Engaging directors in clinical governance may be a challenge (Table 12.2), but it is essential.

12.2.2.2 Hard Measurement and Soft Intelligence for Managing Quality Accounts

Measurement is widely held to be essential for quality improvement and is certainly essential for providing the data needed by boards for managing their quality accounts. There are many sources of relevant information, including self-reporting by clinicians (of which incident reporting is one example), notifications by clinicians about problems with other clinicians or the system more generally, complaints from patients, collection and analysis of outcome data, analysis of data from claims (or closed claims) analysis, and so

Table 12.2 Some key requirements for clinical governance in healthcare organizations. Even if all these requirements were in place, it would still be a challenge in many organizations to get safe medication management in the perioperative period onto the board of directors' list of priorities – but without them, there will no reasonable basis for doing so.

- A belief by directors of the organization that clinical governance is a core part of their fiduciary obligations and that addressing this will improve patient outcomes without damaging the financial performance of the institution

- A reasonable level of knowledge by at least a fair proportion of the directors of healthcare in general and of the principles of quality improvement in particular; training for directors in these areas should be available, and participation in such training should be expected

- The incorporation of quality on the agenda of every board meeting, with reporting against identified quality priorities for the organization and with quality accounts given the same importance as financial accounts

- The identification of explicit priorities for quality improvement

- A formal framework for measuring the quality of the organization's services

- A method of including informal or "soft intelligence" from frontline healthcare workers and patients/consumers into the board's deliberations, which allows them to triangulate with more formal sources of information – this intelligence is like radar for warning of impending problems

- Executive accountability for ensuring that the agreed plans for quality improvement are in fact implemented effectively

Source: Modified from discussion by Bismark et al. 2013 (32) and from Conway 2008 (25).

forth. Any of these sources can provide information relevant to medication safety. Importantly, the type of information received varies according to the process used (36), so triangulation between sources is important.

Retrospective chart review has been used in various studies of adverse events and can identify adverse medication events but is resource intensive and subject to considerable interobserver variability. Trigger tools go some way to addressing these limitations and have greater potential for institutional use to monitor adverse medication events (30,37,38).

For many surgeons in the United Kingdom and some states of the United States, individualized data on the outcomes of surgery are now publicly available. Patients' ratings of the sur-

geons (and other physicians) may also be available. The requirement for this has been externally imposed by surgical organizations and by governments. The internal use of such data by institutions is clearly important but not straightforward (39). It is a reasonable assumption that safer medication management might manifest in better patient outcomes, so it is interesting to ask whether a similar approach should be taken to the measurement and public publication of outcome data for anesthesiologists or other relevant physicians (e.g., intensivists and internists). In fact, patients' outcomes reflect the overall care provided by entire teams of clinicians working in the context of particular institutions, and it has been recommended that a better approach is to make outcome data publicly available at the unit level as part of the monitoring of standard of care, but also to require boards of directors to attest to the presence of (confidential) internal processes to assure that all their clinicians are functioning at an acceptably safe standard (39). The latter requirement could extend to attesting that they have invested in appropriate initiatives to enhance medication safety and that they have a system to ensure that their clinicians are engaging with these. We think institutions should embrace this general approach, whether required to or not. In fact many go some distance toward doing this, but as discussed earlier, the missing component is the systematic assurance of compliance with safe practices by staff.

An important drawback of most metrics used to monitor quality is that they tend to be lag indicators – they give a picture of what quality was like at some point in the past. Imagine an approach like that in aviation defense – the critical breakthrough provided by radar in the Second World War was that it gave warning of impending problems (in the form of air raids) before they actually manifested themselves (albeit only just in time). A second drawback is that most metrics in common use only reflect things that have already been identified as worthy of measuring. Our example of the cases of sepsis arising from contaminated propofol is exactly the sort of thing that directors or senior hospital managers are unlikely to see coming – the failures in safe practice leading to this problem were identified through the systems of surveillance and follow-up of the microbiology department, but unfortunately only after serious harm had occurred to three patients. A third drawback is that many directors are poorly equipped for evaluating the quality proposals put in front of them and deciding which ones really do constitute priorities. As indicated, education is part of the solution, but in reality, for most directors, the expertise gap is unbridgeable. It is a real challenge for directors to evaluate and check the advice they are receiving from diverse experts, some of whom may be self-styled rather than genuine.

An idea that has recently been adopted by the Health Quality and Safety Commission in New Zealand is that of "soft intelligence" (40). This idea has been the subject of a qualitative study by Waring and Bishop, as "knowledge from the backstage" (41). In essence, the idea is that clinicians (and others) at the workface know what is happening and that their informal conversations at the water cooler, in the breakroom, or in the corridors are an important form of early warning about present or impending problems. This idea aligns with the concept of director and chief executive officer "walk-arounds" and with the importance of having a low threshold for receiving input from staff and patients to the business of boards of directors. In our three examples of aseptic management of medications, the implication would be that some communication would take place between the frontline clinicians who have safety concerns and the board of directors (perhaps through the chief executive officer) of the institution. The directors would not necessarily accept all communications of this type on face value, but they should at least consider the matters they raise and also integrate the information with more formal sources of information. We can see that a board that had already identified medication safety and hospital-acquired infections as priorities (as in the findings of Bismark et al. [32]) would be able to use this more spontaneous source of information to reaffirm the importance of these priorities. Importantly, this type of information would assist them in evaluating whether their programs were in fact appropriately targeted or whether there were gaps that still needed to be addressed. Information of this type would also serve to alert directors to pending problems that had not hitherto been considered (see Table 12.2).

Notifications from staff members about concerns with the system or about colleagues are another potential source of information for the management and governance of healthcare institutions. In fact, such notifications may be the only source of information about certain problems during anesthesia.

However, notwithstanding legal obligations to do this in some countries and an arguable ethical responsibility to do so whatever the law, many physicians are reluctant to criticize their colleagues (at least through formal processes) (42). In the context of medication error, this may be a missed opportunity for improvement. One might contrast commercial pilots, who we doubt would tolerate violations of accepted procedures on the part of their copilots, with anesthesiologists (and surgeons and nurses as well), who clearly are often reluctant to criticize the practices of colleagues even when they believe these to be somewhat unsafe.

12.2.2.3 Information from Patients
Information about adverse events, and certainly about near misses, is rarely documented in patients' records. For example, in 2003 Weissman et al. surveyed a random sample of patients after discharge from hospitals in Massachusetts and also reviewed the medical records of consenting participants. Many additional serious and preventable adverse events were identified by the surveyed patients to those identified by review of the medical notes (43). Similarly, in 2001 in Boston, Weingart et al. identified almost twice as many adverse events and near misses by interviewing consenting patients as by reviewing their medical records (44). It follows that patients themselves are an important source of information on adverse events, errors, near misses, and other failures in the care they have received. We live in an era in which feedback from consumers through formal and informal mechanisms is increasingly the norm. This culture of feedback is progressively infiltrating healthcare. It is not unexpected that patient and family reviews of healthcare may be discordant with formal assessment by published standards (45). Many healthcare institutions are now conducting patient experience surveys and collecting patient-reported outcome measures as part of their quality assurance programs. Such surveys should include questions that explicitly address important aspects of medication safety, including an invitation to report any failures in care experienced by the patient.

Similarly, many healthcare institutions have also invested considerably into processes for receiving, considering, and responding to complaints. A formal complaint by a patient is somewhat different from a response to a survey or a request to be interviewed and may produce more targeted information about problems. On the other hand, it seems (anecdotally at least) that many people are reluctant to complain, particularly if they perceive an actual or potential need to continue receiving treatment from the clinician or institution in question. Even in well-resourced settings, a further barrier to laying a complaint lies in knowing how to do this. Therefore, in some countries (e.g., New Zealand), there is a legal requirement for patients to be informed about their right to complain and about how to do this.

An assumption about patient complaints and notifications by members of staff is that something will be done about them. Also, it may be that feeding information from patients back to practitioners and management is likely to motivate them to embrace and invest in safer medication practices. On the other hand, the assumption that complaints in general facilitate better quality in healthcare has been challenged. Cunningham has pointed out that the positivist construct on which this belief is based may be flawed. His study (with Dovey) in 2000 showed that complaints had marked short- and long-term effects on doctors, which he summarized as a "shame" response. He argues that complaints may serve to promote defensive rather than high-quality practices (46,47). Similar concerns may well apply to notifications to management from staff about concerns about colleagues.

Interestingly, it seems that complaints frequently relate to the way in which staff (including anesthesia staff) have interacted with patients (i.e., problems with communication, including the style of communication) as much as to the fact that harm has occurred (48). In particular, one study showed that medication errors are more likely to be identified through incident reporting than through complaints (36). This may be, in part, because (as discussed earlier) patients are seldom told about medication errors unless the impact of the error is obvious, but this may also be a matter of the threshold for laying a complaint. We suspect patients know about medication errors far more often than they complain about them, so, as indicated, patient surveys should include explicit questions about medication events (43).

12.3 National and International External Regulation of Medication Safety

Some institutions in the United States, the United Kingdom, and many other countries have achieved effective levels of clinical governance, reflecting boards that are highly engaged in the quality of the services they provide and who use broadly based systems of monitoring that provide information across the entire range of the provided services. However, as we have seen, the extent and effectiveness of clinical governance are variable, and even in well-governed institutions, medication safety in the specific context of anesthesia and the perioperative period may not be seen as a particular priority when compared with other challenges for the provision of safe, high-quality care. What then is the role of external regulation within countries in ensuring that all institutions adopt acceptable standards of clinical governance (with all that that implies) and, furthermore, that they address specific areas of practice of this type? And is there any form of international regulation that can influence the safety of medication practices in institutions within countries that do not have effective national regulation of the quality and safety of healthcare?

12.3.1 Accreditation

12.3.1.1 National Nongovernmental Agencies

In the United States and many other countries, the Joint Commission (TJC: see www. jointcommission.org/, accessed January 21, 2020), an independent nonprofit organization founded in 1951, plays a key role in accrediting healthcare organizations. TJC adopted total quality improvement (TQI) as a "new paradigm" as long ago as 1989 (49). Its work includes the provision of resources for patients, on the principle that health literacy and engagement with one's own care are key elements of assuring quality. For example, they provide a series of "Speaking Up" videos (available on the website: www.jointcommission.org/, accessed January 21, 2020) including one called "Take Medication Safely." The focus of TJC is broad, and many aspects of accreditation can be expected to improve the overall capability of an institution to manage medications safely through the perioperative period (Table 12.3).

Table 12.3 Some aspects of medication safety addressed by the Joint Commission (TJC) through its accreditation processes (this list is not exhaustive)[a]

- The labeling of medications once they leave the original container and are transferred to another container, unless immediately administered, is addressed under National Patient Safety Goals

- TJC's Medication Management standards require that medications be stored on the basis of manufacturers' recommendations, including the use of warmers, monitoring temperatures, and proper changes in expiration dating

- TJC requires processes be developed and implemented related to safe storage and administration of high-alert and high-risk medications, such as paralytic agents

- TJC requires a process be put into place to address record keeping and antidiversion strategies of medications

[a] For assistance in preparing this list, we are grateful to Robert Campbell, PharmD, Director, Clinical Standards Interpretation Hospital/Ambulatory Programs and Director, Medication Management, The Joint Commission.

However, it seems (understandably) that their accreditation processes do not seek to explicitly and comprehensively address medication management during anesthesia and the perioperative period. In addition, a recent Harvard Global Health study found that TJC-accredited hospitals had no better patient outcomes than did state- or other agency-accredited hospitals, raising the concern that the resources expended on obtaining and maintaining TJC accreditation may not result in improved patient safety (50).

Also, in the United States, the Institute for Healthcare Improvement (IHI: www.ihi.org/, accessed July 14, 2020), founded in 1991, has become hugely influential in advancing QI. On its website, three phases of focus are described: the identification and spread of best practices in its first decade; innovation, research and development, and the discovery of new solutions to old problems in its second decade; and addressing healthcare as a complete social and geopolitical enterprise in its third decade. In its second decade, it launched two major campaigns to spread best practices. In line with the focus of the third decade, the IHI created the Triple Aim, described as "a framework for optimizing health system performance by simultaneously focusing on the health of a population, the experience of care for individuals within that population, and the per capita cost of providing that care." This framework has been very influential. For example, a modification for local priori-

ties has been adopted in New Zealand and linked to the dual objectives of "doing the right thing" and "doing things right first time" (51). On its website, the IHI lists topics alphabetically. These include "Medication Reconciliation to Prevent Adverse Drug Events," "High-Alert Medication Safety," and "Surgical Site Infection," all of which are relevant to perioperative management of medications. Thus, engagement in IHI programs, as with TJC accreditation, is likely to enhance medication safety in the perioperative period, in the United States and internationally. Again, this is likely to occur more indirectly than directly, particularly with the IHI's third-phase shift to a more capability-focused social construct of quality improvement. A further issue is that there is no compulsion and relatively little incentive to engage with IHI, other than an institution's commitment to QI, and perhaps because of a perceived value in doing so for institutional reputation. The same applies to TJC accreditation in countries other than the United States, but in the United States, formal accreditation by TJC or an equivalent agency is required to receive payment from the federally funded Medicare and Medicaid programs, so it is in effect mandatory.

12.3.1.2 National Governmental Agencies

In recent years, many governments have established departments or semi-independent organizations to advance CQI, sometimes on its own (with QA managed separately) and sometimes within a TQI framework. For example, the Australian Commission on Safety and Quality in Health Care (see www.safetyandquality.gov.au/, accessed January 21, 2020) was set up in 2006 "to lead and coordinate national improvements in safety and quality in health care" but has subsequently shifted its focus to include the development of standards and accreditation of organizations against them. Medication safety is an explicit focus for this body. Work of relevance to this chapter includes the development and promulgation of national inpatient medication charts, medication reconciliation, and joint statements with the Australian and New Zealand College of Anaesthetists (ANZCA; see: www.anzca.edu.au/, accessed January 21, 2020) on the topical application and accidental injection of chlorhexidine and on neuraxial connectors. The joint statements are recommendations rather than legislated requirements, but they can be expected to be of considerable influence and would also be taken into account by the courts in cases of civil litigation. The Health Quality and Safety Commission (see www.hqsc.govt.nz/, accessed January 21, 2020) was set up by the Government of New Zealand in 2010 to monitor and improve the quality of health and disability services. It has few explicit powers but considerable influence. In its early years, coordinating and advancing aspects of medication safety nationally was one of its main priorities. Aspects addressed included medicine reconciliation on admission and discharge from hospital, a standardized medication record, and adverse medication event reporting. Again, these would all advance medication safety during anesthesia or the perioperative period, but these aspects of medication management were not addressed explicitly. Somewhat in line with the IHI, the commission has shifted the focus for its limited resources to capacity development and to population-level challenges to the quality of healthcare, notably inequity between groups in access to services. However, it still has a substantial program dedicated to improving surgical site infection, which includes assuring the timely administration of antibiotics and the effective use of the WHO Surgical Safety Checklist (which in turn includes checks for patients' allergies.) These efforts have been associated with a worthwhile reduction in the rate of postoperative *Staphylococcus aureus* infections in patients undergoing hip and knee arthroplasties (40). In the United Kingdom, the National Institute for Health and Care Excellence (NICE: see www.nice.org.uk/, accessed January 21, 2020) was established in 1999 (as the National Institute for Clinical Excellence) and has evolved to becoming a Non Departmental Public Body, accountable to government but independent of it. NICE "provides national guidance and advice to improve health and social care." Its advice is highly respected, and it has influence internationally. It has statements on various aspects of the safe use of medicines, some of which are relevant in the perioperative period, but again, there seems to be no explicit focus on this part of the patient's journey.

There are many other examples of organizations of this kind. In addition, most countries have licensing bodies for healthcare practitioners that have increasingly embraced the need for practitioners to develop continued competence as well as for initial qualifications to enter practice. These bodies

typically regulate individual practitioners rather than institutions. One might envisage, for example, that a medical practitioner whose poor aseptic practice in the management of propofol resulted in the sepsis of a patient could end up appearing before the disciplinary branch of such a licensing authority, facing sanctions that might vary from censure to loss of license to practice. These bodies variably also promulgate ethical guidance on practice. For example, both the General Medical Council in the United Kingdom (see www.gmc-uk.org/, accessed January 21, 2020) and the Medical Council of New Zealand (see www.mcnz.org.nz/, accessed January 21, 2020) have published statements on good practice in prescribing medicines. These are relevant to physicians who practice perioperatively but do not provide comprehensive guidance on medication management during this period. The Medical Councils of Canada (see https://mcc.ca/about/, accessed January 21, 2020) and Australia (see www.amc.org.au/, accessed January 21, 2020) function in broadly similar ways. In the United States, the licensure of medical and other health professionals is done by each state, and there are many variations on these themes within the 195 countries of the world.

12.3.1.3 Specialist Colleges and Other Training and Professional Organizations

A potentially very effective (if incidental) source of regulation of many aspects of safe medication practice in the perioperative period is to be found in the accreditation of institutions for the training of specialist doctors in countries such as England, Ireland, Canada, Australia, and New Zealand, notably those involved with anesthesia, surgery, and nursing. Details vary, but an excellent binational example can be found in Australia and New Zealand.[1] The Australian Medical Council (AMC) and the New Zealand Medical Council (NZMC) assess and accredit specialist medical education and professional development programs in Australia (see www.amc.org.au/, accessed January 21, 2020) and New Zealand. These programs are mandatory in both countries and set standards for specialist medical

---

[1] We are grateful to Dr. Leona Wilson, executive director of professional affairs and former president of ANZCA, for her helpful comments in regard to ANZCA's processes.

training, which lead to qualifications for practice in recognized medical specialties. Requirements for these programs are that "the provider has a clear process and criteria to assess, accredit and monitor facilities and posts as training sites" (52). To this end, the colleges develop and promulgate guidelines or other documents on standards of practice, including both structure (i.e., physical requirements, including equipment, the area around beds in postoperative care units, and so forth) and process in their *professional documents* (in effect, guidelines). These colleges have well-developed processes by which their professional documents are regularly reviewed and updated. Many of the ANZCA professional documents deal in detail with various aspects of safe medication management in the perioperative period (Table 12.4). Furthermore, ANZCA liaises with other bodies when relevant to produce joint statements: PS09 on sedation for diagnostic and interventional procedures (see Table 12.4) is a prime example and represents a statement of broad consensus on safe practice in the administration of sedative agents whether by anesthesiologists or any other health professionals. Notably, these documents contain various provisions that would explicitly address the propofol contamination reported from Turkey: PS51 (53), clause 5.6.1 states that "The time interval between drawing up a drug and administering

it should be as short as practicable." In addition, in PS28 (54), section 4.4 deals with avoiding the contamination of medications. Both documents also specify that the contents of any one ampule should only be administered to one patient. The point, of course, is that these standards explicitly address not just the use of propofol but safe medication management in the operating room more generally. In fact, many aspects of pre- and postoperative medication management are also covered by these resources, particularly if one includes the parallel contributions of other colleges and organizations such as the Royal Australasian College of Surgeons (RACS: see www.surgeons.org/, accessed January 21, 2020), the College of Intensive Care Medicine in Australia and New Zealand (see www.cicm.org.au/, accessed January 21, 2020), the Faculty of Pain Medicine of ANZCA (see http://fpm.anzca.edu.au/, accessed January 21, 2020), and various nursing and pharmaceutical organizations and registration bodies.

ANZCA and the other listed colleges conduct regular formal visits to accredit hospitals for anesthesia training, predicated on the notion that the training of specialists in anesthesia can only be done in the context of an excellent and safe clinical service. Much of the process is accrediting the service, although some explicitly focuses on the education of the trainees. If expected standards are not met, a

Table 12.4 A selection of guidelines of the Australian and New Zealand College of Anaesthetists related to the perioperative management of medications

Guideline number and title, as a link to the guideline itself
PS01 Recommendations on Essential Training for Rural General Practitioners in Australia Proposing to Administer Anaesthesia
PS03 Guidelines for the Management of Major Regional Analgesia
PS07 Guidelines on Pre-Anaesthesia Consultation and Patient Preparation
PS09 Guidelines on Sedation and/or Analgesia for Diagnostic and Interventional Medical, Dental or Surgical Procedures[a]
PS18 Guidelines on Monitoring During Anaesthesia
PS28 Guidelines on Infection Control in Anaesthesia
PS41 Guidelines on Acute Pain Management
PS51 Guidelines for the Safe Management and Use of Medications in Anaesthesia
PS53 Statement on the Handover Responsibilities of the Anaesthetist
PS54 Statement on the Minimum Safety Requirements for Anaesthetic Machines and Workstations for Clinical Practice
PS60 Guidelines on the Perioperative Management of Patients with Suspected or Proven Hypersensitivity to Chlorhexidine

Source: Available from www.anzca.edu.au/resources/professional-documents, accessed January 21, 2020.
[a] This document has been endorsed by the Australasian College for Emergency Medicine, the College of Intensive Care Medicine of Australia and New Zealand, the Gastroenterological Society of Australia, the New Zealand Society for Gastroenterology, the Royal Australasian College of Surgeons, the Royal Australian and New Zealand College of Psychiatrists, and the Royal Australian and New Zealand College of Radiologists.

meeting is held with the senior management of the institution (usually the chief executive officer and the chief medical officer), and a plan is formulated to address the deficiencies over a reasonable time frame. Most institutions cooperate proactively, but this process has teeth – hospitals of any size depend on trainees for many reasons, and the withdrawal of the privilege to provide training is taken very seriously. Furthermore, considerable adverse publicity and reputational damage inevitably accompany a notice of the intention to withdraw training privileges. Thus, a regulatory framework is in place in Australia and New Zealand that goes a reasonable distance toward the proactive achievement of safer medication practice in the perioperative period. Furthermore, this process exemplifies the type of accountability proposed by Wachter and Pronovost (discussed earlier) but applied to institutions rather than to individuals.

The College of Anaesthesiologists of Ireland (see www.anaesthesia.ie/, accessed January 21, 2020) appears to run a similar program to that of ANZCA (see www.anaesthesia.ie/training/ hospital-accreditation/, accessed January 21, 2020). In the United Kingdom, somewhat comparable processes have evolved through various phases over time.[2] In 2010, the Postgraduate Medical Education and Training Board (PMETB), the nondepartmental public body responsible for postgraduate medical education and training in the United Kingdom, was merged with the General Medical Council (GMC: see www.gmc-uk.org/, accessed January 21, 2020). The GMC is now responsible for all undergraduate and postgraduate training, maintaining the medical, specialist, and general practitioner register and regulation. Colleges write curricula (which are approved by the GMC), administer examinations, and supervise the progress of individuals via a network of college tutors. However, Health Education England (HEE) (see www.hee.nhs.uk/, accessed January 21, 2020) allocates trainees to and responds to any concerns about training in an individual hospital. HEE can act by reducing numbers or removing tiers of trainees from a specialty or the entire hospital, either for a limited time to allow improvement,

or permanently. However, this process seems less grounded in assuring the fundamentals of sound practice than the one in Australia and New Zealand. There are of course many other intertwined regulatory processes in the United Kingdom, but it is not clear whether any are likely to penetrate deeply enough into the details of day-to-day clinical practice to explicitly address more than the higher-level aspects of the safety of perioperative management of medications. Like ANZCA, the Royal College of Anaesthetists (see www.rcoa. ac.uk/, accessed January 21, 2020), which also has a Faculty of Pain Medicine (see www.rcoa.ac.uk/ faculty-of-pain-medicine, accessed January 21, 2020), produces practice guidelines and runs an accreditation program for hospitals, but participation in this is voluntary.

In the United States, the situation is somewhat different. The Accreditation Council for Graduate Medical Education (ACGME), an independent, not-for-profit, physician-led organization, sets and monitors the professional *educational standards* for all of the 11,200 residency and fellowship programs in 180 specialties, at 830 institutions in the United States. While ACGME does set institutional standards and monitors hospitals to ensure that the appropriate culture and climate exist for effective training, they do not set specific guidelines for any area of clinical practice, leaving that to the hospital accrediting bodies. Accreditation by an entity such as TJC is a requirement for establishing a training program, and if a hospital should lose their accreditation, they would immediately lose their credentialing for any training programs as well.

The specific requirements for anesthesiology training, as well as the examinations to achieve board certification are set by the American Board of Anesthesiology (ABA). Like other specialty boards, the ABA sets criteria for and oversees all training programs for anesthesiologists; it also oversees the progression toward certification of individual trainees. Unlike ANZCA, however, the ABA specifies essentially no standards for the clinical service provided by accredited training programs, leaving those standards to be set primarily by the American Society of Anesthesiologists. The ABA focuses primarily on examining the adequacy of the basic science and clinical knowledge base of trainees and very little on the clinical setting in which that knowledge is attained, again, leaving most of that to the ACGME.

---

[2] We are grateful to Dr. Andrew Hartle, formerly president of the Association of Anaesthetists of Great Britain and Ireland (now renamed the Association of Anaesthetists), for his explanation of the system in the United Kingdom.

In the United States and in other countries, various colleges, societies, and other organizations promulgate guidance and set standards in various ways, notably the Anesthesia Patient Safety Foundation (see www.apsf.org/, accessed January 21, 2020) in the United States, which has a strong focus on medication safety in the perioperative period and publishes a highly influential newsletter.

12.3.1.4 Global Organizations

The World Health Organization (see WHO: www.who.int/, accessed January 21, 2020) has various guidelines and resources that influence practice through governments and more generally. The WHO specifically has issued documents on improving medication safety as well as a manual and a tool to assess local knowledge of medication administration safety (see www.who.int/patient-safety/education/curriculum/who_mc_topic-11.pdf, accessed January 21, 2020). The Surgical Safety Checklist (55) is an example of a WHO resource, and some of the items on this list directly address medication safety during anesthesia and postoperatively. The World Federation of Societies of Anaesthesiologists (see WFSA: www.wfsahq.org/, accessed January 21, 2020) also develops and endorses guidelines and resources, of which the most relevant is the International Standards for a Safe Practice of Anaesthesia, endorsed by both WFSA and WHO (56). The WFSA also provides a facility assessment tool (available on the website) based on these standards, which cover many important aspects of safe anesthesia care, including a list of essential medications.

Without question, these various organizations all contribute to promoting patient safety in general, and medication safety in anesthesia and the perioperative period more particularly. Many of the guidelines are mandated, whether directly through legislation or indirectly through funding arrangements (as with TJC), but even when they are entirely voluntary, they are resources that can inform and be integrated into institutional processes and can influence governments. They may also serve as references to acceptable standards of care for the courts. This possibility may be seen as an unwanted threat, but it should be remembered that the organizations reviewed here usually take great care in developing and promulgating guidelines and other resources and in ensuring their reasonableness. Thus, from the perspective of reg-

ulation, the possibility that they might be used to inform civil or criminal actions is probably positive on balance and may serve to increase the regulatory effectiveness of these documents.

12.4 Civil Litigation and No-Fault Systems of Compensation

In Chapter 11, we discussed the question of compensation for preventable adverse medication events, and indicated that civil litigation is primarily predicated on the notion that such compensation is appropriate and should be provided. We also explained that, in practice, civil litigation almost always also serves to provide retribution in one way or another.

It is quite difficult to find data on the details of specific cases of litigation involving adverse medication events. The American Society of Anesthesiologists maintains a database of all malpractice suits that resulted in a claim for the plaintiff, called the Closed Claims Project. Data from this project provide some indication of the likely amounts of such damages in the United States (Box 12.1). The median payment for a medication-related claim was US$76,313. Data from the Medical Protection

Box 12.1 Damages paid for medication events in surgical/procedural, obstetrics, and acute pain claims (chronic pain medicine not included) for events occurring between 2005 and 2014, recorded in the Anesthesia Closed Claims Database (N = 1293 for the period and 11,032 for the entire database) analyzed by primary damaging event code. Payments have been adjusted to 2017 US$.

Events:
- All medication events: n = 71 (5.5%)
  - Wrong dose or medication specifically classified in 42 (3.2%)

Payments (all parties):
- 80% of all medication events were settled with a payment to the plaintiff (patient).
- When paid, the median (25–75 percentile) payment of a medication event on behalf of all defendants was $76,313 ($27,448–$468,850).
- The total amount of payments for all medication events by all defendants during this time period was US$21,090,585 in 2017.

Source: Data kindly provided by Dr. Karen B. Domino.

Society (MPS) provide a similar insight for the United Kingdom. For example, a recent report indicates that out of 3000 claims analyzed, there were only a small number for awareness, all of which were settled. The highest total payment was £44,000 (48). Claims were also made for wrong-sided blocks, failure to provide adequate sedation, and nerve damage during the administration of regional or central blockade. No separate category of medication events is provided by the MPS, but it seems that direct medication errors in the form of syringe swaps or dosage errors do not form a large proportion of these claims. Even when a patient dies in association with a medication error, the amount awarded in damages may be surprisingly modest – the data in Table 12.5 suggest an average award of just under £30,000 over a 10-year period. Interestingly, costs amounted to almost 40% of the total paid, and these claims represented a very small proportion of the total cost of National Health Service (NHS) litigation. Thus, it may be that the direct cost of settling claims for avoidable adverse medication events is not so large as to be a major driver for the investment decisions of any particular institution, in either the United States or the United Kingdom. On the other hand, reputational costs may be more compelling, both for institutions and for individuals.

Exemplary damages add a punitive element to the damages awarded in the civil courts in cases where it is perceived that the behavior of the sued person or organization has been particularly egregious. Such damages substantially increase the cost implications of a lost lawsuit, and they also explicitly increase the adverse impact on reputation. It is difficult to know how commonly exemplary damages have been awarded for medication errors.

As we argued in Chapters 7, 8, and 11, deterrent influences cannot be expected to prevent errors, but they may well reduce violations. Also, institutions may choose to invest in safety as part of a general strategy to enhance their reputation, as well as because it is the right thing to do. Thus, we accept that there is at least some truth in the proposition that civil litigation may play a worthwhile role in increasing medication safety. The contrary viewpoint is that the fear of being sued may instead serve primarily to promote defensive medicine. If we return to the specific example of aseptic practices in relation to propofol, it does seem that the potential threat of a civil action against an institution might gain the attention of senior managers and clinicians and provide motivation for change in situations of this sort. On the other hand, there is also an argument that such an action might be

Table 12.5 Clinical claims for damages against the National Health Service (NHS) received from 2006 to 2016 (as of December 31, 2016) where one of the causes was medication error and one of the injuries was fatality. For comparison, the total cost of NHS litigation was £2000,000,000 in 2017–2018 (NHS Resolution Annual Report and accounts 2017–2018).

NHSLA notification year	Number of claims	Damages paid (£)	Defense costs paid (£)	Claimant costs paid (£)	Total paid (£)	Total damages (£)	Total claim (£)
2006/07	19	425,900	47,584	282,406	755,890	425,900	755,890
2007/08	19	561,500	73,810	347,847	983,157	561,500	983,157
2008/09	25	1,348,000	112,366	714,100	2,174,466	1,348,000	2,174,466
2009/10	24	623,304	143,999	522,245	1,289,548	623,304	1,289,548
2010/11	25	732,903	71,131	459,312	1,263,345	732,903	1,263,345
2011/12	39	3,597,171	189,760	1,164,836	4,951,768	3,632,171	5,148,239
2012/13	20	543,250	102,623	350,449	996,322	1,043,250	1,728,992
2013/14	40	759,526	257,662	784,962	1,802,150	759,526	1,876,988
2014/15	49	1,221,416	201,997	429,313	1,852,726	2,321,416	3,905,498
2015/16	50	600,398	152,950	133,865	887,212	1,743,898	3,049,918
Total	352	10,418,518	1,385,638	5,190,834	16,994,990	14,850,018	25,040,518

Source: Information kindly provided by Mr. John Mead, NHS Litigation Authority, through Professor Robin Ferner.

less than just for a practitioner unfortunate to be the first individual caught up in a sequence where medication practices that were widespread in their country resulted first in patient harm and then in a lawsuit. This argument, however, is much weaker for civil lawsuits than it is for the criminal law. Unfortunately, at least in the United States, the civil lawsuit process is so difficult, tortuous, and lengthy that many patients who have been harmed by a preventable medication error, choose not to sue their physician. In addition, hospitals may prevail in their defense even in the face of a clear error, through sophisticated arguments brought by their lawyers, or through missteps by the plaintiff's lawyers. Indeed, in one study of 20 years of litigated cases, plaintiffs won only 50% of the jury trials even when other physicians rated the care as "poor" (57). As noted in Chapter 4, this often leaves patients without the financial compensation that they need to recover from physical and emotional harm. It is clear that a "full disclosure and rapid compensation" practice, as promoted by the University of Michigan (58), and now many other institutions, is a far more just and appropriate mechanism than a battle in the courts.

In Chapter 11, we explained that the most important disadvantage of tort law is the requirement for patients to actually prove fault. For this and other reasons, national no-fault systems of compensation have been established in the Nordic countries and in New Zealand. Even in these countries, some element of fault is typically implicitly or explicitly required. It is accepted that not all harm from healthcare can be compensated – to do so would be completely unaffordable and would also go beyond any reasonable requirement for social justice. Nevertheless, the burden of *proof of fault* has been alleviated. This has led to some widening of the boundaries between what can and cannot be compensated. For example, in New Zealand at the time of writing, many postoperative infections are classified by this country's Accident Compensation Corporation (ACC: see www.acc.co.nz/, accessed January 21, 2020), the agency responsible for compensating all forms of accident, as "treatment injuries." As such, they are eligible for compensation. This is a generous approach, and it is hard to see how a civil suit for a postoperative infection would succeed in any country in the absence of clear evidence of some failure in treatment. The lack of such evidence does not, how-

ever, necessarily mean that no such failure occurred – and the Keystone ICU project referenced earlier has shown that it is possible to virtually eliminate all of at least one type of infection, namely, CLABSI. Indeed, at least some infections would have arisen (at least in part) from things such as failures in administering prophylactic antibiotics when indicated, in the aseptic technique of the surgical team, or in the hand hygiene of any of the people involved in the patient's postoperative care. We are not clear on the reasoning behind the New Zealand approach, but it does seem to strike a balance between compensating some patients in whose care no fault has occurred with making sure that those for whom fault was a factor are in fact compensated – even if the particular fault cannot be identified. It is perhaps also consistent with the notion that current rates of postoperative infection (like CLABSI) should not be accepted as an inevitable consequence of surgery. More generally, it does seem that patients covered by systems of this type would be less likely to find themselves in a position where they are left to bear the costs of harm arising from failures in medication practices than they would be in systems that depend on tort law, and this appears to be the case (59). The social context is relevant – New Zealand, like the Nordic countries (and others), has a publicly funded hospital system in which the consequences of adverse medication events would be treated anyway, without cost to the patient, so the issue of which division of the government ultimately pays becomes somewhat moot.

Importantly, as mentioned earlier, the right to sue for accidents, including accidents in healthcare, has been removed in New Zealand as part of the social contract under which no-fault compensation was introduced (a principal exception being that it is possible to take the ACC itself to court). In the Nordic countries, it is still possible for patients to sue, but very few patients appear to choose this route over the less adversarial approach of using their no-fault compensation systems. Removing the need to prove fault from the process by which patients obtain compensation means that some of the barriers to open disclosure and transparency have also been removed, and the primary focus of all concerned can be on the well-being of the patient. Also, prevention can be built into the system – for example, the ACC has a prevention arm that seeks to improve safety proactively. This arm has engaged in initiatives to reduce postoperative infection in general but has not substantially engaged with the question of medication safety. The overall costs to society are likely to be lower with no-fault systems of this sort than with tort law – there are substantial administrative costs, but they seem to be considerably less than those associated with civil litigation. It is sometimes suggested that these systems are, nevertheless, more expensive than litigation because they more widely open the door to compensation. The converse view is that patients who are avoidably injured by healthcare should be compensated, and also that governmental systems can limit individual payments to reasonable levels. Furthermore, the amount of compensation paid for a particular type of injury can be somewhat standardized, in contrast to the substantial variation seen in settlements awarded by the courts. No-fault systems seem also to be less stressful for patients to negotiate than the law courts.

Unfortunately, no system is perfect. The reality is that only a minority of patients who are injured from any aspect of healthcare do receive compensation, whatever system is in place (60,61). Notwithstanding these and other limitations, Bismark and Paterson recently came to the following conclusion: "Compared with a medical malpractice system, the New Zealand system offers more-timely compensation to a greater number of injured patients and more-effective processes for complaint resolution and provider accountability" (59).

It seems unlikely that a country such as the United States would adopt a national no-fault approach to compensation of iatrogenic harm in any foreseeable future. However, institutions can choose to operate under a system of tort law in various ways, some of which can (and do) draw on principles similar to those underpinning the Nordic and New Zealand systems. Many claims can be (and are) settled out of court through negotiation. This can save years of anguish for all parties, and considerable expense. The settlement process is typically managed within a branch of the risk management division of the institution in question and may be integrated into an overall strategy for enhancing patient safety and experience. Clearly this provides an opportunity to reduce the costs and reputational consequences of litigation while at the same time providing compensation to a greater proportion of patients who seek it, albeit probably at lower levels than

might be obtained by some individuals through successful lawsuits. Anecdotally, even the potential of civil litigation to promote defensive medicine may be reduced by such approaches: It seems that the risk of actually ending up in court facing a civil action is quite low for individual practitioners who work in high-caliber institutions that have excellent risk management divisions, perhaps in part because the standard of care in such institutions is likely to be high. This sort of integrated approach may also provide ways to inform programs of CQI and may motivate insistence by the institution that practitioners do in fact engage in such programs. In addition, patients who have genuine cause to complain and seek compensation are likely to respond well to having their concerns taken seriously from the outset by the practitioners and the institution, and to being offered a straightforward route to resolution. In the end, the best strategies for managing the medicolegal risks of healthcare are first to manage the risks of healthcare itself and then to treat patients as one would want to be treated oneself – and many excellent institutions around the world have embraced these principles, regardless of the wider system in which they function.

12.5 Criminal Law

We opened this chapter with brief reference to several cases in which doctors, including anesthesiologists, have been prosecuted because a patient has died following a failure in some aspect of medication management in the perioperative period. Three fundamental assumptions and/or objectives underlie prosecutions of this type. First that a patient has died through negligence, therefore someone should be punished because, as a matter of justice, that person deserves to be punished. The second is that such punishment is declarative and makes clear to all that the failure in contention is viewed by the courts as unacceptable in the context of the social values pertaining to that society at that time. The third is that it is hoped that a conviction and punishment will deter others from doing the same thing (or similar things) again. These ideas are superficially attractive, and it has been suggested that in England the use of the criminal law in response to cases of inadvertently caused avoidable harm to patients may be increasing (62).

The various regulatory and prosecutor responses involving Dr. Bawa-Garba after the death of Jack

Adcock have been unfolding over recent years, have been subject to much analysis and commentary, and have prompted two major policy reviews. The context was not the perioperative period, but it was an acute care (pediatric) setting that has much in common with acute perioperative medicine. In particular, the case involved aspects of the management of medications commonly used or encountered in the perioperative period (an antibiotic and an angiotensin-converting enzyme [ACE] inhibitor). It illustrates many important points relevant to the regulation of medication safety in general, not just by means of the criminal law, so it is worth reviewing in some detail.

12.5.1 The Case of Jack Adcock

Jack Adcock's story was described in detail elsewhere (63). He was taken to a general practitioner by his mother on February 18, 2011. He was 6 years old and had Down syndrome. He had undergone previous heart surgery as a small baby and continued to have heart problems for which he was taking enalapril (an ACE inhibitor that works by reducing vasoconstriction and lowering blood pressure). He had been unwell since the night before his admission, with vomiting and diarrhea. He was referred directly to the children's assessment unit at Leicester Royal Infirmary.

Dr. Hadiza Bawa-Garber, a well-regarded pediatrics registrar (i.e., a resident) with a previously unblemished record, was born in Nigeria but moved to the United Kingdom when she was 13 years old. She had recently returned to work after 13 months of maternity leave. Before her leave, she had been working in a community setting, managing children with nonacute conditions. Nevertheless, on this particular day, because of staffing shortages, she agreed to cover the hospitals' acute pediatric services. There were also shortages that affected the provision of nursing care. In addition, the consultant (i.e., the attending) who was meant to be on call that day appears to have overlooked teaching commitments elsewhere and so had arranged for a colleague, who had other duties, to cover his work.

At 10:30 a.m., Dr. Bawa-Garba was called to assess Jack, who was obviously dehydrated and very unwell – notably he did not flinch when an intravenous cannula was inserted. She ordered a chest radiograph and some blood tests. She made a presumptive diagnosis of viral gastroenteritis and

elected not to begin antibiotics. She also decided to omit Jack's enalapril, presumably because of concern that it might further reduce Jack's already low blood pressure. Therefore, she deliberately left it out of the list of medications that she charted for Jack. However, she seems to have not documented the reasons for this (appropriate) decision or to have explained these to either Jack's mother or to the nurses (or at least not to the nurses who were later involved in Jack's care on the ward).

Jack's first blood results were highly abnormal (pH 7.0 and lactate 11 mmol/liter). Dr. Bawa-Garba responded by giving Jack more intravenous fluid. An hour later, Jack seemed to have become more responsive, and his pH had improved to 7.24, but this second blood sample was of inadequate volume for a repeat lactate to be measured. About this time, the hospital computer system went down, making it difficult or impossible to access further results. At around 3 p.m., Jack was apparently sitting up in bed and drinking. Dr. Bawa-Garba, who had been busy with other patients, finally managed to review the radiograph of Jack's chest. This showed changes consistent with infection, so she began antibiotics. The basis for the criminal prosecution included (among other matters) the assertion that this radiograph should have been reviewed earlier and that if antibiotics had been started earlier Jack would have been less likely to die.

No more senior doctor reviewed Jack at any time during this admission. The first time Dr. Bawa-Garba presented the information about Jack to a senior doctor was at 4:30 p.m., when her on-call consultant arrived in the hospital. She later said that she assumed he would go and review Jack, but this did not happen. He in turn later asserted that she did not make her expectation of this clear.

At about 7 p.m., Jack was moved to one of the hospital wards, where his mother noticed that his enalapril had been omitted, and she asked the nurses about this. The nurse explained that she was unable to administer the medication because it had not been prescribed on the medication chart. However, she suggested to Jack's mother that she could do so, as she would on any other day, at home. On the strength of this advice, which must have appeared entirely reasonable to her, Mrs. Adcock gave Jack his normal dose of enalapril.

Quite soon after this, just after 8 p.m., Jack collapsed. After a brief period of confusion over mistaken identity, resuscitation was attempted but was unsuccessful. A postmortem concluded that Jack had died of a streptococcal infection that had led to sepsis.

The subsequent legal and regulatory responses involved internal institutional processes, an external review of the hospital trust, reflective learning under the United Kingdom's requirements for the continuous professional development of doctors, an inquest, a review by the Medical Practitioners Tribunal Service (MPTS), an appeal by the GMC, several hearings in the criminal courts, and two national reviews. It took many years.

The hospital processes included an apology to Jack's mother and an internal inquiry. Also, in the United Kingdom, doctors are expected by the GMC to partake in reflective learning and to document this. Dr. Bawa-Garba had begun writing her own reflections on the case. Then, in a meeting with her on-call consultant, a list of reflections was made that seems to have included everything either of them thought she might have done better. At any rate, Dr. Bawa-Garba did not agree with all of the points and declined to sign the document. Notwithstanding some commentary to the contrary, it is reasonably clear that this document was subsequently used by the prosecution to inform its questioning of Dr. Bawa-Garba.

The hospital took Dr. Bawa-Garba off the call roster and allocated her to the pediatric intensive care unit. Apparently, this was in recognition of her need for further training, to provide her with the opportunity to see many more children with sepsis, under close supervision.

The hospital conducted an internal investigation that led to a report in August 2011, updated 6 months later. This report noted errors made by Dr. Bawa-Garba (including failing to recognize the severity of Jack's illness) and by the nursing staff, but it also identified a series of "system failings" including six root causes for Jack's death. It made 23 recommendations including 79 actions to minimize the risk of another child dying under such circumstances.

In February 2012, the police laid charges of manslaughter against Dr. Bawa-Garba. However, 7 weeks later she was told that these charges would not proceed.

In July 2013, the inquest into Jack's death began. During these proceedings, it was suggested that enalapril may have contributed to Jack's death. The coroner dismissed this, on the basis that it had not been mentioned in the report from the pathologist or from toxicology. Expert evidence suggested that if Jack had received the right treatment (including but not only in respect to antibiotics), he might well have survived. The inquest was adjourned shortly after this evidence and the case referred back to the Crown Prosecution Service, which in December 2014 again laid criminal charges against Dr. Bawa-Garba and also two of the nurses involved with Jack's care.

Over this period of time, an external review of the University Hospitals of Leicester NHS Trust found evidence of many deficiencies in care, including insufficient numbers of staff, inadequate supervision of junior doctors, and errors in the care of many patients which had the potential to cause harm.

The criminal trial began in October 2015 – more than 4 ½ years after Jack's death. The issues presented to the jury were very complicated, with many conflicts between the expert evidence introduced by the prosecution and that introduced by the defense. These have been summarized elsewhere (64). On November 4, 2015, Dr. Bawa-Garba was convicted of manslaughter with a 2-year suspended jail sentence. One of the nurses was found not guilty, but the other (an agency nurse) was similarly convicted and received the same sentence (among other things it was found that this nurse had failed to make regular recordings of Jack's vital signs and of his fluid balance) (65,66). Dr. Bawa-Garba applied for leave to appeal, but this was denied.

In June 2017, the MPTS, having reviewed the case, suspended Dr. Bawa-Garba from practice for a year. They found that her actions had fallen "far below the standards expected of a competent doctor," but they had taken into account other factors, including the fact she had learnt from her errors and had a previously unblemished record, and also the numerous system failures identified at the Leicester Royal Infirmary. The GMC proceeded to appeal this decision, successfully. This may seem surprising, because the MPTS is a statutory committee of the GMC, accountable to the GMC Council as well as Parliament. However, such appeals are permissible specifically because of arrangements to ensure that the MPTS is independent from the GMC in its decision-making and that it is at arm's length from the investigatory role of the GMC. At any rate, in January 2018, Dr. Bawa-Garba was struck off the medical register, with the implication that she could never work again as a doctor in the United Kingdom. This development led to widespread criticism from the medical profession in the United Kingdom and internationally, notably (but by no means only) in the specialty of pediatrics. A crowdfunding campaign facilitated another appeal, and on August 13, 2018 (7½ years after Jack's death), three senior judges, headed by the Lord Chief Justice, unanimously restored the MPTS's original decision, allowing for Dr. Bawa-Garba to be reinstated on the medical register (67).

On February 6, 2018, the Secretary of State commissioned a rapid policy review by Professor Sir Norman Williams into gross negligence manslaughter in healthcare (68). This made several important recommendations (Table 12.6).

The GMC has also initiated a review into gross negligence manslaughter (and culpable homicide in Scotland). Among the many observations made in this review, the following comments are worth quoting: "Although the criminal investigation and prosecution of doctors is extremely rare, the effect of just one case has been palpable and profound across the medical profession. Many doctors feel unfairly vulnerable to criminal and regulatory proceedings should they make a mistake which leads to a patient being harmed." And, "But the decisions of a regulator when things go wrong are

Table 12.6 Some recommendations of the Williams review of particular relevance to the perioperative management of medications (shortened from the original)

- That systemic issues and human factors should be considered alongside other matters when errors lead to a death, ensuring that the context of an incident is understood and taken into account.

- That better support should be provided to bereaved families, including timely information and the opportunity to be actively involved throughout investigative and regulatory processes.

- That the GMC should no longer be able to require registrants to provide reflective material when investigating fitness to practice cases.

- That concerns about the overrepresentation of Black, Asian, and minority ethnic healthcare professionals in fitness to practice cases should be investigated and addressed.

Source: Williams 2018 (68).

only the final stage of a complex series of processes which begin with the healthcare service provider and which may stretch over many years. Those processes often do not serve the needs of doctors or patients and their families" (69).

12.5.2 The Role of Criminal Law in Responding to Failures in the Management of Perioperative Medications

The complicated matter of the general question of the role of the criminal law in responding to failures in the provision of healthcare, and while undertaking socially important but dangerous services more generally, has been extensively reviewed and discussed elsewhere (70–73). So has the particular case of Jack Adcock, for example in Ameratunga et al. (64). It is important to appreciate that there is a definitive difference between civil litigation and prosecution. As we have explained, the former is a normal transaction between members of society in which the primary intent is loss adjustment rather than punishment. The latter is an action by the state against an individual with the explicit objective of punishment within a framework of justice. In practice, the latter implies such things as being formally arrested (often with the application of handcuffs), having to supply fingerprints and photographs to the police, potential or actual loss of liberty, and a strong association with other crimes, such as assault, rape, robbery, and so forth. The reputational consequences are an order of magnitude more serious than those of a civil lawsuit.

If we return to the three objectives of criminal prosecution, we can see that criminal prosecution clearly achieves the first objective, that of punishment – and this is true whether the accused doctor is convicted or not, or even culpable or not, although obviously conviction (and perhaps also sentencing) substantially increases the severity of the punishment. However, we do not agree with the assumption that such punishment is necessarily just. For the reasons outlined in Chapters 7 and 8, we view prosecutions arising primarily out of genuine errors rather than serious violations as fundamentally unjust. This is particularly true when an individual is prosecuted in circumstances in which other people, and failures in the system, have also contributed in one way or another to the failures in question. We think the death of Jack

Adcock provides a good example of such a case, as evidenced by the two inquiries into the hospital's processes. Another good example is the case of Drs. Prentice and Sullman who injected vincristine into the cerebrospinal fluid of a patient instead of methotrexate. The judge, in summing up, made two points: He said, "It seems to me you could have been helped more than you were helped." He also said, "You are far from being bad men; you are good men who contrary to your normal behaviour on this one occasion were guilty of momentary recklessness" (74). The role of character in relation to criminal prosecutions is beyond the scope of this chapter (75), other than to note that we accept that a previously blameless life does not excuse a serious crime. However, the key point here is the complete lack of any element of *mens rea*.[3] All three of these doctors were not only good doctors, they were conscientiously trying to do the right thing when they made the errors in the management of medications. This does not seem to be a good basis for convicting them of manslaughter.

The second purpose of criminal prosecution is declarative. One can understand that a grieving parent might well appreciate this aspect of a successful criminal prosecution. However, we are not sure the declarative element in these cases actually goes to the heart of the failings that led to the tragedies. The message surely should not be about never making a medication error but rather about the adequacy of systems, supervision, and levels of staffing, and the overall commitment to quality and safety expected of any healthcare system. A clearly distinguishing feature between these medication errors and many other major crimes is that the perpetrators of the latter are seldom in doubt about the egregious nature of their actions, whereas in these cases, the doctors were all actually trying to do the right things for their patients. These were deaths that arose from slips, lapses, and mistakes, not from any element of deliberate violation on the part of the charged doctors. The substantial protest against the actions of the GMC by doctors in the United Kingdom suggests that in

the case of Dr. Bawa-Garber, many believed that (in effect) "There but for the grace of God go I." That should certainly not be true for a criminal prosecution. Interestingly, if the fundamental implication of a criminal conviction were correct, namely, that the doctor had committed a serious crime, then the actions of the GMC were logical: such a doctor should not be allowed to practice. Yet the MPTS (the GMC's own tribunal) found that the circumstances did not warrant permanent deregistration, and certainly the vast majority of medical sentiment seems to support the latter view. We suggest that the declarative element in this case was primarily an expression of outrage that a child died, avoidably. Actually, we agree that there is considerable value in a really strong statement to the effect that avoidable deaths (or other serious harm) attributable to error should not occur. However, we are not convinced that a criminal prosecution of a junior doctor is the best way to express this point. For one thing, the proportion of criminal prosecutions of health professionals which have resulted in a not-guilty verdict is quite high (higher than would normally be expected for prosecutions for manslaughter). Such verdicts often reflect technical legal issue more than fundamental questions about the standard of care. For example, inadvertently substituting one medication for another is a failure in the administration of an intended treatment, whether harm occurs or not, and if harm occurs, whether a conviction ensues or not. A decision by a public or crown prosecutor to lay criminal charges is likely to raise expectations from families that justice will be manifest through conviction and a harsh penalty. A not-guilty verdict, or a light sentence, may well leave the family with the sense that the accused has been vindicated, or let off, and thus the declarative value of the process may well be diminished. Furthermore, as we have noted for both these objectives, there is a lack of proportionality between the punishment of a fatal error, and the typical complete lack of punishment for exactly equivalent errors that turn out by good fortune not to cause harm. This is particularly true for avoidable adverse medication events (of all kinds), which as we have repeatedly observed, are very common. It is clear that the punishment of these events reflects their outcome, not the underlying processes that lead to them.

---

[3] *Mens rea* translates as "guilty mind" and in the context of medication error would imply some knowledge that the decision of action in question was wrong at the time it was made or taken, and a lack of concern about that. It is widely (but not universally) held that *mens rea* ought to be a requirement for criminal convictions.

Alternatively, more consistent means are needed to achieve this declarative objective. It has been suggested that the charge of corporate manslaughter might be more appropriate in this regard, but there are numerous barriers to the success of such charges, and we are not drawn to this suggestion (70).

The third of the objectives we listed is that of deterrence, to prevent future occurrences of similar failings. In Chapters 7 and 8, we discussed the general point that deterrence may be effective for violations and for systemic factors, but not for genuine errors, as illustrated by the inadvertent cases of intrathecal injection of vincristine which continued to occur despite the high-profile conviction of Drs. Prentice and Sullman (76). A more specific issue, however, is that a criminal prosecution does not typically provide the sort of sophisticated analysis required to identify the numerous elements that need to be addressed if prevention of future failures in medication management is to be achieved. Indeed, it can hardly do so, because the processes of justice limit the focus substantially to the elements of practice considered to amount to a crime, notably the presence and degree of negligence involved and the certainty that this negligence contributed to the death. A further issue is that junior doctors (or any other junior doctors whose minds might have been focused by the deterrent effect of a criminal conviction of one of their colleagues) have little if any power to change the system that set up the circumstances in which errors of this sort were likely to occur. To be effective in bringing about systemic change, deterrence must (among other things) influence those who have the authority to institute such change. In our vincristine cases, the failure lies at least in part in the decision of pharmacy directors not to provide vincristine in 50 mL minibags, and methotrexate in a syringe. No pharmacy directors have been held responsible for any of the vincristine deaths. As indicated in the previous section, the argument for a deterrent value is much stronger in relation to litigation directed at an institution.

A particularly interesting point in the report of the three cases of sepsis from Turkey (8) is that none of these patients died. Thus, a criminal prosecution would not be likely at this stage in any country and certainly could not be brought for manslaughter. This is another major limitation of the criminal law in driving improvement in healthcare. In some countries, such as France, this limitation is reduced by a broader, more proactive and inquisitorial approach to the use of the criminal law in the regulation of healthcare (77). We have already discussed the potential value of alternative possibilities of civil actions, particularly those directed against the institution.

We see very little role for criminal law in the regulation of medication safety. However, it is essential that alternative mechanisms are adequate and are seen to be so by the wider public. The fact that failures in medication administration may have serious, and sometimes fatal consequences is not in itself a reason to punish such errors but definitely is a reason to address the factors in the system that predispose to them. In the case of Jack Adcock, there were many such factors. There are many other mechanisms for responding to deaths of this sort, many of which have been discussed in this chapter. The real challenge, however, is to ensure the effectiveness of these processes in avoiding tragedies of this type in the first place.

In Table 12.7, we provide some commentary on the case of Dr. Bawa-Garba in relation to the various processes and mechanisms that might potentially have played a role in preventing the death of Jack Adcock in the first place. We see it as a sad reflection on the current state of the regulation of healthcare that a case of this sort could actually occur in a well-resourced country within a system as highly respected as the NHS. Perhaps the single factor most likely to have changed the outcome in this case would have been much closer supervision of this junior doctor whose recent (and perhaps total) experience did not adequately equip her to manage such a challenging day's work on her own. Ameratunga et al. commented on the importance of "a cultural commitment by consultants to appropriate supervision as a cornerstone of high quality medicine" (64) and suggested that this probably was present in most United Kingdom hospitals. As illustrated in Table 12.7, such a commitment needs to be matched by thoughtful allocation of junior doctors to particular duties, and by adequate numbers of staff at all levels and in all disciplines. Furthermore, the nature of the complexity of medication management in acutely ill patients, such as those undergoing surgery and perioperative care, means that the solution to one medication failure

Table 12.7 Commentary on some aspects of the care of Jack Adcock, on the more general implications for safe medication practice in the perioperative period (and more generally), and on some possible regulatory mechanisms that might be relevant to avoiding a tragedy of this type in the first place

Comment on the specific case of Dr. Hadiza Bawa-Garba	Comment on implications for medication safety in the perioperative period	Possible regulatory considerations that might have helped avoid this tragic event
Dr. Bawa-Garba was well motivated – she agreed (indeed, we understand she even offered) to cover a staffing deficit and take on the acute work that needed doing on February 18, 2011, even though this extended her abilities beyond the area of practice in which she was most experienced, particularly in light of recent maternity leave.	Risk is created when staffing shortages are covered by people ill equipped to do the required work. This occurs frequently with anesthesia residents, as they move from one unit or specialty area to another and certainly to staff (senior or junior) returning to work after significant periods of absence. Orientation, retraining, and closer than normal supervision should be provided as appropriate.	Institutional boards of directors should regularly review approaches to junior doctor staffing rosters and allocation to areas of work; concerned individuals (staff or patients) should elevate the issues to their institution's board. Accreditation by external agencies (notably the process carried out by ANZCA), has the potential to address safe levels of staffing.
Nursing shortages, poor monitoring of Jack's condition on the ward by an agency nurse, and a poor decision by nursing staff to encourage Jack's mother to administer an uncharted medication may have contributed to the outcome in this case.	Stable and experienced nursing staff contribute substantially to medication safety on the wards and should be seen as part of any systematic approach to safe medication management.	Institutional boards of directors should consider and ensure safe levels of stable and appropriately qualified staff – concerned individuals (staff or patients) should elevate the issues to their institution's board. Accreditation by external agencies (including or with input from nursing organizations) has the potential ability to address safe nursing requirements.
Dr. Bawa-Garba was very lightly supervised, particularly given the point made earlier. If a senior doctor had been involved in checking and reviewing cases as they were admitted, different decisions might well have been made, or if not, the same decisions would have been far more defensible, so that Jack's mother could have been much more confident that reasonable judgments had been made.	Supervision of junior doctor's (and of junior nurses, or, as in this case, agency nurses without relevant local experience) is critically important for safety in general and for medication safety in particular.	Professional bodies, such as specialty colleges, should provide clear guidance on supervision (and many do). Accreditation by external agencies (notably the process carried out by ANZCA), has the potential to ensure that appropriate supervision is indeed provided. Institutional boards of directors should consider these issues and address them – concerned individuals (staff or patients) should elevate the issues to their institution's board.
The decision regarding use of antibiotics in a child thought to have viral gastroenteritis may involve a tension between the urgency with which serious bacterial infections should be treated and a desire to avoid overuse of antibiotics for viral infections (which are common).	Many decisions about medications in the perioperative period are difficult and need to be made in a timely fashion. This requires expertise but also often warrants consultation with a colleague (even in the case of senior doctors).	The involvement of a second, perhaps more senior physician is critically important in difficult cases, but one that is not easily covered by regulation. Nevertheless, guidance is available from some professional bodies on the importance of consultation by any doctor, and particularly by junior doctors.

The administration of enalapril may have been inadvisable in a critically unwell child, which is consistent with Dr. Bawa-Garba's decision not to order it. On the other hand, this might have been avoided had she been more effective in "sharing her mental model" and communicating the importance of her decision to the nursing staff (at least) and to Jack's mother as well. We note that she was very busy, but we also note that these important safety points received very little attention in the criminal proceedings, particularly the point about communication.	Failures in communication underlie many avoidable adverse medication events – notably but not only between residents and attendings working together in the operating room, and between doctors and nurses on the wards. The importance of documenting and sharing important information for the ongoing management of medications cannot be overstated. In the ward context, there is a very strong case for keeping family members closely informed about medication plans or concerns.	The general issue of communication is enormously important but difficult to regulate. Adequate documentation is expected by disciplinary authorities and the courts, but this particular failure is arguably not covered by the strictly understood requirements for prescribing medications. Institutional boards of directors should consider investing in various forms of communication training, and this should be (and is) encouraged by various professional organizations such as colleges and the Anesthesia Patient Safety Foundation.
Over the course of these proceedings, Dr. Bawa-Garba will have spent considerable time away from work, including during the 12-month suspension. This is not a good way to deal with areas where competence needs to be improved – indeed it is likely to exacerbate any deficiencies arising from other periods of leave from work, such as her maternity leave.	We have discussed the issue of punishments that are both proportionate (which, arguably, does apply to a year's suspension in this case) and also likely to address the particular behavioral or educational need of the doctor in question (which clearly does not apply). Actually, total loss of licensure would remove an incompetent or poorly motivated doctor from practice, and might be more effective than by temporary suspension in some cases, but we agree with the Medical Practitioners Tribunal Service that this would not have been a proportionate punishment in this case.	Reform and widely reaching education are needed in this regard. More appropriate forms of punishment need to be found for those relatively rare cases when punishment is actually deserved.
The cost of these proceedings has been considerable, from both sides.	This money would have been far better invested into addressing the many shortcomings identified in the hospital's reviews to avoid the occurrence of problems of this sort, rather than after the event.	The problem of the opportunity costs inherent in the reactive and adversarial nature of many legal responses to inadvertent iatrogenic harm has been discussed in detail elsewhere (70). We are a long way from moving to proactive and less adversarial alternatives.
The proceedings will inevitably have damaged Dr. Bawa-Garba's confidence as a doctor.	As discussed earlier in the text, practitioners are likely to feel shame about any form of discipline or complaint, and indeed about any adverse event for which they feel responsible. The extent of such feelings would presumably be much greater after a criminal conviction, and the consequent loss of confidence may impact on a doctor's subsequent ability to practice. We have discussed these issues of the "second victim" and the potential for a "third victim" – a patient injured by a doctor who is performing poorly after a major adverse event – in Chapter 5. Specific proactive counseling, carefully supervised relevant training, and support to address this aspect of safety is warranted in circumstances of this kind.	Reform and widely reaching education are needed in this regard. Again, the provision of such support is a matter that Institutional Boards of Directors should consider.
We would not wish to comment on Jack's mother's feelings about this case, but it would be entirely understandable if, after 8½ years, any mother was frustrated and dissatisfied with the processes and would prefer a harsher and more definitive outcome.	At the heart of any adverse event is a patient and that patient's family. Addressing their needs as early and as effectively as possible should be a top priority after any adverse event. One of the more important recommendations from the Williams report addresses this point (see Table 12.5).	Ultimately, the best response to avoidable adverse medication events (including those of omission or timeliness) is to avoid them, by proactively improving the quality and safety of care.

will not necessarily be the solution to the next one. Even well-supervised and competent doctors make mistakes, as well as slips and lapses. Thus, training and supervision need to be supplemented by good systems and a commitment to engage in safe practices.

12.6 Conclusions

In this chapter and Chapter 11, we considered legal and regulatory responses to avoidable adverse medication events. This is a very broad topic and, in the wider context of healthcare more generally, has been the subject of entire books (71). The picture that emerges from this chapter is that of a wide range of poorly interlinked regulatory processes. We noted some similarities but also considerable variation between countries. Some approaches are proactive in their effect, while others are reactive, and serve primarily to provide compensation after an avoidable adverse event or to punish those perceived as responsible.

Regulation can assist in promoting medication safety. Regulation can operate through influence and through compulsion, both of which have advantages and limitations. What is really required is the wholehearted engagement of everyone in the organization in the substance of the accreditation process and the mission of achieving safe, high-quality patient care. In no small part this comes back to the need for ongoing professionalism and self-regulation by physicians, not in place of recent trends to less physician-centric methods of regulation, but in parallel to these and in alignment with the internal processes of their institutions. At the same time, we see a critical role for boards of directors in setting priorities and driving a just culture in which no such distinction is made between different professional groups, and in which genuine accountability for safe practices is expected.

There is undoubtedly a role for the civil law in providing compensation for patients injured through avoidable adverse medication events and also in providing some degree of declarative retribution. We think litigation is likely to be most effective in promoting safe medication management when it is directed against institutions and will serve patients best when the response is based on "full disclosure and rapid compensation" practices, like that of the University of Michigan. By contrast, we see almost no place for criminal action in the regulation of safe medication practices in the

perioperative period, except where recklessness is involved (leaving a patient unattended during an anesthetic or working while under the influence of alcohol or other cognition-affecting drugs, for example), or where deliberate malfeasance is a factor.

References

1. Pronovost P, Needham D, Berenholtz S, et al. An intervention to decrease catheter-related bloodstream infections in the ICU. *N Engl J Med.* 2006;355(26):2725–32.

2. Bowdle TA, Jelacic S, Nair B, et al. Facilitated self-reported anaesthetic medication errors before and after implementation of a safety bundle and barcode-based safety system. *Br J Anaesth.* 2018;121(6):1338–45.

3. Merry AF, Gargiulo DA, Bissett I, et al. The effect of implementing an aseptic practice bundle for anaesthetists to reduce postoperative infections, the Anaesthetists Be Cleaner (ABC) study: protocol for a stepped wedge, cluster randomised, multi-site trial. *Trials.* 2019;20(342). Accessed January 18, 2020. https://trialsjournal.biomedcentral.com/articles/10.1186/s13063-019-3402-8

4. Wachter RM, Pronovost PJ. Balancing "no blame" with accountability in patient safety. *N Engl J Med.* 2009;361(14):1401–6.

5. Wahr JA, Abernathy JH 3rd, Lazarra EH, et al. Medication safety in the operating room: literature and expert-based recommendations. *Br J Anaesth.* 2017;118(1):32–43.

6. Merry AF, Webster CS, Hannam J, et al. Multimodal system designed to reduce errors in recording and administration of drugs in anaesthesia: prospective randomised clinical evaluation. *BMJ.* 2011;343:d5543.

7. Bennett SN, McNeil MM, Bland LA, et al. Postoperative infections traced to contamination of an intravenous anesthetic, propofol. *N Engl J Med.* 1995;333(3):147–54.

8. Cilli F, Nazli-Zeka A, Arda B, et al. *Serratia marcescens* sepsis outbreak caused by contaminated propofol. *Am J Infect Control.* 2019;47(5):582–4.

9. Sakuragi T, Yanagisawa K, Shirai Y, Dan K. Growth of *Escherichia coli* in propofol, lidocaine, and mixtures of propofol and lidocaine. *Acta Anaesthesiol Scand.* 1999;43(4):476–9.

10. Merry AF, Webster CS, Mathew DJ. A new, safety-oriented, integrated drug administration and automated anesthesia record system. *Anesth Analg.* 2001;93(2):385–90.

11. Merry AF, Hannam JA, Webster CS, et al. Retesting the hypothesis of a clinical randomized controlled trial in a simulation environment to Validate Anesthesia Simulation in Error Research (the VASER study). *Anesthesiology*. 2017;126(3):472–81.

12. Jensen LS, Merry AF, Webster CS, Weller J, Larsson L. Evidence-based strategies for preventing drug administration errors during anaesthesia. *Anaesthesia*. 2004;59(5):493–504.

13. Eichhorn JH. APSF hosts medication safety conference: consensus group defines challenges and opportunities for improved practice. *APSF Newsletter*. 2010;25(1):1–7. Accessed January 3, 2020. https://www.apsf.org/article/apsf-hosts-medication-safety-conference/

14. Allegranzi B, Gayet-Ageron A, Damani N, et al. Global implementation of WHO's multimodal strategy for improvement of hand hygiene: A quasi-experimental study. *Lancet Infect Dis*. 2013;13(10):843–51.

15. Cohen J, Vincent JL, Adhikari NK, et al. Sepsis: a roadmap for future research. [Review]. *Lancet Infect Dis*. 2015;1(5):581–614.

16. Executive Board. *Improving the Prevention, Diagnosis and Management of Sepsis*. Geneva: World Health Organization; 2017. Accessed January 18, 2020. https://apps.who.int/iris/handle/10665/275534

17. Floros P, Sawhney R, Vrtik M, et al. Risk factors and management approach for deep sternal wound infection after cardiac surgery at a tertiary medical centre. *Heart Lung Circ*. 2011;20(11):712–17.

18. Graf K, Ott E, Vonberg RP, et al. Economic aspects of deep sternal wound infections. *Eur J Cardiothorac Surg*. 2010;37(4):893–6.

19. Arduino MJ, Bland LA, McAllister SK, et al. Microbial growth and endotoxin production in the intravenous anesthetic propofol. *Infect Control Hosp Epidemiol*. 1991;12(9):535–9.

20. Munoz-Price LS, Bowdle A, Johnston BL, et al. Infection prevention in the operating room anesthesia work area. *Infect Control Hosp Epidemiol*. 2019;40:1–17.

21. Jelacic S, Bowdle A, Nair BG, et al. A system for anesthesia drug administration using barcode technology: the Codonics Safe Label System and Smart Anesthesia Manager. *Anesth Analg*. 2015;121(2):410–21.

22. Loftus RW, Koff MD, Birnbach DJ. The dynamics and implications of bacterial transmission events arising from the anesthesia work area. *Anesth Analg*. 2015;120(4):853–60.

23. Scally G, Donaldson LJ. The NHS's 50 anniversary. Clinical governance and the drive for quality improvement in the new NHS in England. *BMJ*. 1998;317(7150):61–5.

24. Clinical Governance. *Guidance for Healthcare Providers*. Wellington, New Zealand: Health Quality and Safety Commission; 2017. Accessed January 18, 2020. https://www.hqsc.govt.nz/publications-and-resources/publication/2851/

25. Conway J. Getting boards on board: engaging governing boards in quality and safety. *Jt Comm J Qual Patient Saf*. 2008;34(4):214–20.

26. The Secretary of State. *Statutory Instruments 2010 no. 279: The National Health Service (Quality Accounts) Regulations*. London: HMSO; 2010. Accessed January 18, 2020. https://www.ncepod.org.uk/pdf/reporters/QualityAccountsRegs.pdf

27. Imperial College Healthcare, NHS Trust. *Quality Account 2018/19*. London: Imperial College Healthcare, NHS Trust; 2019. Accessed January 18, 2020. https://www.imperial.nhs.uk/about-us/news/trust-annual-report-2018-19-is-now-available

28. Health Quality and Safety Commission New Zealand. *Quality Accounts. A Guidance Manual for the New Zealand Health and Disability Sector*. Wellington: Health Quality and Safety Commission; 2014. Accessed January 18, 2020. https://www.hqsc.govt.nz/assets/Health-Quality-Evaluation/PR/QA-guidance-manual-May-2014.pdf

29. Brilli RJ, McClead RE Jr, Crandall WV, et al. A comprehensive patient safety program can significantly reduce preventable harm, associated costs, and hospital mortality. *J Pediatr*. 2013;163(6):1638–45.

30. McClead RE Jr, Catt C, Davis JT, et al. An internal quality improvement collaborative significantly reduces hospital-wide medication error related adverse drug events. *J Pediatr*. 2014;165(6):1222–9.e1.

31. O'Dowd A. NHS quality accounts are failing to tell the whole story. *BMJ*. 2011;342:d91.

32. Bismark MM, Walter SJ, Studdert DM. The role of boards in clinical governance: activities and attitudes among members of public health service boards in Victoria. *Aust Health Rev*. 2013;37(5):682–7.

33. Martin L, Mate K. *IHI Innovation System*. Boston, MA: Institute for Healthcare Improvement; 2018. IHI White Paper. Accessed January 8, 2020. https://www.ihi.org/resources/Pages/IHIWhitePapers/IHI-Innovation-System.aspx

34. Daley U, Gandhi T, Mate K, Whittington J, Renton M, Huebner J. *Framework for Effective Board Governance of Health System Quality*. Boston, MA: Institute for Healthcare Improvement; 2018. IHI White Paper. Accessed January 8, 2020. http://www.ihi.org/resources/Pages/IHIWhitePapers/Framework-Effective-Board-Governance-Health-System-Quality.aspx

35. Jha A, Epstein A. Hospital governance and the quality of care. *Health Aff (Millwood)*. 2010;29(1):182–7.

36. Hogan H, Olsen S, Scobie S, et al. What can we learn about patient safety from information sources within an acute hospital: a step on the ladder of integrated risk management? *Qual Saf Health Care*. 2008;17(3):209–15.

37. Rozich JD, Haraden CR, Resar RK. Adverse drug event trigger tool: a practical methodology for measuring medication related harm. *Qual Saf Health Care*. 2003;12(3):194–200.

38. Resar RK, Rozich JD, Classen D. Methodology and rationale for the measurement of harm with trigger tools. *Qual Saf Health Care*. 2003;12(suppl 2):ii39–45.

39. Hamblin R, Shuker C, Stolarek I, Wilson J, Merry AF. Public reporting of health care performance data: what we know and what we should do. *N Z Med J*. 2016;129(1431):7–17.

40. Health Quality Intelligence. *A Window on the Quality of New Zealand's Health Care*. Wellington, New Zealand: Health Quality and Safety Commission; 2018. Accessed January 20, 2020. https://www.hqsc.govt.nz/our-programmes/ health-quality-evaluation/publications-and-resources/publication/3364/

41. Waring JJ, Bishop S. "Water cooler" learning: knowledge sharing at the clinical "backstage" and its contribution to patient safety. *J Health Organ Manag*. 2010;24(4):325–42.

42. Aasland OG, Forde R. Impact of feeling responsible for adverse events on doctors' personal and professional lives: the importance of being open to criticism from colleagues. *Qual Saf Health Care*. 2005;14(1):13–17.

43. Weissman JS, Schneider EC, Weingart SN, et al. Comparing patient-reported hospital adverse events with medical record review: do patients know something that hospitals do not? *Ann Intern Med*. 2008;149(2):100–8.

44. Weingart SN, Pagovich O, Sands DZ, et al. What can hospitalized patients tell us about adverse events? Learning from patient-reported incidents. *J Gen Intern Med*. 2005;20(9):830–6.

45. Johari K, Kellogg C, Vazquez K, et al. Ratings game: an analysis of Nursing Home Compare and Yelp ratings. *BMJ Qual Saf*. 2018;27(8):619–24.

46. Cunningham W, Dovey S. The effect on medical practice of disciplinary complaints: potentially negative for patient care. *N Engl J Med*. 2000;113(1121):464–7.

47. Cunningham W, Wilson H. Complaints, shame and defensive medicine. *BMJ Qual Saf*. 2011;20(5):449–52.

48. Mounsey H, Jolly J. Learning from cases – anaesthesia. *Med Prot Soc*. 2019. Accessed May 6, 2019. https://www.medicalprotection.org/uk/ articles/learning-from-cases---anaesthesia

49. Appel F. From quality assurance to quality improvement: the Joint Commission and the new quality paradigm. *J Qual Assur*. 1991;13(5): 26–9.

50. Lam MB, Figueroa JF, Feyman Y, et al. Association between patient outcomes and accreditation in US hospitals: observational study. *BMJ*. 2018;363:k4011.

51. Health Quality and Safety Commission. *Statement of Intent 2017–21*. Wellington, New Zealand: Health Quality and Safety Commission; 2017. Accessed January 18, 2020. https://www.hqsc.govt .nz/publications-and-resources/publication/2971/

52. Specialist Education Accreditation Committee. *Standards for Assessment and Accreditation of Specialist Medical Programs and Professional Development Programs by the Australian Medical Council*. Kingston, ACT: Australian Medical Council Limited; 2015. Accessed January 3, 2020. https://www.amc.org.au/accreditation-and-recognition/accreditation-standards-and-procedures/

53. Australian and New Zealand College of Anaesthetists. *Guidelines for the Safe Management and Use of Medications in Anaesthesia*. Melbourne: Australian and New Zealand College of Anaesthetists; 2018. Policy document *PS 51; 2018*. Accessed January 18, 2020. https://www.anzca .edu.au/resources/professional-documents

54. Australian and New Zealand College of Anaesthetists. *Guidelines on Infection Control in Anaesthesia*. Melbourne: Australian and New Zealand College of Anaesthetists; 2015. Policy document *PS 28*. Accessed January 18, 2020. https://www.anzca.edu.au/resources/professional-documents

55. World Health Organization. *The WHO Surgical Safety Checklist [Revised January 2009]*. Geneva: World Health Organization; 2009. Accessed January 3, 2020. http://whqlibdoc.who.int/ publications/2009/9789241598590_eng_ Checklist.pdf

56. Gelb AW, Morriss WW, Johnson W, Merry AF; International Standards for a Safe Practice of Anesthesia Workgroup. World Health Organization–World Federation of Societies of Anaesthesiologists (WHO-WFSA) International Standards for a Safe Practice of Anesthesia. *Anesth Analg*. 2018;126(6):2047–55.

57. Peters PG Jr. Twenty years of evidence on the outcomes of malpractice claims. *Clin Orthop Relat Res*. 2009;467(2):352–7.

58. Kachalia A, Kaufman SR, Boothman R, et al. Liability claims and costs before and after implementation of a medical error disclosure program. *Ann Intern Med.* 2010;153(4):213–21.

59. Bismark M, Paterson R. No-fault compensation in New Zealand: harmonizing injury compensation, provider accountability, and patient safety. *Health Aff (Millwood).* 2006;25(1):278–83.

60. Brennan TA, Leape LL. Adverse events, negligence in hospitalized patients: results from the Harvard Medical Practice Study. *Perspect Healthc Risk Manage.* 1991;11(2):2–8.

61. Bismark MM, Brennan TA, Davis PB, Studdert DM. Claiming behaviour in a no-fault system of medical injury: a descriptive analysis of claimants and non-claimants. *Med J Aust.* 2006;185(4):203–7.

62. Ferner RE, McDowell SE. Doctors charged with manslaughter in the course of medical practice, 1795–2005: a literature review. *J R Soc Med.* 2006;99(6):309–14.

63. Cohen D. Struck off for honest mistakes. *BBC News.* 2018. Accessed January 3, 2020. https://www.bbc.co.uk/news/resources/idt-sh/the_struck_off_doctor

64. Ameratunga R, Klonin H, Vaughan J, Merry A, Cusack J. Criminalisation of unintentional error in healthcare in the UK: a perspective from New Zealand. *BMJ.* 2019;364:l706.

65. Jack Adcock death: Nurse Isabel Amaro struck off register. BBC News. August 4, 2016. Accessed January 3, 2020. https://www.bbc.com/news/uk-england-leicestershire-36978810

66. Nurse Isabel Amaro who left Down's syndrome boy to die in his bed is struck off. Health Medicine Network. 2018. Accessed January 3, 2020. http://healthmedicinet.com/i/nurse-isabel-amaro-who-left-downs-syndrome-boy-to-die-in-his-bed-is-struck-off/

67. Dyer C. Hadiza Bawa-Garba wins right to practise again. *BMJ.* 2018;362:k3510.

68. Williams N. *Professor Sir Norman Williams Review: Gross Negligence Manslaughter in Healthcare. The Report of a Rapid Policy Review.* London: Department of Health and Social Care; 2018. Accessed January 18, 2020. https://www.gov.uk/government/publications/williams-review-into-gross-negligence-manslaughter-in-healthcare

69. Hamilton L. *Independent Review of Gross Negligence Manslaughter and Culpable Homicide.* London: General Medical Council; 2019. Accessed January 3, 2020. https://www.gmc-uk.org/about/how-we-work/corporate-strategy-plans-and-impact/supporting-a-profession-under-pressure/independent-review-of-medical-manslaughter-and-culpable-homicide

70. Merry AF, Brookbanks W. *Merry and McCall Smith's Errors, Medicine and the Law.* 2nd ed. Cambridge, UK: Cambridge University Press; 2017.

71. Quick O. *Regulating Patient Safety: The End of Professional Dominance?* Cambridge, UK: Cambridge University Press; 2017. Laurie G, Ashcroft R, eds. *Cambridge Bioethics and Law.*

72. Merry AF. How does the law recognize and deal with medical errors? *J R Soc Med.* 2009;102(7):265–71.

73. Merry A. When are errors a crime? Lessons from New Zealand. In: Erin C, Ost S, eds. *The Criminal Justice System and Health Care.* Oxford, UK: Oxford University Press; 2007:67–97.

74. *R v Prentice* [1993] 3 WLR 927.

75. Quick O. Medical manslaughter and expert evidence: the roles of context and character. In: Griffiths D, Sanders A, eds. *Bioethics, Medicine and the Criminal Law.* Vol. 2. Cambridge Bioethics and Law. Cambridge, UK: Cambridge University Press; 2013:101–16.

76. Berwick DM. Not again! *BMJ.* 2001;322(7281):247–8.

77. Kazarian M, Griffiths D, Brazier M. Criminal responsibility for medical malpractice in France. *J Prof Neg.* 2011;27(4):188–99.

13 Barriers to Improving Medication Safety
Why Is Patient Safety So Hard?

13.1 Introduction

The title of this chapter should actually simply be "Why is safety so hard?" as countless industries have struggled with safety over the past centuries. Indeed, safety did not really exist as a social construct prior to the mid-1800s, but came into public consciousness with the Industrial Revolution. As more and more jobs became mechanized, the possibilities for injury and harm increased, as did the public's awareness of them. As noted earlier, some industries have done an exceptional job of safety, with countless hours, weeks, and years without a nuclear power event and millions of flights without a crash (39 million flights in 2019 worldwide – 106,000 flights *per day*: see www.statista.com/statistics/564769/airline-industry-number-of-flights/, accessed January 21, 2020). But these industries at one time also struggled with achieving safety goals even as healthcare struggles today and the barriers have often been the same. The dynamic tradeoffs between productivity and safety, the costs of safer technologies, and a lack of perceived risk are common themes. But perhaps even more than these barriers, which are discussed later in this chapter, safety at its core is beset by paradoxes, as described in detail by James Reason (Box 13.1) (1). These paradoxes may lead well-meaning institutions toward worse rather than better safety and are worth exploring in some detail.

13.2 Safety Paradoxes
13.2.1 Measuring Safety via the Absence of Safety

For most of the past 20 years, the primary measure of safety has been some measurement of "serious safety events," better-termed "unsafe events" (Figure 13.1 [2]). While examination of unsafe events can elucidate better defenses, processes, and procedures, the absence of an infrequent event over a period of time does not necessarily indicate better

---

Box 13.1 Safety paradoxes

- Safety is often defined and measured more by its absence than by its presence.
- Measures designed to enhance a system's safety – defenses, barriers, and safeguards – can also bring about its destruction.
- Many organizations seek to limit variability of human action, but it is the same variability – in the form of timely adjustments to unexpected events – that maintains safety in a dynamic and changing world.
- An unquestioning belief in the attainability of absolute safety (zero accidents or target zero) can seriously impede the achievement of realizable safety goals, while a preoccupation with failure can lead to high reliability.
- In healthcare, safety is only one element of quality; lack of access to essential medications and other treatment is a major cause of harm, so a balance needs to be struck between safety and affordability.
- Incident analysis typically focuses on individual human error, when many errors are team failures.

Source: Modified and expanded from Reason 2000 (1).

---

safety. There were many launches of the space shuttle without a serious event prior to the Challenger disaster, but commentators such as Professor Diane Vaughan do not believe that the NASA culture during that period was safe (3). Over a 2-year period, engineers repeatedly brought forward concerns with the design of the O ring apparatus, including evidence that the O rings had partially failed on 7/9 launches prior to Challenger's last launch (there was evidence of corrosion or hot gas blowby after launch). These concerns were generally ignored as leadership continually moved further and further from previously specified safety limits; eventually leadership gave the go ahead to launch despite an ambient temperature of 36°, a full 18° lower than

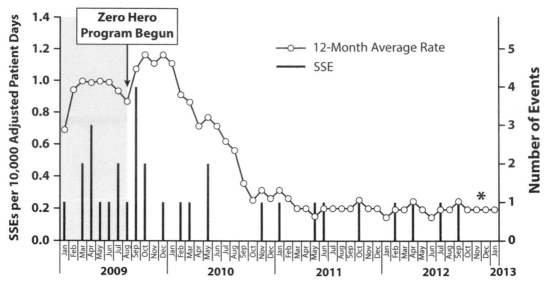

Figure 13.1 Serious safety event (SSE) rate, and number of SSEs before and after introducing a comprehensive, hospital-wide patient safety program). *Significant decrease (P < 0.001). Bars represent number of monthly SSEs and the line represents the 12-month rolling average of SSEs per 10,000 adjusted patient days. Reprinted with permission from Brilli et al. (2).

the previous lowest launch temperature and far below the safe limit set by the manufacturer. This "normalization of deviance" had been uneventful for 2 years (3).

In addition, as safety efforts have their desired effect, fewer and fewer events occur, so there is less and less to study and fewer data to assess whether safety is present or not. As fewer events occur, teams are also likely to become complacent, thinking that no events mean that safety has been achieved. In reality, as Reason states, "no news really is just no news" rather than "good news" and requires "vigilance and heightened defensiveness" (1). Indeed, the trait among high-reliability organizations (HROs) of "preoccupation with failure" illustrates that these organizations achieve success by focusing on the possibility of failure, rather than on the absence of it. This is not to say that we should not continually measure and track medication incidents; it just means that absence of a serious adverse medication event (AME) for a period of time does not necessarily indicate a safer environment for our patients. Certainly, as much attention should be placed on the presence of safety traits (e.g., how often a provider uses barcode technology prior to medication administration) as on adverse events. Another more appropriate measure of safety may be that of "safety climate" (4–6).

13.2.2 Dangerous Defenses

Defenses against medication harm can result in unintended consequences, where the "improvement" actually increases errors. For example, implementation of computerized order entry systems increased medication errors in some units in the short term (7,8); every change to an "improved and safer" syringe pump carries the risk of errors due to unfamiliarity; and changing to International Organization for Standardization (ISO) certified color-coded syringe labels in Ireland led initially to a sharp increase in errors (9).

In addition, well-meaning rules and regulations may either contravene safety or simply shift the risk ("risk displacement"): requiring road workers in England to wear protective hearing devices eliminated the ability of the workers to hear approaching traffic (10); time-consuming double checks may slow resuscitation of a rapidly deteriorating patient. Increasing numbers of defenses may lead to a sense of complacency. For example, managers may feel safe because "we have a policy for that" – but a policy will be ineffective without the commitment of frontline workers to adhere to it. Multiple layers of defenses may result in the identification of increasing numbers of near misses[1] or

---

[1] See footnote e in Chapter 1 about the term "near miss."

precursor events, leading to celebration over the presumed success of the defenses, when in reality, the near misses are indicating a system issue that should be addressed. Again, increased defenses can lead to complacency and shift the focus away from the potential for failures.

13.2.3 Rigid Consistency versus Flexible Variability

One of the primary approaches promulgated for enhancing safety is the reduction of variation. There is little doubt that too much variation exists in healthcare. For example, in Chapter 6 we mentioned the variation between countries in Europe in the use of colored labels for syringes (11). In Chapter 5 we drew attention to a lack of consistency in the way investigations are carried out in the NHS (12). These are areas where one would expect greater standardization. However, a slavish adherence to a set protocol without consideration of the complexities of the situation or patient involved can lead to worse outcomes. Medication overdoses or interactions can easily occur if a protocol is applied without thorough evaluation of the appropriateness of each of its elements in relation to each individual patient. In addition, elimination of all variability would remove an important safeguard, to wit, that "processes remain under control due to compensations by human components" (1). Weick et al. state, "reliability is a dynamic non-event" rather than a static adherence to routines and activities and that unvarying performance cannot cope with the unexpected (13). In many disasters, there is the element of chance, the unforeseen risk that requires immediate human compensation to return the situation to normal (1); everyday life brings issues that are not addressed by guidelines or protocols. Again, from Weick et al., what is needed is "a state of collective mindfulness that creates a rich awareness of discriminatory detail and facilitates the discovery and correction of errors capable of escalation into catastrophe" (13).

13.2.4 Setting a Goal of Zero Events

In much of healthcare, the focus on an unattainable goal of zero adverse events is typified by the Joint Commission's use of the term "never events." At first blush, this seems entirely appropriate – how can one justify accepting even one adverse event or setting a goal that allows even one patient to be harmed? But target zero programs have hidden deficiencies. The

first is that there is typically no specified period of time over which this goal is to be achieved; without this, how can the team measure their progress toward the goal? As Perrow (14) and Reason (1) argue, even in the safest of organizations, new hazards will arise, nasty surprises are inevitable, and one cannot ever achieve a true rate of zero adverse events. Although it is entirely possible, through safety efforts and mindfulness, to significantly lengthen the duration between such events, one can never be assured that the goal of zero has been attained (14). The second deficiency in a target zero approach is that such a goal intuits that a decisive victory can be achieved and the war for safety won, while in reality, HROs "see the 'safety war' for what it really is: an endless guerilla conflict" (1). In part, this guerilla conflict arises from the inevitable tension between production and protection. If a hospital never admits a patient, it will never have an adverse event. At the other end of the spectrum, increases in cost associated with an increase in safety may create a barrier to access essential healthcare for some people. Thus, paradoxically, too great an emphasis on safety may indirectly lead to harm. On the other hand, if production is the primary goal, safety will necessarily suffer: Lower staffing ratios for nurses and pharmacists certainly reduce expenses but will also increase the rate of preventable adverse events, which themselves carry human, financial, and reputational costs. Thus, there is a dynamic and complex relationship between protection and productivity that must be acknowledged and understood (15). The precise cost at which access to healthcare becomes problematic depends on the available resources. For a nation, this will depend on its wealth (usually measured as gross domestic product [GDP] per capita) and its political decisions on the prioritization and distribution of expenditure. For an individual hospital, context will vary enormously. For many hospitals, market forces and the need to make a profit (or at least to avoid losing money) will be a big driver. Some hospitals will aim to provide the highest possible standards of care for an elite group of "customers" able to afford this. Others will have wider social responsibilities. For most, it will be necessary to find a balance that allows them to achieve adequate productivity affordably, with the lowest event rate possible (1). For these reasons, the Health Quality and Safety Commission in New Zealand has chosen to use the term "always report and review" rather than "never" to refer to very serious preventable adverse events (see https://www.hqsc.govt.nz/our-programmes/adverse-events/publications-and-resources/publication/2936/, accessed January 21, 2020).

13.2.5 Concentrating on Individual Human Error versus Team Error

As discussed in Chapter 6, there is a strong tendency to explain error in terms of decisions and actions by individuals, yet our most serious safety events usually follow failures in teamwork. Over the past 10 years of analyzing sentinel events, the Joint Commission has found that the most common source of failure is either communication or leadership. As explained in Chapters 6 and 7, these failures typically feed into classic constructs of human error (such as the Reason-Rasmussen General Error Model [16]) through their influence on the mental models of the members of the team and the extent to which these are both shared and accurate (17). It seems that many safety investigations focus on an analysis of a single human's error, when in reality we should be considering how and why teams fail and also, in the construct of Safety II (18), how and why they usually succeed (19–21). Some failures in communication can actually be seen as failures to complete a process and therefore as action errors. An example would be prescribing a new medication without teaching a patient about it. Similarly, an example discussed in Chapter 11 involved deciding to stop a medication (enalapril in the Jack Adcock case) without informing the pediatric patient's mother or the nursing staff of the reasons for doing so or documenting these reasons in the patients' notes.

This emphasis on the team (including the patient) may seem to be of less importance to medication errors in anesthesia than to many other contexts because a single human frequently appears to be the source of these errors. This is certainly not the case – teamwork, communication, and the sharing of mental models between different members of the operating room team (17) are very important for medication safety in anesthesia. For example, failures in communication between attending and resident anesthesiologists or at handoffs between anesthesiologists during the care of a patient may lead to errors, and so might a failure to communicate to a surgeon that protamine is being given to reverse the effects of heparin or a failure to convey to a nurse in the postanesthetic care unit that a particular medication has (or has not) been given. Furthermore, as discussed in Chapters 11 and 12, the wider culture and regulatory environment in which practitioners care for patients may make a substantial difference to the amount of investment into making the system for medication administration safer, and to the extent to which individuals engage in practices designed to promote safety. Culture is itself a manifestation of teamwork. More research is needed to further inform how and why team failures contribute to medication errors (22).

In the following sections, we explore some specific barriers to achieving medication safety; each should be interpreted in light of the safety paradoxes outlined earlier.

13.3 Culture
13.3.1 Leadership Voids, Lack of Training

As described in Chapters 9 and 11, all safety efforts begin with institutional leadership. Unwillingness by the leadership of an institution to commit to the effort and costs of improving patient safety means that this will not happen. Unfortunately, although patient safety cannot occur without full commitment by the frontline personnel, it cannot be achieved from "grassroots" effort alone. Healthcare leaders find their time and energy divided between many different and demanding projects, and safety often becomes an easy thing to commit to verbally without a genuine will to make it happen. A brief survey of course work listings for a variety of Master's in Healthcare Administration (MHA) programs found few that included courses on patient safety. Quality Improvement was frequently listed, but not formal training in the science of patient safety. There are exceptions to this – for example, the Master of Health Leadership program at the University of Auckland (see www.auckland.ac.nz/en/study/study-options/find-a-study-option/master-of-health-leadership-mhlthld.html, accessed January 21, 2020) includes two papers explicitly addressing patient safety at the individual and systems level, respectively, but these papers are optional.

Much of the training for any MHA degree is about finances, and much of healthcare leadership is preoccupied with profitability, rather than safety. This is not only dangerous, but it may ignore the very thing that could improve productivity. When Paul O'Neill gave his first speech after taking the helm of Alcoa (a major producer of aluminum), he did not address the faltering product lines, or the unprofit-ability of the company, but rather focused on one and only one thing – worker safety. This focus spooked Wall Street, but within a year profits and productivity were at an all-time high. When asked whether the workers so appreciated the focus on safety that they responded willingly when asked to increase productivity, Mr. O'Neill simply said, "I never had to ask."[2]

It is obviously important for patient safety to be integrated into the curricula of medical, nursing, and pharmacy schools (23). An initiative by the World Health Organization has provided resources to facilitate and inform the former objective (24), but the extent and success of such training is variable (25,26). Given the importance of teamwork for safety, the biggest gap in the training of any of these groups of professionals lies in the siloed way in which each group is trained (i.e., nursing students with nursing students, medical students with medical students, etc.). Interprofessional training initiatives with a focus on safety are still somewhat exceptional (27,28) and typically postgraduate (29,30).

13.3.2 Power, Hierarchy, and Disruptive Behavior versus a Culture of Respect

In the cockpit recording of the horrific crash of two fully loaded jumbo jets on the runway at Tenerife, the copilot can be heard asking the pilot twice whether the PanAm aircraft had cleared the active runway. It had not, the pilot ignored the copilot, and 582 people lost their lives (31). That event, and several others where the pilot continued what the airline industry calls a "controlled descent into terrain" despite warnings by copilots, occurred in large part because of the hierarchy that used to prevail in the cockpit, where, traditionally, the copilots (being more junior) could not disagree with or challenge the captain. Nearly 25 years ago, Geert Hofstede described the concept of power distance: "The power distance index is defined as 'the extent to which the less powerful members of organizations and institutions (like the family) *accept and expect* [authors' emphasis] that power is distributed unequally" (32). It is important that this concept is grounded in the fact that the lower-status individuals accept, and thus do not challenge, the power structure, even when they know their superior to be wrong. In healthcare, despite considerable progress over recent years in improving this aspect of culture in

many institutions, power distance remains substantial and widely accepted: Nurses often do not question physicians, or residents challenge their seniors. Institutions that have a more hierarchical structure also tend to have lower safety climate ratings (33,34).

The airline industry has successfully moved to a culture where anyone who has a concern is expected to, and can, voice it and stop a plane from taking off (35). In medicine, we are far from this ideal. There are institutions in which the safety culture is excellent, but this is far from universal. There have been countless medication errors where a nurse, pharmacist, or resident recognized the error but did not speak up because of previous humiliating encounters with disrespectful physicians, or with senior colleagues in their own discipline. The near continual shaming and demeaning of nurses, of junior faculty, and of physicians in training is cited by Lucien Leape and his coauthors as the number one deterrent to achieving patient safety (36). These authors point out that "a single disruptive physician can poison the atmosphere of an entire unit." They describe six categories of disrespectful behavior in the healthcare setting (Box 13.2) and argue that, perhaps worst of all, a pervasive culture of disrespect to colleagues leads to a disrespect of patients and dismissal of their (often correct) concerns that things are not going well.

Leape et al. summarize the implications of disrespect as follows:

Disrespect is a threat to patient safety because it inhibits collegiality and action essential to teamwork, cuts off communication, undermines morale, and inhibits compliance with and implementation of new practices. Nurses and students are particularly at risk, but disrespectful treatment is also devastating for patients. Disrespect underlies the tensions and dissatisfactions that diminish joy and fulfillment in work for all health care workers and contributes to turnover of highly

---

> **Box 13.2 Six categories for classifying disrespectful behavior in the healthcare setting**
>
> - Humiliating behavior
> - Demeaning treatment of nurses, residents, and students
> - Passive-aggressive behavior
> - Passive disrespect
> - Dismissive treatment of patients
> - Systemic disrespect
>
> *Source*: From Leape et al. 2012 (36).

---

[2] Personal communication, J.W.

qualified staff. Disrespectful behavior is rooted, in part, in characteristics of the individual, such as insecurity or aggressiveness, but it is also learned, tolerated, and reinforced in the hierarchical hospital culture. (36)

Disruptive behavior has long been pervasive throughout healthcare. For example, in a 2008 survey, 77% of respondents reported witnessing disruptive behavior in physicians, and 65% reported witnessing disruptive behavior in nurses. Two-thirds agreed that these behaviors were linked to adverse events, including mortality (37). More recently, an expert advisory group on bullying and sexual harassment commissioned by the Royal Australasian College of Surgeons (RACS) found widespread problems with the safety culture in surgery, in and beyond the operating room, which were not confined to surgeons or to Australia (38,39). RACS responded proactively with a "Let's Operate with Respect" campaign underpinned by training, and that work is ongoing.

We know that double checks can reduce medication errors: these checks can be via computerized order entry systems, or between clinicians, or by pharmacists checking a physician's orders. However, a physician can carelessly, or arrogantly, override computer alerts, and if a pharmacist or nurse is browbeaten repeatedly, they may become less and less likely to question the appropriateness of a dose or medication. An illustrative case of an unsafe practice leading to a death is one where a minibag of antibiotics and a minibag of bupivacaine intended for epidural infusion were removed from the medication cabinet at the same time and the bupivacaine was, fatally, given intravenously. On this obstetrics suite, the nurses had taken to bringing the epidural infusion into the room (against policy) prior to the anesthesiologist's arrival, because of repeated complaints and admonitions by the anesthesiologists over having to wait for the bupivacaine to arrive (40). Physicians may be completely unaware of how their behavior can set the climate for unsafe acts. From Leape et al. again,

Creating a culture of respect requires action on many fronts: modeling respectful conduct; educating students, physicians, and non-physicians on appropriate behavior; conducting performance evaluations to identify those in need of help; providing counseling and training when needed; and supporting frontline changes that increase the sense of fairness, transparency, collaboration, and individual responsibility. (41)

Unless executive leadership sets the tone, moves quickly to correct any disruptive behavior by any team member, and continually ensures accountability, patient safety efforts will falter.

13.3.3 Barriers to Incident Reporting: Fear of Retribution, Blame, or Shame

As discussed earlier in this book, a robust, local incident reporting framework is critical to understanding vulnerabilities to error and identifying areas for improvement in safety. Unfortunately, our reporting structures and procedures often create an atmosphere in which frontline staff are afraid to report. As a young researcher, Amy Edmondson had the theory that units with high teamwork qualities would also have low reported error rates. To her surprise, she found something quite different – the ward with the highest rate of *reporting* errors also had a very high teamwork score, and vice versa (42). A deeper understanding of safety has come about through her realization that when nurses felt valued and respected and had great respect for and trust in their managers, they felt safe when reporting errors and therefore reported often (43–45). Comments from the nurses from high reporting and high teamwork wards and those from low reporting, low teamwork wards are starkly different (Table 13.1). Clearly, local culture can significantly influence error reporting; unless senior managers and executives are in touch with their staff (e.g., via regular frontline walks), they "may not know which group has which culture" (44) and be unable to assess whether reporting rates represent a just and safe culture or whether reporting is low because of a culture of blame and shame. Dr. Edmonson's work provides a stark imperative to those setting up incident reporting systems to also provide a setting of "psychological safety": nonpunitive, respectful, encouraging, and affirming. This can be difficult to do, as many healthcare workers see errors as stemming from breaches of standard practice (46) and blame themselves rather than seeking to discover system changes that would prevent such an error from harming a patient. We know many more errors occur than are reported (47), indicating that this is a very real barrier to patient safety.

Even when leadership acts in a nonpunitive fashion, role-specific cultural norms can significantly affect reporting (48). Nurses and pharmacists appear to be far more likely than physicians to

Table 13.1 Attitudes to medication error and reporting of errors on hospital wards

Hospital ward	University 1 and Memorial 1	Memorial 4	University 2	Memorial 3
Detected error rate[a]	23.68 17.23	11.02	8.6	2.34
Rating of openess	High	Medium	Low	Very low
Attitude to errors	Learn	Blame, fear	Blame, fear	Blame
Nurse manager style	Hands off but approachable	Hands on, controlling	Hands off	Hands off and controlling
Nurse manager view of staff	They are too hard on themselves They are capable and seasoned	Nurses are nervous and defensive about mistakes	Nurses are always assessing and judging each other	Treats residents and nurses as kids who need discipline
Staff view of nurse manager	A superb nurse and leader A counselor, not a boss	Controlling and overbearing Makes you feel guilty and want to cover your butt	Punitive Gives you the silent treatment Makes you feel guilty	Treats you as guilty if you make an error Treats you like a 2-year-old
Staff view of errors	Natural, normal, important to document	Reluctant to report; people get in trouble	The environment is unforgiving Heads will roll	You get put on trial

Source: Excerpted from Edmondson 2004 (44).
[a]Detected error rates were those errors reported to the study team by the ward nurses.

report errors (49). While pharmacists view error reporting to be part and parcel of their daily work, physicians are more likely to view an error as a failure, to be anxious about loss of esteem from colleagues, and to be reluctant to report (50). In a study of two hospitals (one academic, one community), 1000 reported incidents were examined: 87% of the reports were filed by nurses, 1.9% by physicians, and 8.9% by other staff (51). In this analysis, voluntarily reported events involved surgical patients only about 15% of the time, but chart reviews from New York (52) and from Colorado and Utah (53) found that surgical events were responsible for nearly half of all adverse events within hospitals. Clearly, voluntary reporting captures a different spectrum of errors than chart reviews or prospective observational studies. Other studies show that physicians often do not perceive reporting as part of their duties and that they fear being shamed. Shame has long been pervasive in physician training (36) and likely contributes to physicians' reluctance to report even incidents that do not reach patients. Reporting by physicians may increase when the system is purpose-built to serve their particular specialty: for example, in Australia and

New Zealand, the WebAIRS reporting system set up by anesthesiologists for anesthesiologists (54) has now received over 8000 reports, almost all from anesthesiologists. A similar level of engagement was seen in its predecessor, the Australian Incident Monitoring Study (55).

13.4 Financial Barriers

One of the difficulties in implementing interventions to prevent medication errors is that many low- and middle-income countries (LMIC), and even underresourced hospitals in high-income countries, simply do not have the money to invest in technological solutions. We have discussed this question in relation to LMIC in Chapter 10, but even in high-income countries, the question turns to the opportunity costs associated with proposed safety initiatives. Safety is not the only element of quality in healthcare: In *Crossing the Quality Chasm*, the Institute of Medicine also listed timeliness, efficiency, effectiveness, equity, and patient centeredness, collectively captured by the acronym STEEEP (56,88). There is no value in a healthcare service that is perfectly safe but too expensive to be accessible to the patients that need it, and also no ethical basis for pursuing such an objective. Unfortunately, very few healthcare systems are sufficiently well resourced to avoid the need to strike a balance between the relative value of investing in each of the different elements of quality.

It follows that it is trite to make comments like "safety first" and "safety is priceless." Cost is a relevant consideration when evaluating a proposal to institute initiatives to improve patient safety. A business case for such proposals is appropriate. What this means precisely may vary, but as a minimum the following would typically be expected:

- The likely costs both of initiation and of ongoing maintenance of the change
- The expected gains in both human and financial terms
- The risks of the proposal
- The risks of not implementing the proposal
- The expected return on investment (ROI)

Initiatives to improve medication safety are often expensive, and their total costs are often poorly appreciated; often there is no obvious immediate ROI, unlike investments in MRI scanners or robotic surgical systems that may generate income directly.

13.4.1 The Costs of Safety

It can be difficult to accurately estimate the true costs of investing in safety. While the costs of technology are obvious and quantifiable, the costs of nontechnology solutions can be more obscure. It is worth considering some examples.

13.4.1.1 Electronic Health and Pharmacy Systems

According to Becker's Hospital Review (see https://beckershospitalreview.com, accessed January 21, 2020), implementation of an Epic electronic health record (EHR) system has cost anywhere from $43 million for a single hospital, to $1.2 billion for HealthPartners, a Boston-based health system with at least 11 hospitals and hundreds of clinics and nursing homes. The costs of this type of software vary widely depending on the number of locations and units involved, the modules provided or chosen, and the brand. Specifically for medication safety, EHR systems can include a completely networked pharmacy system with inventory control, computerized order entry, automated dispensing cabinets, medication reconciliation and barcode medication administration – or only a select few of these modalities. As noted earlier, only a handful of operating rooms around the world have barcode-aided dispensing/labeling/administration systems despite evidence of improved safety with these (57,58). This may reflect a perception that the risks of medication error are relatively low, and that therefore the potential benefits do not justify the substantial costs.

13.4.1.2 Prefilled Syringes

There is a cost to buying prefilled syringes, or to having them made in hospital pharmacies. Many of the medications that one might wish to place in these syringes are off patent and very inexpensive. On the face of things, putting these medications into prefilled syringes may increase their cost many times over. In one exercise in a New Zealand setting, the cost of a particular intravenous medication was about US25 cents and that of supplying this medication in prefilled syringes more than US$2.50 per syringe. The conclusion from hospital administrators was that the use of prefilled would increase the cost of medications used in anesthesia 10-fold. Not surprisingly, the proposition was deemed to be insupportable.

We suggest this framing of the situation is too simplistic. The cost to consider should be the overall cost of delivering an anesthetic, or even that of the entire surgical procedure, including salaries and infrastructural costs. This will usually run to thousands of dollars, and in this context, the cost of prefilled syringes becomes a very small percentage of the total. In addition, there are considerable cost savings with prefilled syringes, which we outline in Chapter 9.

13.4.1.3 Frontline Staffing

Multiple studies have shown a clear correlation between both nursing and pharmacist staffing levels and medication errors, as well as mortality (59–63). Despite this clear correlation, staffing levels are typically the first thing to be impacted when a hospital faces a budget shortfall. Unlike high-reliability industries, hospitals often have little sensitivity to the impact of operational decisions of this sort on safety and continue to believe that the work can be done with fewer workers simply by increasing efficiency. All too often, convincing evidence of the very real patient harm that occurs through cost cutting is simply ignored or blamed on individual failures, rather than a failure of the system.

13.4.1.4 Comprehensive Quality and Safety Programs

Effective quality and safety programs require dedicated staff for safety and team training, for quality audits, and for managing incident reporting systems. The investment must be made up front, and it can be 12–18 months before a significant effect is seen in patient outcomes. Introduction of an intensive patient safety program in the Nationwide Children's Hospital (2) included increasing patient safety team members from 8 to 33 and increasing the annual budget from $690,000 to $3.3 million. Serious safety events fell by 82% and mortality fell from 1% to 0.75% ($p < 0.001$, see Figure 13.1). The calculated savings, however, were only $1.8 million and did not cover the ongoing costs of the initiative. Financial calculations do not, of course, adequately account for the human costs, to patients and to their loved ones, and (as discussed in Chapter 4) to the clinicians whose care inadvertently resulted in these deaths or other forms of harm. Nevertheless, the fact that the direct ROI was negative could lead some chief financial officers, who may see their primary responsibility as that of saving money, to consider such programs as poor investments.

A further cost of any comprehensive safety program is training in patient safety behaviors and tools as well as teamwork skills. Effective team training may require blocks of operating rooms to be "offline" for 3- to 4-hour periods on a regular basis, so that surgeons, anesthetists, nurses, and technicians can all attend a multidisciplinary program (64), or to allow for in situ simulation training (20,65). Alternatively, it may include regular exercises in dedicated simulation facilities, which removes staff from their clinical duties. And single training episodes are not enough – there must be continual, ongoing, quarterly or biannual refresher courses to sustain improvements (66,67). Although many institutions (e.g., the Veterans Health Administration, the University of Michigan) have committed to team training programs, others have deemed the cost prohibitive. It is interesting to contrast this situation with that in the airline industry, where regular participation by pilots in simulation training is seen as essential, and as "business as usual." A commercial pilot who failed

to complete assigned simulation training would be removed from the cockpit and required to retrain and pass the relevant evaluation before being allowed to fly again.

13.4.1.5 Productivity versus Safety

Demands for increased productivity in healthcare typically imply increased speed in the form of faster turnover times in the operating room facilitated by quicker drawing up of vials into syringes in anesthesia, less thorough checks, and multitasking to "improve efficiency." Mandating increased productivity and speed may lead to shortcuts or skipping steps that the same managers have required by policy. As discussed in Chapter 8, a common theme explaining violations is that violating is sometimes seen as the only way to get the job done. Room turnover is faster when some surfaces are not wiped, and central line placement is quicker using three little blue towels than full barrier protection. Thus, executive leadership may inadvertently drive unsafe practices when the focus is more on productivity than on safety.

13.4.1.6 Balancing One Cost against Another

It is not only financial officers and other healthcare managers who have a responsibility to manage the overall cost of healthcare in a fiscally responsible fashion. Every clinician should be engaged in finding ways to make healthcare more affordable, and therefore more accessible. There may be many opportunities to save money in ways that will have little impact on the delivery of safe healthcare, and doing this can offset the costs of safety initiatives. For example, Tabing et al. implemented an intervention in their institution that required the approval of the attending anesthesiologist before the use of remifentanil and dexmedetomidine during a case (68). They concurrently removed desflurane vaporizers from the main operating rooms, rendering desflurane available only on request. They chose these three agents for their intervention because of their relatively high costs. Data were analyzed from over 24,000 cases. They achieved a mean cost saving of $10.95 per case for anesthetic medications. They found no difference in the incidence of patient recovery time, unplanned intubations, and reintubations, but postoperative nausea and vomiting decreased after the intervention.

Unfortunately, barriers to this sort of approach are quite common. One lies in a reluctance on the part of senior hospital management to devolve budgetary control in this way and a corresponding suspicion on the part of clinicians that if they do save money in one area it will be diverted by management from their safety priorities to the hospital's bottom line. Such suspicions are not without foundation, and to some extent hospitals do need to balance their overall budgets, but ways have to be found to engage individual departments in this sort of fiscal responsibility. A second barrier lies in the potential perception that an initiative of this sort is a challenge to clinical autonomy (see the discussion of this issue later). In fact, Tabing's intervention did not actually restrict the autonomy of the participating anesthesiologists to use these three medications if they so choose, it simply created an incentive to consider alternatives. Extending this approach to greater standardization of anesthesia practice in general, through a process of departmental consensus, has potential for savings substantially greater than that achieved in this study (69).

13.4.2 A Broader View of the Financial Benefits of Medication Safety

A whole-of-society view on the cost of adverse medication events is more likely to give a positive ROI at a national level than an analysis confined to the costs saved for a hospital. For example, avoiding even one episode of brain damage or paraplegia will save millions of dollars to the public purse over the life of the injured patient. Health economists attempt to capture these broader aspects of cost in estimates of the dollar value of a lost quality-adjusted life year (QUALI), or a whole life. They may also factor in the cost of lost productivity to society. However, many of these costs fall to the community. The extent to which they may be tied back to the hospital in which the injury occurred or to the clinician involved with the adverse event depends on the wider system in which that hospital is operating. In the United States, for example, the threat of litigation may provide financial justification for investing in safety if it can be shown that an initiative is likely to reduce adverse events. In New Zealand, and in the Nordic countries, national systems for no-fault compensation of accidents have made the potential of lawsuits arising from treatment injury unlikely (70). At any rate, it can be seen that the true cost of an adverse medication event may be difficult to estimate, and only some of the savings actually achieved through investing in safety may be realized in the financial accounts of the healthcare institution itself.

13.5 Human Nature

In the final analysis, patient safety is hard because it ultimately depends on human actions and choices. In Chapters 7 and 8, we discussed how our unconscious patterns of cognition result in error and how our conscious actions also drive either safety or harm. We humans must choose whether or not to follow policies, procedures, and guidelines; we must choose, as chief executive officers or chief financial officers, whether or not to purchase expensive technologies and expand staffing levels among nurses and pharmacists; as leaders at every level, we must choose whether or not to reinforce a just culture and eliminate a culture of disrespect, even when it means doing things that are difficult, such as disciplining a highly productive but disruptive surgeon.

Anyone who has set out to effect a change in personal life or at work has run into the inescapable truth that change is hard. Since most of patient safety involves change – that is, we would not be having this discussion if patients were already acceptably safe – we must accept that we cannot simply write a new policy or procedure and expect all to fall in line. There are reams written about change management, including some books that are easy to grasp (e.g., *Our Iceberg Is Melting*, by Kotter and Rathgeber [71]) and some that are more difficult (e.g., *The New Economics*, by Deming [72]). Edward Deming spent a lifetime helping industries and organizations to change, most notably helping Japan rebuild after World War II, and worked hard in his later years to define a comprehensive theory of management that would enable organizations to become highly reliable. He termed the route to effective transformation "The System of Profound Knowledge," which included four domains that leaders must understand if they are to be successful in driving effective change, including change to improve patient safety:

- A *theory of knowledge*, which addresses questions like the following: How do we know what change will be effective? What do we think will happen when we make these changes? How will we know that a change is truly significant? How do we measure improvement?

- A *respect for systems* that seeks to deeply understand how the system is currently working. What will be the possible unintended consequences of the change? What are the individual process steps that need to change to affect the overall desired improvement?

- An *understanding of variability* – leaders must understand and account for subtle variation in how different teams might approach the change, and how these variations could affect the overall improvement. It also allows for teams to investigate variations in processes between institutions, to understand why and how certain processes work better than others (see the Northern New England Cardiovascular Disease Study Group [73]).

- An *appreciation of the psychology of human nature* – any change agent must have a deep understanding of human nature and how we respond to change, what motivates us to improve, how fear drives actions and data reported, and how we derive joy and satisfaction from our work.

A comprehensive presentation of change theory is beyond the scope of this book. The point here is that resistance to change contributes to making patient safety elusive. Also, it is important to recognize that when we fail to effect the change we desire, the underlying reason might not be that we are inept or that our colleagues are acting badly or are just stubborn, although those are certainly common themes. It may be because of poor change management.

13.5.1 Violations

A major theme of this book is that violations make an important contribution to avoidable adverse medication events. We have therefore dedicated the whole of Chapter 8 to this topic. The failure to address minor violations in healthcare is certainly a major barrier to safe medication management. In a series of 20 simulated anesthetics (74), anesthesia providers committed 35 "events of interest" that had the potential to harm a patient, and 34% of these events were deviations from guidelines. Several themes were identified as to why the anesthesia personnel chose to do these things (Table 13.2). Deviation from protocol is certainly not limited to healthcare, and the themes for deviation or violation cross all industries. Iszatt-White explored the complexity of violation among road maintenance workers and found reasons that go far deeper than being perverse or contrarian. Factors such as risk displacement, where the consequence occurs remote from or long after the violation, the operatives' sense of self-efficacy (i.e., their confidence in their ability to work safely without guidelines), and the need for heedfulness as well as compliance (i.e., at times following a particular policy would be riskier than violating it), need to be considered when attempting to eliminate violations or to establish accountability for things that go wrong (10).

Table 13.2 Reasons that anesthesiologists deviate from accepted medication administration guidelines

Learned behaviors	• Having trained with a senior who deviated from guidelines • Difficulty in switching from prior learned behavior to the new guideline
Personal attitudes to the guidelines	• Both positive and negative views of guidelines in general ("doctors don't become consultants to be told exactly what to do" versus "in an emergency situation, when people are stressed, a protocol is a great thing to follow, because you don't miss the basics") • Uncertainty about when to deviate from the guidelines for individual patients • A belief that variability in practice is a positive attribute that actually improves patient safety (See Box 13.1: Reason's Safety Paradoxes [1])
Issues with guidelines	• Lack of supporting evidence • Poor design that did not reflect clinical reality • Low clinical relevance
Environmental barriers	• Practical issues (unfamiliar with operating room layout, difficulty with barcode scanner, layout of workspace) • Time pressure, excessive workload
Cultural influences	• Top-down influences (positive influence from senior leadership does not always result in change in the workplace) • Influence of peers (normalization of deviance, differing guidelines between institutions, countries, etc.)

Source: Modified from Webster et al. 2015 (74).

13.5.2 "I Won't and You Can't Make Me": The Question of Clinical Autonomy

In Chapters 7 and 11, we discussed the fact that doctors have long cherished their right to make autonomous decisions about the care of their patients, on the basis of the authority arising from their training and positions as registered health professionals and the seniority associated with being an attending physician (for example). Exercise of this autonomy to make the best decisions for each patient is appropriate if it reflects differences between individual patients. Unfortunately, there is considerable evidence to suggest that variation in practice often arises from idiosyncratic differences in the preferences of individual practitioners or institutions rather than from differences between patients (Box 13.3) (75–77). Furthermore, marked variation can be found even in relation to practices about which well-developed and agreed guidelines exist (78,79). A key intervention to reducing medication error is standardization of process, but this is often resisted strongly by physicians who assert their right to retain their idiosyncratic ways of doing things (whether for using a particular cardioplegia solution or a particular method of preparing infusions of medications). These personal preferences are often vigorously defended, and firm leadership is required to establish consensus over standardized approaches to important aspects of medication administration.

In Chapter 8, we discussed the question of hand hygiene in some detail. Like hand hygiene guidelines, techniques to improve communication, and hence safety, such as "speak back" and "read back" and the use of phonetic and numeric conventions, are often simply ignored, and sometimes even scornfully dismissed when other team members attempt to use them. Engagement with technology designed to improve safety may also be variable. In two studies of barcode administration of medications in the operating room conducted in different countries, some anesthesia providers simply would not use the barcode scanners and associated computerized support that had been provided at some cost by their department (57,84). This cherished view of physician autonomy also leads to poor application of evidence-based best practices (85).

13.5.3 Lies, Damn Lies, and Statistics

Best practices in medication processes have been defined through review of data and the development of expert consensus by multiple organizations, and the key messages are remarkably consistent

---

Box 13.3 Variation in healthcare

Variation of all kinds is prominent in the provision of healthcare in general and in the use of medications in particular. Some of this variation has been captured in the *Dartmouth Atlas of Healthcare Variation* and other similar atlases around the world (80–83).

Three categories of care have been described:

- *Effective care*, in which there is a reasonable level of expert agreement on the interpretation of the available evidence, and the choice of treatment aligns with agreed guidelines based on this evidence
- *Preference-sensitive care*, in which there is more than one effective treatment, and a choice is made by the physician and patient together, taking into account factors such as each patient's different circumstances and wishes
- *Supply-sensitive care*, in which the available infrastructure and capacity determine the type and quantity of treatment that is provided

Variation in care is warranted when it reflects differences between individual patients, their comorbidities, their values, and their personal preferences and needs (i.e., when it is preference-sensitive care). Unwarranted variation reflects factors that have nothing to do with the patient: typically, it reflects differences in approach between institutions and between physicians. Some of these differences have their origin in the interpretation of evidence, some arise from commercial drivers in fee-for-service systems, some arise from unconscious bias, and some arise from other factors. For example, medication shortages will force undesired variation in practice from time to time. Conversely, the availability of a new medication or other form of therapy that is effectively marketed may lead to its overuse. However, if a valuable new medication is perceived as very expensive (e.g., as has been the case with sugammadex), this may lead to restrictions being placed by hospital administrators on its supply to clinicians, and therefore (arguably) to its underuse.

(86). Unfortunately, there are few randomized controlled studies and very little outcome data to inform such guidelines. This provides room for some to not adopt the guidance on the grounds of a lack of "real" evidence, or to insist that their idiosyncratic practices have not been shown to be harmful. In addition, the quality of research is variable, and conflicting evidence is common, so a given practitioner can often find at least one article that will support their preferred way of doing things (85). To make matters worse, as discussed in Chapter 11, some of the data that have been used to inform practice over recent decades have turned out to be fraudulent. To our knowledge, fraud has not been prominent in relation to research into medication safety, but the uncertainty of medical knowledge for all the reasons touched on here is a well-accepted problem. To use legal terms, one might say that the arguments for many safe medication practices must be viewed as based on the balance of probability rather than on being beyond reasonable doubt. One should not lose sight of the fact that balance of probability is the legal test for civil liability. We see no grounds for individuals to reject guidelines that are based on expert consensus informed by the best available evidence and then formally adopted by their own institutions or departments. In fact, to do so is to fail to understand the concept of evidence-based medicine, which, as explained in Chapter 9, has never suggested that the only acceptable evidence to inform practice should be outcome data from double-blind randomized clinical trials (87). Sadly, some practitioners will turn any element of uncertainty to the cause of supporting their right to practice as they choose.

13.6 Conclusions

We saw in Chapter 9 that we have many avenues to improve medication safety in anesthesia and the perioperative period, with considerable evidence and expert consensus to support them. However, human nature, just as it leads to errors, also often drives resistance to implementing safety interventions. Achieving improved patient safety requires a deep understanding of not just how things go wrong when error-prone human beings work within complex systems but also why changes that would have a high probability of reducing the risk of errors are so often resisted. This effort to understand why we do not change is absolutely imperative, as our continued refusal to change to safer methods continues to imperil our patients. We have all become familiar with the phrase "to err is human," and some know the full Alexander Pope quote "to err is human, to forgive divine," but the original concept is much older. It was certainly understood by Sophocles, who incorporated it into *Antigone*, where the king Creon, having murdered his competitor for disloyalty, also forbids the dead man's sisters from bringing his corpse home, insisting that a burial would impute honor when none should be given. When Antigone, the dead man's sister, defies him, Creon has her imprisoned. The king's advisor Tiresias counsels him that his refusal to allow burial was an error, but that to persist in that error by then murdering Antigone would damn him, stating, "Think son, think! To err is human, true, but only he is damned who having sinned will not repent, will not repair." We can be forgiven our natural errors, but to persist in behaviors and practices, whether individually or as institutions, that put our patients at unnecessary risk is unforgivable.

References

1. Reason J. Safety paradoxes and safety culture. *Inj Control Saf Promot*. 2000;7(3):3–14.

2. Brilli RJ, McClead RE Jr, Crandall WV, et al. A comprehensive patient safety program can significantly reduce preventable harm, associated costs, and hospital mortality. *J Pediatr*. 2013;163(6):1638–45.

3. Vaughan D. *The Challenger Launch Decision: Risky Technology, Culture, and Deviance at NASA*. Enlarged Edition. Chicago, IL: University of Chicago Press; 2016.

4. Sexton JB, Berenholtz SM, Goeschel CA, et al. Assessing and improving safety climate in a large cohort of intensive care units. *Crit Care Med*. 2011;39(5):934–9.

5. Singer SJ, Gaba DM, Falwell A, et al. Patient safety climate in 92 US hospitals: differences by work area and discipline. *Med Care*. 2009;47(1):23–31.

6. Valentin A, Schiffinger M, Steyrer J, Huber C, Strunk G. Safety climate reduces medication and dislodgement errors in routine intensive care practice. *Intensive Care Med*. 2013;39(3):391–8.

7. Villamanan E, Larrubia Y, Ruano M, et al. Potential medication errors associated with computer prescriber order entry. *Int J Clin Pharm*. 2013;35(4):577–83.

8. Wetterneck TB, Walker JM, Blosky MA, et al. Factors contributing to an increase in

duplicate medication order errors after CPOE implementation. *J Am Med Inform Assoc.* 2011;18(6):774–82.

9. Shannon J, O'Riain S. Introduction of "international syringe labelling" in the Republic of Ireland. *Ir J Med Sci.* 2009;178(3):291–6.

10. Iszatt-White M. Catching them at it: an ethnography of rule violation. *Ethnography.* 2007;8(4):445–65.

11. Wickboldt N, Balzer F, Goncerut J, et al. A survey of standardised drug syringe label use in European anaesthesiology departments. *Eur J Anaesthesiol.* 2012;29(9):446–51.

12. Hamilton L. *Independent Review of Gross Negligence Manslaughter and Culpable Homicide.* London: General Medical Council; 2019. Accessed January 3, 2020. https://www.gmc-uk.org/about/how-we-work/corporate-strategy-plans-and-impact/supporting-a-profession-under-pressure/independent-review-of-medical-manslaughter-and-culpable-homicide

13. Weick KE, Sutcliffe KM, Obstfeld D. Organizing for high reliability: processes of collective mindfulness. In: Sutton R, Staw B, eds. *Research in Organizational Behavior.* Vol. 21. Stamford, CT: Elsevier Science/JAI Press; 1999:81–123.

14. Perrow C. *Normal Accidents: Living with High-Risk Technologies.* New York, NY: Basic Books; 1984.

15. Donabedian A. *An Introduction to Quality Assurance in Health Care.* New York, NY: Oxford University Press; 2003.

16. Reason J. *Human Error.* New York, NY: Cambridge University Press; 1990.

17. Nakarada-Kordic I, Weller JM, Webster CS, et al. Assessing the similarity of mental models of operating room team members and implications for patient safety: a prospective, replicated study. *BMC Med Educ.* 2016;16(1):229.

18. Braithwaite J, Wears RL, Hollnagel E. Resilient health care: turning patient safety on its head. *Int J Qual Health Care.* 2015;27(5):418–20.

19. Lingard L, McDougall A, Levstik M, et al. Representing complexity well: a story about teamwork, with implications for how we teach collaboration. *Med Educ.* 2012;46(9):869–77.

20. Weller J, Civil I, Torrie J, et al. Can team training make surgery safer? Lessons for national implementation of a simulation-based programme. *N Z Med J.* 2016;129(1443):9–17.

21. Merry AF, Weller J, Mitchell SJ. Teamwork, communication, formula-one racing and the outcomes of cardiac surgery. *J Extra Corpor Technol.* 2014;46(1):7–14.

22. Wahr JA, Prager RL, Abernathy JH 3rd, et al. Patient safety in the cardiac operating room: human factors and teamwork: a scientific statement from the American Heart Association. *Circulation.* 2013;128(10):1139–69.

23. VanGraafeiland B, Sloand E, Silbert-Flagg J, Gleason K, Dennison Himmelfarb C. Academic-clinical service partnerships are innovative strategies to advance patient safety competence and leadership in prelicensure nursing students. *Nurs Outlook.* 2019;67(1):49–53.

24. Walton M, Woodward H, Van Staalduinen S, et al. The WHO patient safety curriculum guide for medical schools. *Qual Saf Health Care.* 2010;19(6):542–6.

25. Garden A, Bernau S, Robinson G, Chalmers C. Undergraduate education to address patient safety. *N Z Med J.* 2008;121(1279):119–21.

26. Wong BM, Levinson W, Shojania KG. Quality improvement in medical education: current state and future directions [Review]. *Med Educ.* 2012;46(1):107–19.

27. Horsburgh M, Merry A, Seddon M, et al. Educating for healthcare quality improvement in an interprofessional learning environment: a New Zealand initiative. *J Interprof Care.* 2006;20(5):555–7.

28. Horsburgh M, Merry AF, Seddon M. Patient safety in an interprofessional learning environment. *Med Educ.* 2005;39(5):512–13.

29. Watts BV, Williams L, Mills PD, et al. Curriculum development and implementation of a national interprofessional fellowship in patient safety. *J Patient Saf.* 2018;14(3):127–32.

30. Okuyama A, Martowirono K, Bijnen B. Assessing the patient safety competencies of healthcare professionals: a systematic review. *BMJ Qual Saf.* 2011;20(11):991–1000.

31. Weick K. The vulnerable system: an analysis of the Tenerife air disaster. *J Manage.* 1990;16(3): 571–93.

32. Hofstede G. Measuring organizational cultures: a qualitative and quantitative study across twenty cases. *Adm Sci Q.* 1990;35:286–316.

33. Singer SJ, Falwell A, Gaba DM, et al. Identifying organizational cultures that promote patient safety. *Health Care Manage Rev.* 2009;34(4): 300–11.

34. Hartmann CW, Meterko M, Rosen AK, et al. Relationship of hospital organizational culture to patient safety climate in the Veterans Health Administration. *Med Care Res Rev.* 2009;66(3):320–38.

35. Shappell S, Wiegmann D. A methodology for assessing safety programs targeting human error in aviation. *Int J Aviat Psychol.* 2009;19(3):252–69.

36. Leape LL, Shore MF, Dienstag JL, et al. Perspective: a culture of respect, part 1: the nature and causes of disrespectful behavior by physicians. *Acad Med.* 2012;87(7):845–52.

37. Rosenstein AH, O'Daniel M. A survey of the impact of disruptive behaviors and communication defects on patient safety. *Jt Comm J Qual Patient Saf.* 2008;34(8):464–71.

38. Coopes A. Operate with respect: how Australia is confronting sexual harassment of trainees. *BMJ.* 2016;354:i4210.

39. Royal Australasian College of Surgeons. *Draft Report and EAG Research Results.* Melbourne: Royal Australasian College of Surgeons; 2015. Accessed July 18, 2020. https://anzscts.org/racs-eag-report-on-discrimination-bullying-and-sexual-harassment/

40. Smetzer J, Baker C, Byrne FD, Cohen MR. Shaping systems for better behavioral choices: lessons learned from a fatal medication error. *Jt Comm J Qual Patient Saf.* 2010;36(4):152–63.

41. Leape LL, Shore MF, Dienstag JL, et al. Perspective: a culture of respect, part 2: creating a culture of respect. *Acad Med.* 2012;87(7):853–8.

42. Edmondson A. Learning from mistakes is easier said than done: group and organizational influences on the detection and correction of human error. *J Appl Behav Sci.* 1996;32(1):5–28.

43. Edmondson A. Psychological safety and learning behavior in work teams. *ASQ.* 1999;44(2):350–83.

44. Edmondson AC. Learning from failure in health care: frequent opportunities, pervasive barriers. *Qual Saf Health Care.* 2004;13(suppl. 2):ii3–9.

45. Edmondson AC, Bohmer RM, Pisano GP. Disrupted routines: team learning and new technology implementation in hospitals. *ASQ.* 2001;46(4):685–716.

46. Espin S, Lingard L, Baker GR, Regehr G. Persistence of unsafe practice in everyday work: an exploration of organizational and psychological factors constraining safety in the operating room. *Qual Saf Health Care.* 2006;15(3):165–70.

47. Bayazidi S, Zarezadeh Y, Zamanzadeh V, Parvan K. Medication error reporting rate and its barriers and facilitators among nurses. *J Caring Sci.* 2012;1(4):231–6.

48. Naveh E, Katz-Navon T, Stern Z. Readiness to report medical treatment errors: the effects of safety procedures, safety information, and priority of safety. *Med Care.* 2006;44(2):117–23.

49. Panesar SS, Cleary K, Sheikh A. Reflections on the National Patient Safety Agency's database of medical errors. *J R Soc Med.* 2009;102(7): 256–8.

50. Sarvadikar A, Prescott G, Williams D. Attitudes to reporting medication error among differing healthcare professionals. *Eur J Clin Pharmacol.* 2010;66(8):843–53.

51. Nuckols TK, Bell DS, Liu H, Paddock SM, Hilborne LH. Rates and types of events reported to established incident reporting systems in two US hospitals. *Qual Saf Health Care.* 2007;16(3):164–8.

52. Brennan TA, Leape LL, Laird NM, et al. Incidence of adverse events and negligence in hospitalized patients. Results of the Harvard Medical Practice Study I. *N Engl J Med.* 1991;324(6):370–6.

53. Gawande AA, Thomas EJ, Zinner MJ, Brennan TA. The incidence and nature of surgical adverse events in Colorado and Utah in 1992. *Surgery.* 1999;126(1):66–75.

54. Gibbs NM, Culwick M, Merry AF. A cross-sectional overview of the first 4,000 incidents reported to webAIRS, a de-identified web-based anaesthesia incident reporting system in Australia and New Zealand. *Anaesth Intensive Care.* 2017;45(1):28–35.

55. Webb RK, Currie M, Morgan CA, et al. The Australian Incident Monitoring Study: an analysis of 2000 incident reports. *Anaesth Intensive Care.* 1993;21(5):520–8.

56. Kohn LA, Corrigan JM, Donaldson MS, editors. *To Err is Human: Building a Safer Health System.* Washington DC: National Academy Press; 1999.

57. Merry AF, Webster CS, Hannam J, et al. Multimodal system designed to reduce errors in recording and administration of drugs in anaesthesia: prospective randomised clinical evaluation. *BMJ.* 2011;343:d5543.

58. Merry AF, Hannam JA, Webster CS, et al. Retesting the hypothesis of a clinical randomized controlled trial in a simulation environment to Validate Anesthesia Simulation in Error Research (the VASER study). *Anesthesiology.* 2017;126(3):472–81.

59. Flynn L, Liang Y, Dickson GL, Xie M, Suh DC. Nurses' practice environments, error interception practices, and inpatient medication errors. *J Nurs Scholarsh.* 2012;44(2):180–6.

60. Van den Heede K, Lesaffre E, Diya L, et al. The relationship between inpatient cardiac surgery mortality and nurse numbers and educational level: analysis of administrative data. *Int J Nurs Stud.* 2009;46(6):796–803.

61. Pronovost PJ, Angus DC, Dorman T, et al. Physician staffing patterns and clinical outcomes in critically ill patients: a systematic review. *JAMA*. 2002;288(17):2151–62.

62. Bond CA, Raehl CL, Franke T. Medication errors in United States hospitals. *Pharmacotherapy*. 2001;21(9):1023–36.

63. Bond CA, Raehl CL. Clinical pharmacy services, pharmacy staffing, and hospital mortality rates. *Pharmacotherapy*. 2007;27(4):481–93.

64. Neily J, Mills PD, Young-Xu YN, et al. Association between implementation of a medical team training program and surgical mortality. *JAMA*. 2010;304(15):1693 700.

65. Weller J, Cumin D, Torrie J, et al. Multidisciplinary operating room simulation-based team training to reduce treatment errors: a feasibility study in New Zealand hospitals. *N Z Med J*. 2015;128(1418):40–51.

66. Pronovost PJ, Goeschel CA, Colantuoni E, et al. Sustaining reductions in catheter related bloodstream infections in Michigan intensive care units: observational study. *BMJ*. 2010;340:c309.

67. Armour Forse R, Bramble JD, McQuillan R. Team training can improve operating room performance. *Surgery*. 2011;150(4):771–8.

68. Tabing AK, Ehrenfeld JM, Wanderer JP. Limiting the accessibility of cost-prohibitive drugs reduces overall anesthetic drug costs: a retrospective before and after analysis. *Can J Anaesth*. 2015;62(10):1045–54.

69. Merry AF, Hamblin R. Curtailing the cost of anesthetic drugs: prudent economics or an infringement of clinical autonomy? *Can J Anaesth*. 2015;62:1029–33.

70. Merry AF, Brookbanks W. *Merry and McCall Smith's Errors, Medicine and the Law*. 2nd ed. Cambridge, UK: Cambridge University Press; 2017.

71. Kotter JP, Rathgeber H. *Our Iceberg Is Melting: Changing and Succeeding under Any Conditions*. New York, NY: St. Martin's Press; 2006.

72. Deming WE. *The New Economics*. Cambridge, MA: Massachusetts Institute of Technology, Center for Advanced Engineering Study; 1994.

73. O'Connor GT, Plume SK, Olmstead EM, et al. A regional intervention to improve the hospital mortality associated with coronary artery bypass graft surgery. The Northern New England Cardiovascular Disease Study Group. *JAMA*. 1996;275(11):841–6.

74. Webster CS, Andersson E, Edwards K, et al. Deviation from accepted drug administration guidelines during anaesthesia in twenty highly realistic simulated cases. *Anaesth Intensive Care*. 2015;43(6):698–706.

75. Wennberg JE, Peters PG Jr. Unwarranted variations in the quality of health care: can the law help medicine provide a remedy/remedies? *Spec Law Dig Health Care Law*. 2004(305):9–25.

76. Fisher ES, Wennberg DE, Stukel TA, et al. The implications of regional variations in Medicare spending. Part 1: the content, quality, and accessibility of care. *Ann Intern Med*. 2003;138(4):273–87.

77. Fisher ES, Wennberg DE, Stukel TA, et al. The implications of regional variations in Medicare spending. Part 2: health outcomes and satisfaction with care. *Ann Intern Med*. 2003;138(4):288–98.

78. McGlynn E, Asch S, Adams J, et al. The quality of health care delivered to adults in the United States. *N Engl J Med*. 2003;348(26):2635–45.

79. Runciman WB, Hunt TD, Hannaford NA, et al. CareTrack: assessing the appropriateness of health care delivery in Australia. *Med J Aust*. 2012;197(2):100–5.

80. DeMott K. Healthcare practices vary widely from town to town: regional Dartmouth Atlas. *Health Syst Lead*. 1997;4(1):2–3.

81. Fisher ES, Wennberg JE. Health care quality, geographic variations, and the challenge of supply-sensitive care. *Perspect Biol Med*. 2003;46(1):69–79.

82. Dartmouth Atlas Project. Centre for the Evaluative Clinical Sciences Staff. *The Dartmouth Atlas of Health Care*. 2004. Accessed January 14, 2020. https://www.dartmouthatlas.org

83. Newman L. New Dartmouth Atlas: improving US cardiac care? *Lancet*. 2000;356(9230):660.

84. Jelacic S, Bowdle A, Nair BG, et al. A system for anesthesia drug administration using barcode technology: the Codonics Safe Label System and Smart Anesthesia Manager. *Anesth Analg*. 2015;121(2):410–21.

85. Reinertsen JL. Zen and the art of physician autonomy maintenance. *Ann Intern Med*. 2003;138(12):992–5.

86. Wahr JA, Abernathy JH 3rd, Lazarra EH, et al. Medication safety in the operating room: literature and expert-based recommendations. *Br J Anaesth*. 2017;118(1):32–43.

87. Sackett DL, Rosenberg WM, Gray JA, Haynes RB, Richardson WS. Evidence based medicine: what it is and what it isn't. *Br Med J*. 1996;312(7023):71–2

88. Institute of Medicine. *Crossing the Quality Chasm: A New Health System for the 21st Century*. Washington, DC: National Academy Press; 2001.

14 Conclusions

We began the introduction to this book with the arresting statement that medication errors are believed to be a leading cause of avoidable harm to patients around the world, with an estimated cost of US$42 billion per year. We introduced the reader to real people who have died due to this harm, and to the providers who, although working hard to do the right thing, inadvertently did the wrong thing, and thus set off a cascade of injury and pain for their patients, and for themselves. We presented multiple interventions believed by experts to reduce harm, and acknowledge the obstacles to putting these interventions into everyday practice. We introduced the World Health Organization's (WHO's) third global patient safety challenge "Medication Without Harm," the goal of which is to reduce the level of severe, avoidable harm related to medications by 50% over 5 years, globally (1,2).

We see medication safety as a Safety II construct, in which there is as much to be gained by learning from things that have gone well as by learning from things that have gone wrong. Nevertheless, much goes wrong with the management of medications in anesthesia and the perioperative period today. In Chapters 2 and 3, we painted a picture of errors, adverse events, and harm, with considerable room for improvement. In Chapters 4 and 5, we described the human dimension of this problem – the patients who are the victims of failures in safe medication management and the clinicians who are also impacted by the consequences of the failures. We challenged the widespread use of the term "second victim," which we think undermines the idea that clinicians have a responsibility to be effective in responding to the needs of their harmed patients directly and through improving the system to reduce the likelihood of such events in the future. Nevertheless, we acknowledged that there are some circumstances when the emotional and professional harm to clinicians involved in adverse medication events is of a magnitude that does justify this term.

In Chapters 6, 7, and 8, we provided a detailed analysis of how and why things go wrong in medication management. Chapter 9 is a review of interventions to improve medication safety, and in Chapter 10 we considered how these apply in special settings and circumstances. In Chapters 11 and 12, we then considered in detail the regulatory and legal aspects of ensuring medication safety and conclude that a new and more proactive approach is required. We emphasized the need for a restorative solutions-oriented response when good people who work to help patients end up inadvertently harming them. Depressingly, Chapter 13 provides an outline of the many barriers to progress in improving medication safety.

How do we bring all of this together in a way that allows individual clinicians, hospital leadership, and national funding and quality improvement agencies to overcomes these barriers?

14.1 The Big Picture

One key to success in efforts to substantially improve medication safety lies in an appreciation of the limitations of linear approaches to managing a complex system. Ensuring good process management for those aspects of the system that are linear is, of course, essential, but safe medication management also requires dynamic control of all the interacting elements of the system at multiple levels. Systems theoretic process analysis (STPA) (3) offers some promise in this regard. STPA does not begin with an assumption that adverse events are the consequences of linear sequences of events. Instead, it seeks to understand how to constrain the behavior of the system within safe limits across its different levels.

14.1.1 The Global Level

The third WHO Global Patient Safety Challenge: *Medication Without Harm* (4), is an authoritative call for international action on medication safety. The strategic framework of this challenge identifies

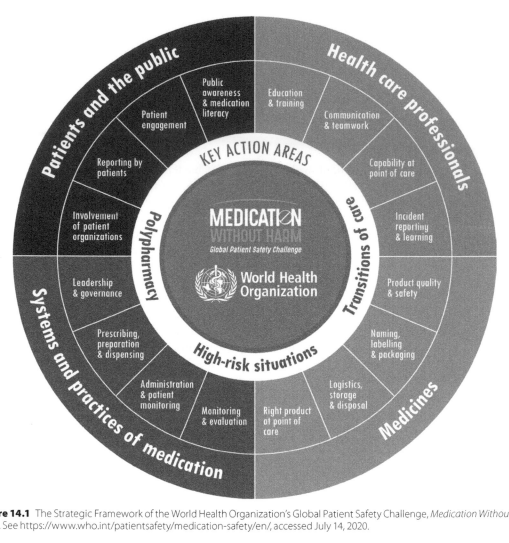

Figure 14.1 The Strategic Framework of the World Health Organization's Global Patient Safety Challenge, *Medication Without Harm*. See https://www.who.int/patientsafety/medication-safety/en/, accessed July 14, 2020.

three key action areas: transitions of care (discussed in Chapters 2 and 3), high-risk situations (clearly anesthesia and the perioperative period qualify), and polypharmacy (which applies directly to many patients undergoing surgery and which could also be extended to encompass the point that a great number of medications are involved during anesthesia and the postoperative care of surgical patients). Four domains of the challenge are described: patients and the public, healthcare professionals, medicines and systems, and practices of medication, with four subdomains for each domain (Figure 14.1).

14.1.2 The National Level

Ideally, governments should respond to this challenge by requiring, coordinating, funding, and supporting improvements to medication safety

in general, including during anesthesia and the perioperative period. In many countries, this has happened to a varying degree (see, for example, the national medication safety program of the Health Quality and Safety Commission in New Zealand [5]), but in many the call has fallen on deaf governmental ears.

14.1.3 The Institutional and Departmental Level

It follows from the previous comment that the drive for change will need to come from institutions, and indeed, probably from within institutions at the level of the department. These levels can be considered together because it is essential that they are aligned. We think there is a responsibility for clinicians at the workplace to respond to the challenge, but senior leadership must also be involved – and this sentence could equally well be rephrased in the reverse order. The imperative on all concerned is. to act, rather than to wait for someone else to take the initiative.

Many of these subdomains of this framework have been discussed within earlier chapters of this book. Other, more targeted frameworks, such as that of the Anesthesia Patient Safety Foundation, can be integrated into this overarching WHO framework to inform the priorities for attention in specific contexts, such as during anesthesia, for example. In this conclusion, we do not repeat the detail that has been covered elsewhere. Rather, we emphasize the need for a commitment by institutions to adopt a strategically comprehensive approach to the continuous improvement of medication safety in anesthesia and the perioperative period.

As discussed in Chapter 9, measurement is fundamental to quality improvement, and although it is not explicitly mentioned in Figure 14.1, it must be included in any serious approach to improving medication safety. Similarly, culture is key to safe medication practice (see Figure 9.2) and must be addressed at all levels of the institution. In fact, ensuring a cultural commitment to safety should be the primary focus of any response to the WHO challenge. The culture of any organization or department is set by its leadership and is also strongly influenced by the wider prevailing culture of the country in which the institution functions. As one example of this, there is a substantial difference between countries in the extent to which corruption is permitted to flourish (see www.transparency.org/, accessed January 20, 2020). Corruption is very corrosive to the advancement of high-quality healthcare, and an assessment of its potential influence should be included, and taken into account, in any plan for improving medication safety.

14.1.4 Patients and the Public

One of the four domains of the WHO challenge is that of patients and the public. This is a domain that has been insufficiently considered in much of the literature on medication safety in anesthesia, and perhaps also on medication safety more generally. Improving the medication literacy of patients as part of their overall health literacy clearly has considerable potential to increase the safety of the way in which they use the medications that they have been prescribed to take, but there may be a greater role for patients to be included in understanding and checking the medications administered to them on the ward and in the codesign of interventions to improve medication safety (6). Beyond that, mobilizing public awareness on the issue of medication safety and enlisting their support in requiring and funding ways of improving practice in this regard may have considerable potential to advance this cause.

14.2 Last Words

By this point in this book, it must be very clear to any reader that we ("we" the authors and "we" in the more general sense) do not know all the answers to the challenge of improving medication safety in anesthesia and perioperative medicine. However, it should also be clear by now that to do nothing is unacceptable. Furthermore, it should also be clear that the situation is far from hopeless – there is a great deal that can be done. Thus, the imperative is to act, not just as individual practitioners but collectively, within and beyond institutional boundaries, in a coordinated, committed, and sustained manner.

We hope this book will be of use to those who do indeed choose to respond to the "Medication Without Harm" Global Patient Safety Challenge of the WHO, particularly in the context of anesthesia and perioperative medicine, and perhaps more generally as well.

References

1. Donaldson LJ, Kelley ET, Dhingra-Kumar N, Kieny MP, Sheikh A. Medication without harm: WHO's third global patient safety challenge. *Lancet*. 2017;389(10080):1680–1.

2. WHO Global Patient Safety Challenge: Medication Without Harm. Geneva: World Health Organization; 2017. Available from: https://www.who.int/patientsafety/medication-safety/medication-without-harm-brochure/en/. Accessed January 18, 2020.

3. Leveson N. *Engineering a Safer World: Systems Thinking Applied to Safety*. Cambridge, MA: MIT Press; 2011.

4. World Health Organization. *WHO Launches Global Effort to Halve Medication-Related Errors in 5 Years*. Geneva: World Health Organisation; 2017. Accessed January 18, 2020. https://www.who.int/mediacentre/news/releases/2017/medication-related-errors/en/

5. Health Quality and Safety Commission New Zealand. *Haumaru rongoā – Medication Safety.* Wellington: Health Quality and Safety Commission; 2019. Accessed January 18, 2020. https://www.hqsc.govt.nz/our-programmes/medication-safety/

6. Khodambashi S, Haugland D, Ellingsberg A, et al. An experimental comparison of a co-design visualizing personal drug information and patient information leaflets: Usability aspects. *Stud Health Technol Inform.* 2017;245:748–52

Index